Introduction to

Public Health

3e

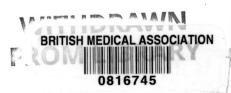

Introduction to

Public Health

3e

Mary Louise Fleming PhD, MA, BEd, Dip Teach
Professor, Head of the School of Public Health and Social
Work at the Queensland University of Technology,
Brisbane, Queensland

Elizabeth Parker EdD, MSW, BA
Adjunct Associate Professor, School of Public Health
and Social Work at the Queensland University of
Technology, Brisbane, Queensland

ELSEVIER

ELSEVIER

Elsevier Australia. ACN 001 002 357
(a division of Reed International Books Australia Pty Ltd)
Tower 1, 475 Victoria Avenue, Chatswood, NSW 2067

This publication has been carefully reviewed and checked to ensure that the content is as accurate and current as possible at time of publication. We would recommend, however, that the reader verify any procedures, treatments, drug dosages or legal content described in this book. Neither the author, the contributors, nor the publisher assume any liability for injury and/or damage to persons or property arising from any error in or omission from this publication.

National Library of Australia Cataloguing-in-Publication entry

---

Fleming, Mary Louise, author.

Introduction to public health / MaryLou Fleming; Elizabeth Parker.

Third edition.

9780729542036 (paperback)

Public health.

Parker, Elizabeth, author.

362.1

Content Strategist: Melinda McEvoy
Content Development Specialist: Natalie Hamad
Project Manager: Anitha Rajarathnam
Edited by Kate Stone
Proofread by Teresa McIntyre
Index by Robert Swanson
Typeset by Toppan Best-set Premedia Limited
Cover and internal design by Natalie Bowra
Printed in China by China Translation and Printing Services

Last digit is the print number: 9 8 7 6 5 4 3 2 1

Contents

Introduction

Why is public health important?

Introduction to Public Health is about the discipline of public health, the nature and scope of public health activity, and the challenges that face public health in the twenty-first century. The book is designed as an introductory text to the principles and practice of public health. This is a complex and multifaceted area. What we have tried to do in this book is make public health easy to understand without making it simplistic. As many authors have stated, public health is essentially about the organised efforts of society to promote, protect and restore the public's health (Brownson et al. 2011, Last 2001, Schneider 2011, Turnock 2012, Winslow 1920). It is multidisciplinary in nature, and it is influenced by genetic, physical, social, cultural, economic and political determinants of health.

How do we define public health, and what are the disciplines that contribute to public health? How has the area changed over time? Are there health issues in the twenty-first century that change the focus and activity of public health? Yes, there are! There are many challenges facing public health now and in the future, just as there have been over the course of the history of organised public health efforts, dating from around 1850 in the Western world.

Of what relevance is public health to the many health disciplines that contribute to it? How might an understanding of public health contribute to a range of health professionals who use the principles and practices of public health in their professional activities? These are the questions that this book addresses. *Introduction to Public Health* leads the reader on a journey of discovery that concludes with an understanding of the nature and scope of public health and the challenges facing the field into the future. In this edition we have included one new chapter, 'Public health and social policy', in order to broaden our understanding of the policy influences on public health.

The book is designed for a range of students undertaking health courses where there is a focus on advancing the health of the population. While it is imperative that people wanting to be public health professionals understand the theory and practice of public health, many other health workers contribute to effective public health practice. This book would also be relevant to a range of undergraduate students who want an introductory understanding of public health and its practice.

Public health is an innately political process. As we discuss in this book, there is a clear relationship between disease and the way in which society is structured. Income distribution, the allocation of resources to ensure sufficient infrastructure for transport, housing and education, and how much political support there is to provide adequately for these fundamental services, all impact on our health. They particularly impact on the health of certain groups within the population who do not have the financial, social and political resources to advocate for change. Why is it that we still have such disparities in health? For example, the poor health of Aboriginal and Torres Strait Islander peoples, especially with respect to risk factors and chronic disease, is clearly related to the distribution of, and inequities in, economic, political and social status (Australian Institute of Health and Welfare (AIHW) 2014). In an egalitarian society such as Australia, which prides itself on a 'fair go for all', should this be acceptable? In this book, we discuss the political, social and economic determinants of health, as well as the physical and environmental issues that impact on population health.

Defining and understanding 'public health'

Defining 'public health' is not an easy task. This is because not everyone who works in public health agrees on a single definition. Definitions also vary from country to country. For example, the American Public Health Association (APHA) classifies public health into prevention, policy development and population health surveillance activities. It concludes:

> Public health is the practice of preventing disease and promoting good health within groups of people, from small communities to entire countries. Public health professionals rely on policy and research strategies to understand issues such as infant mortality and chronic disease in particular populations. (American Public Health Association 2008)

More recently, at a forum on Innovating, Leading and Moving Public Health Forward (2013), public health practitioners, policymakers and advocates argued for a renewed commitment to placing the population at the centre of the process.

> Everything about how we do our work should have, at its center, a focus around the populations we are serving (American Public Health Association 2013)

In the United Kingdom, the Public Health Association believes that public health deals with a wide range of issues, as identified below. Public health:

- is an approach that focuses on the health and wellbeing of a society and the most effective means of protecting and improving it
- encompasses the science, art and politics of preventing illness and disease and promoting health and wellbeing
- addresses the root causes of illness and disease, including the interacting social, environmental, biological and psychological dimensions, as well as the provision of effective health services
- addresses inequalities, injustices and denials of human rights, which frequently explain large variations in health locally, nationally and globally
- works effectively through partnerships that cut across professional and organisational boundaries, and seeks to eliminate avoidable distinctions
- relies upon evidence, judgement and skills and promotes the participation of the populations who are themselves the subject of policy and action. (United Kingdom Public Health Association 2011)

As pointed out above, public health is essentially about the organised efforts of society to promote, protect and restore the public's health (Brownson et al. 2011, Last 2001, Schneider 2011, Turnock 2012, Winslow 1920). It is both a science and an art, in that it relies on evidence, skill and judgement, it examines the contribution of a range of factors to improving population health, it addresses inequalities, and it is based on partnerships. These elements of public health will be discussed throughout the book, particularly in terms of their application to public health practice. We will be asking you to think about how you might define public health within the context of your own developing professional understanding.

To understand public health we also need to think about the contribution of both the 'art' and the 'science' of improving the health of the population. Throughout this book, you will see many examples of how the science is used to make evidence-based decisions that lead to improvements in the health of the population.

The *science* of public health is about understanding the determinants of health, what works and in what circumstances. It is about using evidence as a basis for decisions about selecting interventions that work with the hard-to-reach and the economically and socially isolated. The 2014 Australian Institute of Health and Welfare report *Australia's Health* identifies a range of risk factors that impact on our health, including the rise in overweight and obesity, harmful smoking rates, and harmful drinking rates. These risk factors also need to be addressed to contribute to meeting 'Closing the Gap' targets for Aboriginal and Torres Strait Islander peoples (AIHW 2014). Each of these issues will be a major challenge for public health and the health workforce well into the future (AIHW 2014).

The *art* of public health has more to do with the practice of public health, and how the science is interpreted and implemented according to population needs and circumstances.

Health practitioners who work in public health also need a vision about what public health could look like in the future. As practitioners, we need to be vigilant to changing circumstances and issues. In addition, we need a set of values and ethics that underpins our practice to be brought to bear in all our public health dealings.

One final important point should be made about the differences between public health and medical care. Both have an important contribution to make to the health of the population. However, the primary focus of medical care is the individual patient and treating people who are ill, although medical practitioners do have a role in health promotion and screening directed towards the individual's care. Public health focuses on promoting health and preventing illness in the population. The problem for public health in measuring its success is that it often takes many years to see shifts in mortality and morbidity patterns as a result of a range of public health interventions introduced over many years. Take, for example, the case of smoking and cardiovascular disease. We know that cigarette smoking is the single largest preventable cause of death and disease in Australia. It is a major risk factor for cardiovascular disease, as well as a range of cancers and other disabling conditions. International evidence shows that well-funded, comprehensive tobacco control programs can successfully reduce tobacco use. There is also an ongoing need to reinvent smoking promotion programs, as different generations, with changing needs, values and beliefs, require different campaign approaches (AIHW 2014).

In summary, this book covers the history and contemporary elements of public health, it includes a conversation about the determinants of health and how they shape public health practice, it discusses the important role for evidence in underpinning public health practice, and it looks into the future to describe the emerging epidemics, and the achievements and challenges facing public health in the twenty-first century.

How this book is organised

The book is organised into five sections. The five sections, and the 17 chapters within them, are outlined on the book's contents page. Each chapter is organised in the following way:

- a list of learning objectives
- an introduction
- the content of the chapter
- review questions.

The following outlines each section of the book and how each helps you to understand the complex relationships that make up contemporary public health.

Section 1 of the book introduces you to definitions of 'public health', the principles that underpin the discipline, and its multidisciplinary and multisectoral nature. We then examine the range of health professionals working in public health, and why they need to comprehend the nature and scope of public health and its role in promoting, protecting and restoring the public's health. We briefly explore the interesting history of public health over the past 160 years since the inception of organised public health efforts. We paint a picture of the historical issues that have impacted on public health over the years, and how history has always been a good signpost for what public health will be like in the future. Finally, we examine the impact of public health policy and social policy on public health practice. You will have the opportunity to consider how public health and social policy decisions impact on a range of health issues and population groups. You will come to understand the nature and function of state health departments around Australia, and their relationship with the federal Department of Health. We consider the role of not-for-profit organisations, and the contribution of local government to public health.

Section 2 covers the range of factors that impact on health and, consequently, the organised efforts of public health. It lays the foundations for decisions about priorities and strategies for public health interventions. It will provide you with evidence upon which decisions are made about where to intervene, how to intervene, and how to track population health changes. We give you an understanding of the fundamental principles of epidemiology, and how this discipline underpins the activities of public health. An understanding of epidemiology will enable you to make informed decisions about patterns of mortality and morbidity, and where to intervene; and it will help you track health changes in the population and in subpopulations over time. We analyse the determinants of health—genetic, physical, social, emotional, economic and environmental. Clarity regarding the determinants of health will assist you, in turn, to understand and apply the principles of public health in your practice.

Section 3 examines the use of evidence to inform the planning and evaluation of public health activity. We begin this section by considering the ethics of public health practice. Undertaking ethical practice is essential for health professionals, no matter what aspect of health they practise in. Using case study examples, we provide you with a picture of how evidence can inform practice. We examine the nature of the evidence being considered, and discuss the issues practitioners need to understand in order to make evidence-based decisions. The final chapter in Section 3 provides you with advice about public health planning and evaluation models, and the nature and extent of their application in practice, using a range of examples in a variety of public health settings.

Four chapters make up *Section 4*. These chapters focus on a continuum of public health activity, from disease control to health protection and health promotion. One focuses on infectious disease and chronic disease control, monitoring and surveillance. Another examines the development and relevance of environmental health to public health. We trace the development and importance of environmental health and occupational health and safety to population health, and examine the contemporary notion of ecological public health. The third chapter covers issues of importance to contemporary public health—emergency planning and response. We define 'disaster', and examine the principles of disaster management. In this section's final chapter, the importance of health advancement and the promotion of health are discussed. This section should give you a good understanding of the scope of public health interventions and their application in practice.

In the final section of the book, *Section 5*, we examine the future for public health in the twenty-first century. We consider the globalisation of health. Public health is a global issue. With travel around the planet easy and accessible to many, health issues that once might have impacted on the population in a region or country are now being transported around the world. In addition, refugee health has become an important part of contemporary public health activity, particularly in the Asia-Pacific region. We introduce the health of Aboriginal and Torres Strait Islander peoples, and discuss the important role that Indigenous and non-Indigenous health workers can play in 'closing the gap' for Indigenous peoples. In the final chapter of this book we think about the challenges facing public health in the future, such as global warming and environmental sustainability. We also talk about the nature and scope of the public health workforce needed to meet these challenges.

Our conversation about 'grand challenges' for public health at the end of the book gives you a chance to consider the major issues facing public health, where we imagine the discipline might be heading, and what the consequences are for the public's health in the next 50 years.

References

American Public Health Association, 2008. What is public health? Our commitment to safe, healthy communities. Online. Available: <http://www.apha.org/~/media/files/pdf/fact%20 sheets/whatisph.ashx> (1 May 2014).

American Public Health Association, 2013. Innovating, leading and moving public health forward. Online. Available: <http://www.rwjf.org/en/blogs/new-public-health/2013/11/ innovating_leading.html> (30 Apr 2014).

Australian Institute of Health and Welfare, 2014. Australia's Health 2014. AIHW Cat. No. AUS 178. AIHW, Canberra.

Brownson, R.C., Baker, E.A., Left, T.L., et al., 2011. Evidence-Based Public Health. Oxford University Press, New York.

Last, J.M., 2001. A Dictionary of Epidemiology, fourth ed. Oxford University Press, New York.

Schneider, M.-J., 2011. Introduction to Public Health, third ed. Jones and Bartlett Learning, Sudbury, MA.

Turnock, B.L., 2012. Essentials of Public Health, second ed. Jones and Bartlett Learning, Sudbury, MA.

United Kingdom Public Health Association, 2011. UKPHA definition of public health. Online. Available: <http://www.ukpha.org.uk/about-us.aspx> (1 May 2014).

Winslow, C.E.A., 1920. The untilled field of public health. Science 9, 23–33.

About the authors

Mick Adams

Dr Mick Adams is a Research Fellow with the Australian Institute of Aboriginal and Torres Strait Islander Studies (AIATSIS) and an Adjunct Professor with the Faculty of Health, Queensland University of Technology. Mick has held a range of positions with Aboriginal and Torres Strait Islander community organisations, representative organisations and government departments, including Chairperson of the National Aboriginal Community Controlled Health Organisation (NACCHO) (2007–2009). Mick has contributed to the advancement of Aboriginal and Torres Strait Islander health for over 30 years.

Catherine Bennett

Professor Catherine Bennett is the foundation Chair in Epidemiology at Deakin University, and Head of the School of Health and Social Development. She specialises in communicable disease epidemiology and teaching research methods. Catherine also has experience working in the government sector. She is engaged in a number of large research programs funded by the National Health and Medical Research Council (NHMRC). She established and leads a NHMRC-funded research program on the epidemiology of community-onset *Staphylococcus aureus* (superbug, MRSA) infections, with collaborators in the United States. Catherine is President of the Council of Academic Public Health Institutions Australia (CAPHIA).

Gerry FitzGerald

Gerry FitzGerald is Professor of Emergency Services in the School of Public Health and Social Work at the Queensland University of Technology, and is responsible for developing emergency and disaster management education and research programs. He has a Bachelor of Medicine/Bachelor of Surgery degree, a Bachelor of Health Administration, and a Doctor of Medicine.

Mary Louise Fleming

Professor Mary Louise Fleming is Head of the School of Public Health and Social Work at the Queensland University of Technology. She has over 20 years' experience in teaching and research in higher education, as well as public health and health promotion. Her research experience is in: action research; process, impact and outcome evaluation in health promotion; and public health interventions. Mary Louise has worked as a consultant for the World Health Organization and for Commonwealth and state health departments, and has sat on National Health and Medical Research Council (NHMRC) public health project grant review panels. She has been widely published in the area of health promotion.

Bronwyn Fredericks

Bronwyn Fredericks is Professor and Pro Vice-Chancellor (Indigenous Engagement) and the BHP Chair in Indigenous Engagement at Central Queensland University. She is an Adjunct Professor with the Health Faculty at the Queensland University of Technology. Bronwyn has worked in the healthcare and human service arena at federal, state and community sector levels, and has been actively engaged with community-controlled organisations in a volunteer, elected or paid capacity for over 30 years.

Trish Gould

Trish Gould is a research officer in the School of Public Health and Social Work at the Queensland University of Technology. She has experience in public health and health promotion research, project management and coordination, writing, and editing. Trish has a MA in biological anthropology, and her interest areas include ethics, human rights, and the health impacts of migration, acculturation, inequity and discrimination.

Xiang-Yu Hou

Dr Xiang-Yu Hou is an Associate Professor in Epidemiology, and lectures in epidemiology and international health in the School of Public Health and Social Work, Queensland University of Technology. Xiang-Yu has a Bachelor of Medicine degree from Shandong University and a Master of Medicine research degree from Peking University in China. She has published over 65 peer-reviewed research papers and two book chapters. Her main research interests are ambulance services, emergency medicine, acute health system research, and international health.

Vanessa Lee

Vanessa Lee is a Senior Lecturer within the Faculty of Health Sciences, University of Sydney. She is co-chair of the Aboriginal and Torres Strait Islander Special Interest Group (SIG) for the Public Health Association of Australia (PHAA), and is a member of the National Indigenous Public Health Curriculum. Vanessa's research interests are within the Aboriginal and Torres Strait Islander community-controlled health sector.

Ray Mahoney

Ray Mahoney is a Lecturer in Aboriginal and Torres Strait Islander Health, in the School of Public Health and Social Work, Queensland University of Technology. He has previously worked in health for the Queensland, New South Wales and Victorian state governments, and with the Aboriginal Community Controlled Health Service Sector in Victoria. Ray's career in Aboriginal and Torres Strait Islander health spans almost 20 years.

Greg Marston

Greg Marston is a Professor in the School of Public Health and Social Work, Queensland University of Technology. He has an extensive record in applied social policy research. He has led a number of Australian Research Council grant-funded projects on long-term unemployment, disability and employment services, and household debt and the fringe lending industry in Australia. Greg's main research interests are the impact of various social and economic policies on ordinary Australians, comparative social policy, contemporary social theory, the organisational dimensions of human service practice, and the role of social policy in transitioning to a low-carbon society. His latest books are a co-edited collection on the implementation of welfare-to-work in a variety of countries (published by Georgetown University Press, 2013), and another on who benefits from the Australian welfare state (published by Palgrave, 2013).

Elizabeth Parker

Elizabeth Parker is an Adjunct Associate Professor in the School of Public Health and Social Work at the Queensland University of Technology. She has teaching and research experience in public health and health promotion, and was a member of the Editorial Advisory Committee for the *Health Promotion Journal of Australia*. She worked as a senior manager in the Toronto Department of Public Health, and has acted as a consultant on projects for the Australian Government and Queensland Health. She is co-author, with Professor Mary Louise Fleming, of the book *Health promotion: principles and practice in the Australian context*.

Thomas Tenkate

Dr Thomas Tenkate is Director of the School of Occupational and Public Health, Ryerson University, Toronto, Canada. Formerly with the School of Public Health and Social Work, Queensland University of Technology, he has been an environmental health practitioner since 1990. He has also worked for Queensland Health for more than 10 years in a variety of environmental health investigatory, policy and research roles. His main interests are in the areas of exposure and risk assessment (particularly relating to human exposure to UV radiation), food safety and communicable disease epidemiology.

Acknowledgements

Thank you to my family for their ongoing support and patience during the writing of the third edition.

A special thank you to Trish Gould, whose support and assistance with this manuscript has meant that Elizabeth and I could complete the job. Without Trish we would still be completing the manuscript. Thank you, Trish, for all your help and for the quality of your work.

Mary Louise Fleming

A special thank you to Emma and other family, friends and colleagues for their support and encouragement during the writing of this third edition. And a special thank you to Trish Gould for her humour, endless patience and dedicated assistance.

Elizabeth Parker

Reviewers

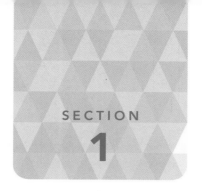

HISTORY AND DEFINITIONS OF PUBLIC HEALTH

- **The first four chapters** in Section 1 of this book provide you with background information about how the discipline is defined, its roles and responsibilities, the history of public health, and its place within the organisational and political structures of the health system in Australia. In the last two chapters there is a discussion about the health and social policy contexts influencing the development and delivery of population health initiatives.

- **Chapter 1 introduces** the nature and scope of public health. In this chapter, we consider various definitions of health, disease and illness, and examine the changing nature of public health definitions. We explore the core functions of public health, and the roles and responsibilities of public health practitioners. In the process, we discuss the way in which public health practitioners do their job, and, in fact, who is the public health workforce and how broadly we might consider that definition. We look briefly at the roles and responsibilities of various levels of government in Australia, and we discuss the role of non-government organisations, associations, community organisations and advocacy groups. At the conclusion of the chapter, we briefly consider the future for public health. This issue is raised again at the end of the book.

- **In Chapter 2 we discuss** the history of public health. This dates essentially from the beginnings of an organised Western public health effort that was focused on containing the spread of disease, with limited knowledge about the natural history of a disease. In more recent times, the complexity of the public health enterprise has become a major focus for public health activity, and it is now clearly evident that there is a need for a multidisciplinary and multisectoral approach to public health endeavours. We trace the evolution of Western public health from its early beginnings to more recent times.

We explore the diversity of thinking that underpinned public health activity, and we trace some of the myths and superstitions that were the forerunners of more contemporary public health activities.

- **Chapter 3 examines** contemporary public health policy, and we present you with information about public health policy and the relationship between public health and the broader health system. We define terms such as 'policy', 'public policy' and 'health policy', and look at the stages and roles in the policy development process. We discuss the basic structure and financing of the health system in Australia, and the role of public health within that context. Discussions take place regarding Australia's national public health priorities and the policy implications. The chapter recognises contemporary international developments in public health and their impact on policymaking in Australia and the health of Australians. We also cover a number of policy initiatives in public health, and consider the range of these policies and the sometimes differing requirements for action within some of the policy statements.

- **In the final chapter** in Section 1, we introduce you to social policy and the implications for public health. We contextualise this discussion around the sociology of health and a conversation about social justice, liberal-democracy, and public versus private providers. The chapter also uses international examples such ObamaCare, and provides a context for a conversation about the history of the welfare state and its impact on health policy, health systems development and the provision of universal healthcare. It examines the notion of 'liberal welfare states' compared with 'social democratic states', and facilitates an understanding of these concepts as they apply to the broad public health context.

- **These four chapters provide** a foundation for the book, in that they define the nature and scope of health and illness and public health, examine its history, its multidisciplinary and multisectoral elements, and its place within the healthcare system, and the broader health and social policy contexts.

Defining health and public health

CHAPTER 1

Mary Louise Fleming

Learning objectives

After reading this chapter, you should be able to:

- define 'health' and 'public health'

- describe why 'health' means different things to different individuals, and be able to consider the range of factors that influence these individual definitions

- recognise and describe how public health is defined, and how each definition has shaped the development and implementation of public health approaches

- describe the major principles underpinning public health

- describe the relationship between public health and other disciplines

- discuss the nature and scope of public health

- provide some examples of public health in practice, as applied to your discipline

- discuss the changing roles of the public health workforce, and the increasing complexity of public health work.

Introduction

What is health? How is it defined and described? What do you mean when you describe yourself as 'healthy'? How is 'public health' defined? What are the fundamental principles of public health? How does public health interact with other disciplines? And how do we describe what public health workers do?

These are many of the questions that will be considered in this chapter and other chapters, which are designed to help you become familiar with the principles and practices of public health. This book is about introductory principles and concepts of public health for students. It is also relevant for health workers from a range of disciplines whose focus ranges from clinical to population health, and who want to understand and incorporate public health principles into their work.

We begin our journey by considering a fundamental issue that underpins the notion of public health—that is, the definition of 'health', and we consider the range and variety of definitions, including those of the general public and professionals.

Defining health and ill health

Complete this simple exercise (Activity 1.1) to help you think about how you and other people define health.

ACTIVITY 1.1 Defining 'health'

- Ask five of your friends, classmates or family members what 'health' means to each of them.
- What common themes have emerged from each of the five definitions of health?
- What was unique about the definitions?
- Do you think they might change over time, and why might this be the case?

REFLECTION 1.1

Keep these five definitions in mind as you read, and compare them with other ways of defining health. How do you think of the term 'health'? Does it mean an absence of illness, or an ability to do all the things you want or have to do every day? Does it have more of a religious, cultural or social significance? The term 'health' is difficult to define. How an individual defines his or her health is sometimes different, compared with a professional's definition of health.

Most health workers see 'health' as central to their work, and believe that the majority of people also hold health to be an important part of their lives. However, we know that this is not the case, as a number of studies (Blaxter 2007, Fleming & Parker 2007, Hanlon et al. 2012a, Huber et al. 2011) have examined the way in which people define health within the context of their daily lives.

Considering the variety of ways in which the term 'health' is defined also enables us to understand the nature and scope of public health in our society. The section that follows discusses general public and professional definitions of 'health' and 'illness'.

Health and illness

Illness is primarily about how an individual experiences disease, and disease itself represents a set of signs and symptoms and medically diagnosed pathological abnormalities.

Illness can be culturally specific, and may also be influenced by social, spiritual, supernatural and psychological factors (Hanlon et al. 2012a). An individual lifestyle perspective has also been seen as an important dimension of health. Introduced initially by the document *A new perspective on the health of Canadians* (Lalonde 1974), the individual lifestyle perspective had as its focus individual behaviours. The World Health Organization (WHO) (defined later in this chapter) subsequently redefined 'lifestyle' to mean behavioural choices made from alternatives that are available to people according to their socio-economic circumstances (Kickbusch 1986). A social view of health considers issues such as the impact of social and economic factors on health, but these dimensions have often been overshadowed by the biomedical view of health. A biomedical model of health predominately has diagnosing diseases as its focus; it does not take into account the role of social factors, and overlooks the notion of disease prevention. In the 1940s, the WHO defined health as 'a state of complete physical, social and emotional wellbeing and not merely the absence of disease or infirmity' (WHO 1948). Some authors have argued that a state of health delineated by this definition is too difficult to achieve or does not relate to the current context of globalisation (Bircher 2005, Huber et al. 2011, Waltner-Toews 2000), but it certainly moved the debate about health away from an exclusively biomedical perspective.

'Health' is difficult to measure because it is a dynamic concept rather than something that is always the same. '[H]ealth cannot be defined without reference to some goals' (Waltner-Toews 2000 p 657), and it is a 'dynamic state of well-being characterised by a physical, mental and social potential' (Bircher 2005 p 335). It is much easier to measure disease or an absence of disease than it is to measure health or wellbeing. Recently, Shilton et al. (2011) proposed a definition of health that included qualities of adaptation and self-management, a human right protected by entitlements, and a 'resource for life that is affected by social, political, economic, and environmental factors' (Shilton et al. 2011 p d5359).

General public definitions of 'health'

General public concepts of health and illness have been extensively researched and discussed. Blaxter (2007), quoting Kleinman, describes three ways in which health and illness have been discussed: professional, alternative and general public. Contemporary scholars prefer to consider public beliefs about health and illness to be defined as 'commonsense understandings and personal experience, imbued with professional rationalization' (Blaxter 2007 p 26). In a seminal study in 1990, Blaxter, while exploring general public definitions of health and illness, found that people define health in a variety of different ways. She suggests that health is defined by people as not being ill or diseased, or as being a reserve against illness. Others define health as a 'healthy life', as physical fitness or as having energy or vitality. Still others take health to mean social relationships; that is, relationships with other people or as a function of the ability to do things. For others, health has meaning as psychosocial wellbeing.

Think back to your earlier activity. How do the definitions of health collected from the five people you have spoken with fit in with the different general public definitions of health and illness discussed above?

The following information introduces you to other dimensions of health that may assist you to understand how complex defining health can be, and how difficult it is to hold a single definition of health that fits with everyone's idea of the dimensions of health.

Collectively, health can be seen to represent the social, cultural and economic context of people's lives—a status, socially recognised and admired. Others believe their health is dominated by religious or supernatural forces (Durie 2004). For some, the centrality of people's relationships to the land, family and community are the central foci for health and wellbeing (Durie 2004, Thompson & Gifford 2000). For Aboriginal and Torres Strait Islander Australians, 'health' is about the totality of their environment.

'"Health" to Aboriginal peoples is a matter of determining all aspects of their life, including control over their physical environment, of dignity, of community self-esteem, and of justice. It is not merely a matter of the provision of doctors, hospitals, medicines or the absence of disease and incapacity' (National Aboriginal Health Strategy Working Party 1989 p ix, National Strategic Framework for Aboriginal and Torres Strait Islander Health 2003–2013). These issues are discussed further in Chapter 16.

A critical perspective

While general public definitions of health have focused on the ways in which health is defined in the day-to-day lives of people, other researchers have examined different contemporary ways of defining health. Table 1.1 summarises some of the ways in which health is defined (Baum 2008, Brown et al. 2005, Hanlon et al. 2012b, Morris 2010, Shilton et al. 2011).

In this chapter we ask you to think about how health is defined, and the limitations of the definitions presented here, so that you can reach your own definition on the basis of your reading of the literature. Health as a term can then be considered in a variety

TABLE 1.1 Contemporary definitions of 'health'

Definitional focus	Application
Defining health in a capitalist society	Defining and controlling mechanism where a person's health is defined primarily through illness.
Health maintenance	Being a good citizen, as becoming ill may mean a person becomes an economic burden on society.
Health as a political perspective	Health is defined by inequities in health status and is influenced by environment, housing and occupational conditions.
Neglecting the complexity of health outcomes	Defined as 'a change in the health of an individual, a group of people or population which is attributable to an intervention or series of interventions', but neglects the complexity of health outcomes (Baum 2002 p 12).
Ecosystem health (Baum 2008, Brown et al. 2005, Morris 2010)	Consideration of the environment and the interdependence of systems within the overall ecosystem in order to achieve long-term sustainability of our planet.
Health is adaptability, self-management and human rights, and is affected by a range of factors	Qualities of adaptation and self-management, a human right protected by entitlements, and a 'resource for life that is affected by social, political, economic, and environmental factors' (Shilton et al. 2011 p d5359).
Global sustainability, equity and wellbeing (Hanlon et al. 2012b)	Public health will play a role in integrating dimensions of life: e.g. the individual and the collective; ecological, equity—human rights and global equity and sustainability; envisioning something better; reflexive and change-focused.

(Summarised from Baum 2008, Brown et al. 2005, Hanlon et al. 2012b, Morris 2010, Shilton et al. 2011)

of different ways, and can be challenged, because sometimes definitions avoid the wide-ranging social, economic and political factors that have a real and sustained impact on the health of the population, as we see in some of the definitions above.

We now turn our attention to consider definitions of 'public health'. The two distinguishing features of almost all definitions of public health are (1) a focus on populations rather than on individuals, and (2) organised and deliberate efforts to promote health, with a focus on collective action.

Defining 'public health': an art and a science?

Public health is based on scientific principles, and it uses a range of disciplines such as epidemiology, biostatistics, biology and biomedical sciences in its analysis of public health problems (Hanlon et al. 2012a; Lin et al. 2014). Public health relies heavily on environmental sciences and the social and behavioural sciences. Public health is also an art, in that it involves applying this scientific knowledge to a range of practical settings that require attention to issues such as selecting intervention strategies and approaches that communities agree to and need. Furthermore, public health deals with social, cultural, political and economic issues, as well as health issues.

Winslow (1920), an American public health leader in the early twentieth century, defined public health as a science and an art:

> … of preventing disease, prolonging life, and promoting physical health and efficiency through organized community efforts for the sanitation of the environment, the control of community infections, the education of the individual in principles of personal hygiene, the organization of medical and nursing services for the early diagnosis and preventive treatment of disease, and the development of the social machinery which will ensure to every individual in the community a standard of living adequate for the maintenance of health. (Winslow 1920 p 24)

In its time, this definition was very forward-thinking, because it identified a number of public health elements that are still considered important. For example, it refers to 'organised efforts', it considers environmental issues and infectious diseases, personal wellbeing, early diagnosis and prevention, and the social dimensions of health. Little did Winslow know that many of the issues that the public health community had controlled or eliminated have re-emerged in the twenty-first century as major challenges.

More recently, the Institute of Medicine (2011) has refined its definition of 'public health' by stressing that population health improvement depends on effectively addressing the multiple determinants of health. The Institute states that large proportions of the US disease burden are preventable, and that the failure of the health system (which includes medical care and public health) to develop and deliver effective preventive strategies is taking a large and growing toll not only on health, but on the nation's economy.

What are some of these emerging threats? They include environmental factors, such as the effects of greenhouse gases and global warming, and HIV/AIDS. Numerous deaths have occurred worldwide from H5N1 avian influenza since the virus first emerged in 2003, and in 2013 a H7N9 strain of avian influenza in poultry emerged which caused human deaths in China. SARS (severe acute respiratory syndrome) and H1N1 (swine flu) remain significant public health issues (McMichael & Butler 2007, US Department of Health and Human Services website 2011). These twenty-first-century challenges require public health to return to its roots to control infectious diseases, as well as be a part of a global effort to sustain the planet and its environment for generations to come (Gostin 2010, McMichael & Butler 2007).

Public health today is recognised as being integral to promoting and sustaining the health of the population. The following definition of public health by Last (2001) supports this approach:

> … the efforts organized by society to protect, promote, and restore the people's health. It is the combination of sciences, skills and beliefs that is directed to the maintenance and improvement of the health of all the people through collective or social actions. (Last 2001 p 145)

Although dated, this definition provides us with a framework from which we can gain a better understanding of the role of public health in our society. It dispels the notion that health is only concerned with curing illness and disease.

Public health is about preventing disease, illness and injury, together with promoting the quality of life of human populations. This is a very complex process, and requires the committed skills and expertise of many different professional disciplines using a range of health approaches from prevention activities to clinical care.

In Australia, similar definitions are used to describe the art and the science of public health. The Public Health Association of Australia (PHAA) discusses public health in terms of going 'beyond the treatment of individuals to encompass health promotion, prevention of disease and disability, recovery and rehabilitation, and disability support. This framework, together with attention to the social, economic and environmental determinants of health, provides particular relevance' and informs the Association's role (PHAA website 2014).

Debates in the literature (Goldberg 2009, Kelly 2011, Rothstein 2009) have focused on how broad and all-encompassing, or narrow, definitions of public health should be. What is common about most of these definitions is the notion that there is an organised desire to improve the health of the population as a whole, a sense of general public interest, and a focus on the broader determinants of health as both risk and protective factors (Beaglehole et al. 2004). It is worthwhile stopping here to consider the meaning of the term 'determinant'. Determinants are discussed in Section Two (Chapters 5, 6 and 7) as both the causes of, and the risk factors for, health events. This requires the elaboration of a causal pathway that begins with the socioeconomic, geopolitical and meteorological determinants, and plotting them to individual and collective health outcomes. It means transcending disciplines as diverse as climatology and sociology, through economics and politics to psychology and biomedicine (Kelly 2011). A wide range of determinants, including physiological, psychosocial, behavioural and risk conditions, 'can work together to influence quality of life, wellbeing, illness and disability. However, the ways in which these determinants manifest themselves in each society would depend on history, culture and politics' (Lin et al. 2007 p 76).

As health workers, your knowledge and understanding of the art and science of public health will be an important element of your professional development. This will enable you to first identify the trends in the health of the population, and, second, demonstrate the skills to appropriately respond to these in restoring, promoting and maintaining the health of the population.

Consider the following scenario to help you think about the contribution of public health to daily life and broaden your understanding of public health (see Case Study 1.1).

CASE STUDY 1.1

A typical morning

You get up in the morning, woken earlier than expected by the waste-disposal truck collecting rubbish outside in your street. Having completed your morning routine (shower, toilet, teeth, etc.), you dress and have a quick look at Facebook. One of your friends has mentioned that it is Breast Cancer Awareness Week. Having realised that you are running late for the first lecture at university, you quickly rush out the door and into the car. Seat belt on, and out into the usual traffic chaos. As you drive past McDonald's, the sign is too enticing, and, remembering you didn't have breakfast at home, you drive through and pick up a muffin and a coffee. Across the road in the local state school you notice the ambulance service has two ambulances on the oval, and school students are climbing in and out of them. Finally arriving at university, you park your car as near as possible to the lecture theatre and walk the short distance to your lecture.

A number of activities we take part in every day affect our health and the public's health collectively. Public health has developed systematic ways of thinking about health issues (Schneider 2006) that enable public health workers to tackle a health issue in a considered and deliberate fashion. However, unless public health has a collective action domain, it will lack a focus on the social and economic issues that are so central to supporting and maintaining the changes that enhance the public's health.

If asked to think about how you might tackle a public health problem, you might think about it in terms of levels of prevention—primary, secondary and tertiary (see Chapter 14 for more detail on these concepts). Primary prevention focuses on maintaining health—for example, school health programs, seat belts in motor vehicles, anti-smoking campaigns, and physical activity and nutrition programs. Secondary prevention aims to minimise the extent of a health problem by focusing on early intervention, such as prostate, bowel and breast screening. Tertiary intervention aims to minimise disability and provide rehabilitation services, such as cardiac rehabilitation.

Another way of dealing with a public health problem is to consider a chain of causation (see Chapter 11), involving an agent, a host and the environment. In this case, prevention is accomplished by interrupting the chain of causation—for example, by providing immunisation, using antibiotics, or purifying water.

For you to gain a more comprehensive understanding of public health, it is vital that you appreciate the underlying vision, values and core components of public health, as they provide the foundations upon which strategies are developed and implemented.

> **ACTIVITY 1.2 Daily life and public health**
>
> - From the scenario above, list the issues that you feel are relevant to public health.

> **REFLECTION 1.2**
>
> Reflect on the issues you have listed above. Did you consider any of the following issues?
>
> - Your access to clean water, sewerage, and rubbish removal and disposal.
> - Your friend's mention of the breast cancer and screening media campaign, which raises your awareness of these issues.
> - Your safety on the road, which is enhanced by legislation such as that of seat-belt wearing, traffic lights and the construction of roadways to maximise safety.
> - Your ability to drive on roads that are maintained for safe use.
> - Your purchase of food, which has been prepared with standards of hygiene that protect your health.
> - The quality of the food you consumed for breakfast.
> - The ambulance service visiting a school to discuss their role.
> - The fact that you parked your car close to the lecture theatre and walked for a short distance to your lecture.

Public health vision and values

Having a vision of where you think public health might be placed in the next 5–10 years is important for the discipline and your practice. A range of factors that impact on health and public health will have a profound effect on the nature and scope of the discipline in the next decade. Globalisation is one of those issues (as discussed in Chapter 15); other issues include the emergence of new virulent infectious diseases, an increase in chronic disease such as diabetes, the ageing population, and the ever-increasing cost and expanding technological sophistication of healthcare. In Chapters 11 to 14 we examine the role of health protection and health promotion in advancing the health of the population, and in Chapter 15 we explore the notion of globalisation and its impact on health.

The traditional values of public health are described by Lawson and Bauman to include:

- using scientific evidence as a basis for action
- focusing on the health of all sections of the population
- emphasising a collective action dimension (Lawson & Bauman 2001 p 5).

Addressing health issues across population sub-groups is also very important, because it affirms the principles of equity and social justice, which are central to public health activity. But it is not always an easy task, because people's lives are complex, and their focus on affordable housing, transport and access to food may mean that health is not a priority. An example of the application of equity and social justice principles to public health can be found in the Victorian Public Health and Wellbeing Plan 2011–2015 (Department of Health, Victoria, 2011). This plan provides the basis for building a statewide prevention system that is complementary to the healthcare system, and that is effective, better coordinated and sustainable over the longer term (Victorian Public Health and Wellbeing Plan 2014).

A 'collective action' dimension, as demonstrated in the Victorian Plan above, tends to be contextualised differently according to the social and cultural aspects of the society in which we live. For example, in the United States there is still a very strong emphasis on individual rights and freedom; in contrast, in Australia there is a notion of the collective good. Applied to public health, this means that the community accepts laws and regulations that limit the individual's freedom, if it protects the health of the population.

Core functions of public health

There are a number of different ways in which the core functions or the focus of public health have been described and defined. Table 1.2 outlines these core functions.

For at least the past 10 years, efforts to define core public health competencies have occurred around the world. In the United States, the United Kingdom and Australia, professional bodies and government instrumentalities have attempted to define the roles and responsibilities of public health workers. In 2000, the National Public Health Partnership (NPHP) (2000) defined core public health functions in Australia.

The *Public Health Education Research Program* (2007), funded by the Australian Government Department of Health, defined public health practice as involving five areas. These are: health monitoring and surveillance; disease prevention and control; health protection; health promotion; and health policy, planning and management. The application of research methods and professional practice form the two underpinning competency groups.

More recently, the then Australian Network of Academic Public Health Institutions (ANAPHI) produced *Foundation competencies for Master of Public Health graduates in Australia* (Genat et al. 2009). The foundation competencies were designed around six

TABLE 1.2 Core functions for public health

Author(s) and categories	Core functions
Lawson and Bauman (2001) Four major task categories	Health promotion and disease prevention; traditional public health functions; monitoring and surveillance; public health policy
Turnock (2001) Seven key practice principles	Social justice; equity of access and equity in health outcomes; links with government; expanding and evolving agenda; preventive focus; balance between science and societal needs; appreciation of the politics of public health
Beaglehole et al. (2004) Five key themes of modern public health theory and practice	Leadership of the health system; collaborative action across sectors; multidisciplinary approaches to all determinants of health; political engagement in the development of public health policy; partnerships with the populations served
Gostin (2004 pp 98–103) Three effective core strategies of public health	Strengthening governmental public health infrastructure; engaging non-governmental actors in partnerships for public health; transforming national health policy—balance between traditional dominant investments in personal healthcare and biomedical research, and investments in the 'multiple determinants of societal health'
Griffiths et al. (2005) Three key domains of public health	Health improvement—focus on reducing inequalities and working with partners outside health; health protection—preventing and controlling infectious diseases, responding to emergencies, and protecting from and dealing with environmental health hazards; health service delivery and quality—evidence-based practice, planning and prioritising and appropriate research, audit and evaluation activities
Hanlon et al. (2012b pp 318–319)	Taking action today to protect and promote health and wellbeing tomorrow through an organised effort that focuses on health improvement, health protection and improving services
Teutsch and Fielding (2013 p 287)	The ability to understand contemporary health problems, to communicate the needs successfully, to identify solutions, and to implement them through programs and policies

areas of practice: health monitoring and surveillance; disease prevention and control; health protection; health promotion; health policy, planning and management; and evidence-based professional population health practice.

Most of the core functions described by the authors in Table 1.2 have common themes that go to the heart of current public health practice. These include collaborative action across sectors, multidisciplinary approaches, establishing partnerships, reducing inequality, and enhancing political support for public health policy. Public health professionals need to work with many other professionals outside as well as inside the health sector, and approach public health issues from a multisector perspective. For example, public health needs to work with government education, housing and transport departments to ensure that these services are available to the whole population in an equitable manner.

What do public health practitioners do?

This question can be considered in two parts. First, who makes up the public health workforce? Second, what role does the public health worker play now and in the future?

Who works in public health? Is it anyone from a health discipline who is involved in some form of public health activity, or is it much narrower, such as a community primary care worker or a public health specialist? Rotem et al. (1995) conducted a study of the public health workforce, and described the workforce as people involved in protecting, promoting and/or restoring the collective health of whole or specific populations.

The authors found that personnel come from a wide range of professional and occupational backgrounds, and that characteristically they are described as having a high degree of versatility and flexibility, and are mature, highly qualified, multiskilled individuals from a variety of backgrounds, who have multiple functions to perform that are not always related to their primary training or occupation (Rotem et al. 1995).

In a New South Wales statewide consultation, a third category of health worker was identified as one with public health components included in their professional practice, such as general practitioners and community health nurses who need an understanding of population health (Madden & Salmon 1999).

For many professions like public health, an expanding scope of practice will increasingly become the focus of professional practice. In rural and remote areas where it is difficult to attract health workers, the potential inclusion of a primary healthcare role for nurses and paramedics already involves a focus on prevention and promotion.

The second question is what does the public health worker do? The role of the public health practitioner, according to van der Maesen and Nijhuis (2000 p 136), involves three important elements:

1   improving social conditions that stimulate health
2   preventing social conditions that threaten health
3   neutralising existing social conditions that cause ill health.

How do you think the three elements listed above relate to the questions in Activity 1.4?

While there are core functions for public health workers, there is a diversity of public health practice. The organisation that employs you, the nature of the position, the organisational philosophy, the governance structure of the organisation, whether it is for profit or not-for-profit, state-based or non-government, all impact on the nature and the scope of the public health work you might be asked to do.

Even though there may be different roles and functions according to the setting in which you work, there are common aspects of practice (see Box 1.1).

BOX 1.1

ROLES AND FUNCTIONS FOR THE PUBLIC HEALTH WORKFORCE

- Understanding the context for public health activity, and its role and functions
- Clarity around political impacts on public health
- Ability to apply a range of methodological approaches to understand data
- A theoretical understanding of the disciplines that underpin public health, and their contribution to strategy selection
- Understanding a range of skills around the surveillance, prevention, promotion and restoration of the population's health
- Developing and analysing policy
- Planning, implementation and evaluation
- Evidence-based practice
- Advocacy, communication and negotiation skills
- Working intersectorally and with multidisciplinary groups
- Ethical practice

Reflecting on the content covered so far, you should now be feeling confident about your understanding of what public health is, and its role and value in today's society. The complexity of public health processes should also be obvious. For public health to be effective, it cannot be undertaken on an 'ad hoc' basis, but must adopt a multidisciplinary approach across a range of professions. Collaborative efforts should engage a number of organisations, both government and non-government. It is also important to include ethics at the forefront of our practice. Chapter 8 examines ethics in public health practice in more detail.

The World Health Organization agenda for public health

We now turn our attention to public health developments that have occurred at an international level. These developments have influenced the public health agenda and given direction to initiatives that have been implemented in Australia.

The WHO has played a significant role in promoting public health, particularly the concept of 'health for all', which has been embraced by countries throughout the world, underpinning their respective health policies. The organisation has a six-point action plan that assists in shaping activity and focus (see Box 1.2).

ACTIVITY 1.4 What do you think public health workers do?

- How would you describe the public health workforce? Would your description be broad and encompassing, or narrow and restrictive? Think back to our discussion of definitions of public health.
- Make a list of the range and scope of activity for the public health worker.
- Select a public health worker—this might be an environmental health officer, a community health nurse, a diabetes educator, or a health promotion practitioner working in the community. Write down what you think a typical day might be for such a worker. Make a list of the roles and responsibilities they might have.
- How does this list relate back to the competencies we discussed earlier in the chapter?

BOX 1.2

WHO'S SIX-POINT ACTION PLAN

1 Promoting development

2 Fostering health security

3 Strengthening health systems

4 Harnessing research, information and evidence

5 Enhancing partnerships

6 Improving performance

(Source: WHO 2011; WHO 2012)

Since the 1970s, the WHO and other substantial international players have had a focus on primary healthcare, prevention and promotion. This has been evident in policy that supports the advancement of promotion and prevention. For example, the WHO *Declaration of Alma-Ata* stressed the importance of a slogan that said 'Health for all by the year 2000' (WHO 1978). This primary healthcare philosophy spoke about the principles of equity, social justice, intersectoral collaboration, community participation and empowerment. It had as its focus the important role of health promotion and disease prevention. (See Chapter 14 for a detailed analysis of health promotion.)

In the 1980s the lifestyle phase became prominent in public health developments. Canada was at the forefront of initiatives to focus on the lifestyles of individuals, but also included social issues. Important considerations involved lifestyle, environment, socioeconomic factors and healthcare system reform.

In more recent times, the global concern for ecosystem sustainability—known in public health circles as 'ecological public health'—has emerged as a prominent theme for public health action. The WHO's *Jakarta Declaration* (1997) went some way towards a focus on sustainability and globalisation. However, in 2005 the WHO *Bangkok Charter for Health Promotion* identified globalisation as a central issue for health promotion endeavours. Participants at the Sixth Global Conference on Health Promotion identified major challenges, actions and commitments needed to address the determinants of health in a globalised world by engaging the many actors and stakeholders critical to achieving health for all. The 8th Global Conference on Health Promotion was held in Helsinki, Finland, in 2013 (WHO 2013). See Chapter 14 for a comprehensive account of the *Ottawa Charter* (WHO 1986) and the other international conferences on health promotion in the evolution of health promotion policy and practice.

The WHO reforecast its endeavours for 'Health for all by the year 2000 and beyond' with the production of 'Health for all by 2010', although some regional areas have targets dated to 2020. The emphasis is on sustainable development, collaboration, protection, prevention, resilience, adaptation, the emergence of chronic diseases and the re-emergence of infectious diseases.

In concert with these activities, the United Nations member states agreed on eight Millennium Development Goals (MDGs), with targets to be achieved by 2015 (United Nations 2013). Four of these goals relate to health outcomes: eradicating extreme poverty and hunger; improving maternal health; reducing child mortality; and dealing

BOX 1.3

FIVE KEY ACTION AREAS FOR THE COMMISSION ON SOCIAL DETERMINANTS OF HEALTH

1 Improving living and learning conditions in early childhood
2 Strengthening social programs to provide fairer employment conditions and access to labour markets, particularly for vulnerable social groups
3 Policies and interventions to protect people in informal employment—that is, those who work without formal contracts or social protections, often in sectors outside government regulation, such as subsistence farming, household-based enterprises, and street vending
4 Policies across sectors to improve living conditions in urban slums
5 Programs to address key determinants of women's health, such as access to education and economic opportunities

(Source: Irwin et al. 2006, p 0750)

with HIV/AIDS, malaria and other infectious diseases (McMichael & Butler 2007). This is a difficult task in the context of the overwhelming range of issues impacting on population health.

In March 2005, the WHO created the Commission on Social Determinants of Health (CSDH) (WHO CSDH website), which operated until May 2008. The components of the CSDH included the commissioners, partner countries, evidence-gathering knowledge networks, civil society organisations and global institutions (Irwin et al. 2006 p 0749). The CSDH developed five action areas, as outlined in Box 1.3.

In 2011, the WHO focused on a global strategy for the prevention and management of non-communicable diseases (WHO 2008). This strategy is a partnership for action to control four diseases—cardiovascular disease, diabetes, cancers, and chronic respiratory diseases—and four shared risk factors—tobacco use, physical inactivity, unhealthy diets and alcohol misuse.

These developments on the international stage are now clearly focused on health inequalities and ecological sustainability. This recognises that inequalities in health are seeded in the structures of society—economically, politically and culturally—and it will take collaborative efforts across sectors to bring good health within the reach of everyone. Chapter 15 covers many of these issues in more detail. Ecological sustainability is considered in Chapters 12 and 17. Most recently, WHO reforms have focused on being better equipped to address the increasingly complex challenges of the health of populations in the twenty-first century (WHO 2014), including improved health outcomes to address global health priorities, and greater coherence in global health to ensure an active and effective role in contributing to the health of all peoples.

It is important to remember that ecological sustainability recognises all components of people's lives, and takes into account the impact that these factors have on the health of populations or subgroups of populations. For example, individuals alone are not totally responsible for their health status. Although they need to adopt positive behaviours in regard to their health, factors such as the environment in which they live, their economic status, and their culture are some of the things which, although they have little or no control over them, can have a significant impact on their health. A focus on sustainable environments for health has evolved as the main focus of public health now and in the foreseeable future.

Public health in the Australian context

In Australia, managing public health activity is multilayered and is influenced by the prevailing political thinking. This chapter introduces you to the systems and organisational arrangements for public health activity. In Chapters 3 and 4 we provide you with more specific information about the healthcare system and its relationship to public health and social policy initiatives impacting on public health.

Responsibility for public health includes the Australian Government Department of Health, state and territory health departments, local government departments, non-government organisations, professional associations, and a range of advocacy groups. In addition, individuals, such as general practitioners and health workers in community health centres, undertake health protection and health promotion roles and responsibilities.

A number of other organisations also play a role. The National Health and Medical Research Council (NHMRC) funds public health research and makes policy statements on health issues; the Australian Institute of Health and Welfare (AIHW) and the Australian Bureau of Statistics (ABS) monitor and report on health data; and universities educate public health, allied health, medical and nursing professionals, and undertake research and consultancy activity in public health. Medicare Locals, to be called primary health networks, play an important role in advancing population health (Australian Government Department of Health 2014a).

AUSTRALIAN GOVERNMENT DEPARTMENT OF HEALTH

The vision of the Department of Health is to achieve better health and wellbeing for all Australians through strengthening evidence-based policy advice, improving program management, research and regulation, and partnerships with other government agencies, consumers and stakeholders (Australian Government Department of Health 2014b). The Population Health Division (Australian Government Department of Health 2014c) and the Office for Aboriginal and Torres Strait Islander Health, within the Department of Health, both play a national leadership role in public health matters, such as infectious diseases, immunisation, nutrition and obesity, physical activity, food policy, smoking, and alcohol and drug abuse. In addition, other offices, such as Health Protection, Mental Health and the Chronic Disease Division, play important roles in prevention. The Population Health Division plays a number of roles in creating and supporting national endeavours in public health. These activities are listed in Box 1.4.

The division has identified a number of broad priorities for public health that focus on identifying and responding to emerging threats and health emergencies, and a focus on prevention, particularly in areas such as nutrition, physical activity, overweight and obesity (see the DoH Population Health Division (PHD) website for a review of current program involvement). The PHD has an emphasis on responding to health issues throughout the lifecourse. In 1996, it established the National Public Health Partnership (NPHP), creating a framework for public health leadership and to strengthen collaboration between stakeholders. The NPHP was disbanded in 2006. More recently, the PHD has been involved in the National Preventative Health Strategy, the National Partnership Agreement on Preventive Health, the Australian Health Survey, and the establishment of the Australian National Preventive Health Agency (disbanded

> **BOX 1.4**
>
> ## ROLE OF THE POPULATION HEALTH DIVISION, AUSTRALIAN GOVERNMENT DEPARTMENT OF HEALTH
>
> - Leadership and coordination of a range of national initiatives
> - Supporting activities aimed at understanding and controlling the determinants of disease
> - Informed decision-making based on effective use of health information, and on the application of research evidence in the design of programs to improve health
> - Relationship building between staff of the department and a range of stakeholders, from states and territories through to academic institutions and non-government organisations
> - Working with these stakeholders to expand their knowledge of factors affecting the health of the population and specific at-risk groups, such as Aboriginal and Torres Strait Islander communities and populations located in rural and remote Australia

in 2014)—all important steps forward in prevention and public health in Australia. Since 2010, successive federal governments have restructured the Department of Health (see Chapter 3 for more details).

In addition, there are a number of federally supported organisations and pieces of legislation that protect and enhance the health of the population. These include the Therapeutic Goods Administration, Food Standards Australia New Zealand, the Australian Radiation Protection and Nuclear Safety Agency, and the Australian Safety and Compensation Council.

To build a prevention agenda in a health system that currently expends the majority of its funds on treatment is an ongoing challenge. As the costs of treatment continue to rise, and health technology becomes more sophisticated and expensive, a focus on prevention has gained modest traction in the health system. The emergence of chronic diseases, such as diabetes, means that people will be living a large part of their lives managing such conditions.

Activity 1.5 asks you to think about the role of the federal government in public health, and about a number of important issues that face the government in the coming years, such as healthcare costs and funding.

> **ACTIVITY 1.5 Advancing public health—the Australian perspective**
>
> - In the past 10 years, what have been the major foci of national developments in public health in Australia?
> - What factors may have influenced national developments? For example, a change of the political party in leadership, health crises, changing patterns of health.
> - What role can non-government organisations play in public health?
> - What role do you think the sustainability and ecological public health movements have had on advancing the activities of public health in the public mind?
> - How do we balance healthcare needs with population health needs in order to be able to fund the health system into the future?

BOX 1.5

STATE/TERRITORY GOVERNMENT FUNCTIONS

- *Health protection*—such as environmental health, drugs and poisons
- *Disease prevention*—examples include surveillance, health education, immunisation, STI (sexually transmissible infection) and cancer screening
- *Health promotion*—including a focus on physical activity, nutrition, maternal and child health, tobacco, drugs and alcohol, and injury prevention
- *Policy and program support*—epidemiology, evaluation, research, workforce development, policy development within and outside the sector impacting on health, and clinical service guidelines

(Adapted from Lin et al. 2014)

REFLECTION 1.5

The federal government, over many years, has played a policy and strategic role in advancing population health. This strategic role has meant an emphasis on policy and the identification of major areas for national development, the detail of which is often translated at state/territory and local government levels. For example, the Population Health Division has set a national agenda for healthy eating and increased physical activity. At the state/territory level that national agenda has been translated into actions that more clearly meet the needs of the population. Do you think that non-government agencies such as the Cancer Fund or the National Heart Foundation have been included in policy initiatives at the federal level? How might you determine whether they have been given a role? How is ecological public health defined? Ask five of your friends if they understand what ecological public health is all about. In Chapter 3 we discuss funding for public health in a healthcare system where the majority of current funds are expended on care and treatment. Can you think of any health professionals who might want funding levels to remain as they are?

State and territory governments

At the state/territory level of public health activity, responsibilities have included: managing public hospitals and community health services; leadership and planning of public health; health surveillance; local government regulation; and health promotion, including working with non-government and other organisations (Baum 2008) (see Box 1.5).

Other roles and responsibilities of public health activity include that of the chief health officer, under whose authority many health activities are located, and who exercises statutory responsibilities. These include environmental protection, occupational health and safety, road and traffic authority, sport and recreation, and consumer affairs. Education departments in each state have a major role to play in promotion and prevention through the health curriculum, health promotion in schools, and a range of other activities, including *Sun Smart, Healthy Tuckshops*, drug and alcohol programs, and driver education. Emergency services departments in each state also play a role in promotion and prevention. For example, with the changing scope of practice, health workers such as ambulance officers play an important role in providing information and education to the general public, and in rural and remote communities, as primary healthcare workers.

In many states a whole-of-government approach is taken where public health and other services form part of a more integrated approach to promotion and prevention, and the multisectoral nature of public health is recognised and supported. The success of any approach depends on political will, interdepartmental collaboration, and positive interaction between all tiers of government.

Local government

Local government has a critical role to play in public health, especially in the area of legislation and creating healthy communities. Local governments' roles in public health activity vary across Australia, but more often than not still include such functions as well-baby clinics, immunisation, food safety, environmental protection, a strong role in cultural and recreational activities and community development, and, importantly, local economic development.

Non-government organisations, community organisations, professional associations, and public health advocacy groups

There is a broad range of organisations and associations that support public health endeavours in Australia. That support comes in a variety of different ways. For example, large well-funded non-government organisations (NGOs), such as the cancer councils, the National Heart Foundation, and Diabetes Australia, have a range of roles—including providing information and education, fundraising, advocacy, lobbying and research—in the promotion of health and the detection and treatment of specific health issues.

Other organisations, such as professional associations, play an important role in lobbying, advocacy and policy development, as well as workforce education through conferences and professional development activities. These associations include the Public Health Association of Australia, the Australian Health Promotion Association, the Australasian Epidemiology Association, and the Australian Institute of Environmental Health.

A third group of organisations are those focused on advocacy and lobbying, including the Women's Health Network, the Consumer Health Forum, and the National Association of Aboriginal Community-Controlled Health Organisations (Baum 2008).

Health promotion foundations are variously integrated into state health departments or have been set up to stand independently of a departmental structure. They have an important role in funding research activities and their application, and, in some jurisdictions, have an advocacy and lobbying role. They do, however, tend to vary in popularity with changing government policy.

To the above list, Baum (2008) adds primary healthcare providers, and universities and research institutions. Primary healthcare providers include general practitioners, who play a role in screening, immunisation and the health education of patients. Universities and research institutes both have education and research functions.

ACTIVITY 1.6 Health in the public arena

- On a regular basis, the media will report on public health issues, initiatives, developments, etc. The newspaper or current affairs programs on television are effective communication vehicles by which the public's awareness may be raised about an issue or an event that directly, or indirectly, impacts on the public's health.

Public health issues in the daily press

Identify and source two articles or reports that comment on a current public health issue. Write a brief review of each newspaper article or television report. Use the following questions to frame your comments:

- Why is it a public health issue? Think about our discussion of definitions of public health.
- Use evidence to decide whether this is an important public health issue. Where should this evidence come from?
- What population or subpopulation is involved?
- What strategies, if any, are being implemented to address the issue or concern?
- What component or components of the public health system would take responsibility? For example, the state health department or a non-government organisation.
- What are the future ramifications if the issue or concern is not addressed?

The future for public health?

There are a number of emerging challenges that public health faces in the twenty-first century. These challenges include the emergence of 'new' infectious diseases, the ongoing presence of HIV/AIDS (particularly in developing countries) and the impact that overweight and obesity have on a range of health issues that influence the population's health. Add to these issues the influence of global climate change and ecological sustainability, and you have a public health system stretched to capacity across a range of fronts.

Throughout the book, we continually return to these themes and issues as we explore the nature and scope of public health.

A final word

In this chapter, we have covered a broad range of issues that are reflective of elements of public health. We have examined definitions of health, both lay and professional; we have considered the definition, vision and values of public health; and the role of a wide range of health workers who play an important role in public health.

We have discussed the role of the WHO in setting a global agenda for public health, and the specific role of governments at three levels in Australia, from federal to state/territory and local government. We introduced you to the range of other associations, community organisations and advocacy groups, who all play important roles in improving the health of the population.

In conclusion, we briefly discussed public health issues emerging in the twenty-first century, and the challenges that face professionals working in the public health field if they are to deal with these issues. We return to these issues in the last chapter of the book.

In the chapter that follows, we look at the history of public health, and see how history provides a good window to the future.

REVIEW QUESTIONS

1 What do you understand by the terms 'health', 'illness', 'disease' and 'public health'?

2 Why should public health have a vision, and what values should public health workers espouse and practise?

3 Write down the core tasks of public health, and think about how these might differ in the future.

4 Who is the public health practitioner, and what do you believe to be the core functions of a public health worker?

5 Make up a table of the three levels of government in Australia, and in each column describe their public health roles and responsibilities.

6 What role do NGOs play in public health?

7 List and briefly comment on the issues you believe will be facing public health in the twenty-first century.

8 How have varying political agendas at state and federal level impacted on public health funding and activity?

Useful websites

- Australian Bureau of Statistics: http://www.abs.gov.au/
- Australian Government Department of Health: http://www.health.gov.au/
- Australian Government Department of Health, Population Health Division: http://www.health.gov.au/internet/main/publishing.nsf/Content/phd-what
- National Health and Medical Research Council: http://www.nhmrc.gov.au/
- United Nations: http://www.un.org/en/
- World Health Organization: http://www.who.int/en/

References

Australian Government Department of Health, 2014a. Primary health networks. Online. Available: <http://www.health.gov.au/internet/main/publishing.nsf/Content/primary_Health_Networks> (22 Aug 2014).

Australian Government Department of Health, 2014b. Overview. Online. Available: <http://www.health.gov.au//internet/main/publishing.nsf/Content/health-overview.htm> (22 Aug 2014).

Australian Government Department of Health, 2014c. Population Health Division. Online. Available: <http://www.health.gov.au/internet/main/publishing.nsf/Content/health-pubhlth-index.htm> (22 Aug 2014).

Baum, F., 2002. The New Public Health, second ed. Oxford University Press, South Melbourne.

Baum, F., 2008. The New Public Health, third ed. Oxford University Press, South Melbourne.

Beaglehole, R., Bonita, R., Horton, R., et al., 2004. Public health in the new era: improving health through collaborative action. Lancet 363, 2084–2086.

Bircher, J., 2005. Towards a dynamic definition of health and disease. Medicine, Health Care, and Philosophy 8, 335–341.

Blaxter, M., 1990. Health and Lifestyles. Routledge, London.

Blaxter, M., 2007. How is health experienced? In: Douglas, J., Earle, S., Handsley, S., et al. (Eds.), A Reader in Promoting Public Health. Sage, London.

Brown, V.A., Grootjans, J., Ritchie, J., et al. (Eds.), 2005. Sustainability and Health: Supporting Global Ecological Integrity in Public Health. Allen and Unwin, Crows Nest.

Department of Health, Victoria, 2011. Victorian Public Health and Wellbeing Plan 2011–2015. Online. Available: <http://www.health.vic.gov.au/prevention/vphwplan.htm> (20 Aug 2014).

Durie, M., 2004. Understanding health and illness. International Journal of Epidemiology 33, 1138–1144.

Fleming, M.L., Parker, E., 2007. Health Promotion: Principles and Practice in the Australian Context, third ed. Allen and Unwin, Crows Nest.

Genat, W., Robinson, P., Parker, E., 2009. Foundation Competencies for Master of Public Health Graduates in Australia. Australian Network of Academic Public Health Institutions (ANAPHI), Brisbane.

Goldberg, D.S., 2009. In support of a broad model of public health: disparities, social epidemiology and public health causation. Public Health Ethics 2 (1), 70–83.

Gostin, L.O., 2004. Health of the people: the highest law? Journal of Law, Medicine and Ethics 32 (3), 509–515.

Gostin, L.O., 2010. Redressing the unconscionable health gap: a global plan for justice. Lancet 375 (9723), 1504–1505.

Griffiths, S., Jewell, T., Donnelly, P., 2005. Public health in practice: the three domains of public health. Public Health 119 (10), 907–913.

Hanlon, P., Carlisle, S., Lyon, A., 2012a. The Future Public Health. Open University Press, Maidenhead.

Hanlon, P., Carlisle, S., Hannah, M., et al., 2012b. A perspective on the future public health: an integrative and ecological framework. Perspectives in Public Health 132 (6), 313–319.

Huber, M., Knottnerus, J.A., Green, L., et al., 2011. How should we define health? BMJ (Clinical Research Ed.) 343, d4163.

Institute of Medicine, 2011. Accountability and for the Public's Health: Revitalizing Law and Policy to Meet New Challenges. National Academies Press, Washington DC.

Irwin, A., Valentine, N., Brown, C., et al., 2006. The Commission on Social Determinants of Health: tackling the social roots of health inequities. PLoS Medicine 3 (6), e106:749–e106:751.

Kelly, M.P., 2011. The future of public health: the lessons of modernism. Commentary. Journal of Public Health 33 (3), 344.

Kickbusch, I., 1986. Lifestyles and health. Social Science and Medicine 22 (2), 117–124.

Lalonde, M., 1974. A New Perspective on the Health of Canadians: A Working Document. Government of Canada, Ottawa.

Last, J.M., 2001. A Dictionary of Epidemiology, fourth ed. Oxford University Press, New York.

Lawson, J.S., Bauman, A.E., 2001. Public Health Australia: An Introduction, second ed. McGraw-Hill, Sydney.

Lin, V., Smith, J., Fawkes, S., 2007. Public Health Practice in Australia: The Organised Effort. Allen and Unwin, Sydney.

Lin, V., Smith, J., Fawkes, S., 2014. Public Health Practice in Australia: The Organised Effort, second ed. Allen and Unwin, Sydney.

Madden, L., Salmon, A., 1999. Public health workforce: results of a NSW statewide consultation on the development of the national public health workforce. NSW Public Health Bulletin 10 (3), 19–21.

McMichael, A.J., Butler, C.D., 2007. Emerging health issues: the widening challenge for population health promotion. Health Promotion International 21 (Suppl. 1), 15–24. doi: 10.1093/heapro/dal047.

Morris, G.P., 2010. Ecological public health and climate change policy. Perspectives in Public Health 130 (1), 34–40.

National Aboriginal Health Strategy Working Party, 1989. A National Aboriginal Health Strategy. Department of Aboriginal Affairs, Canberra.

National Public Health Partnership, 2000. Public Health Practice in Australia Today: A Statement of Core Functions. NPHP, Melbourne.

National Strategic Framework for Aboriginal and Torres Strait Islander Health, 2003–2013. Australian Government Implementation Plan 2007–2013. Australian Government, Canberra.

Public Health Education Research Program, 2007. Proposed Competencies for the Public Health Education Research Program. Australian Government Department of Health and Ageing, Canberra.

Public Health Association of Australia website. Online. Available: <http://www.phaa.net.au/> (25 Feb 2014).

Rotem, A., Walters, J., Dewdney, J., 1995. Editorial: the public health workforce education and training study. Australian Journal of Public Health 19 (5), 437–438.

Rothstein, M.A., 2009. The limits of public health: a response. Public Health Ethics 2 (1), 84–88.

Schneider, M.J., 2006. Introduction to Public Health. Jones and Bartlett Learning, Sudbury, MA.

Shilton, T., Sparks, M., McQueen, D., et al., 2011. Proposal for new definition of health. (Letter) BMJ 343, d5359.

Teutsch, S.M., Fielding, J.E., 2013. Rediscovering the core of public health. Annual Review of Public Health 34 (1), 287–299.

Thompson, S.J., Gifford, S.M., 2000. Trying to keep a balance: the meaning of health and diabetes in an urban Aboriginal community. Social Science and Medicine 61, 1457–1472.

Turnock, B., 2001. Public Health: What It Is and How It Works, second ed. Aspen, Gaithersburg.

United Nations, 2013. The Millennium Development Goals Report 2013. UN, New York.

US Department of Health and Human Services, 2011. FLU.gov website. Online. Available: <http://www.flu.gov/about_the_flu/h5n1/> (3 Apr 2014).

van der Maesen, L.J.G., Nijhuis, H.G.J., 2000. Continuing the debate on the philosophy of modern public health: social quality as a point of reference. Journal of Epidemiology and Community Health 54, 134–141.

Waltner-Toews, D., 2000. The end of medicine: the beginning of health. Futures 32, 655–667.

Winslow, C.E.A., 1920. The untilled fields of public health. Science 51 (1306), 23–33.

World Health Organization, 1948. Constitution. WHO. Online. Available: <http://www.who.int/governance/eb/who_constitution_en.pdf> (3 Apr 2014).

World Health Organization, 1978. Declaration of Alma-Ata. International Conference on Primary Health Care, Alma-Ata, USSR, 6–12 September 1978. Online. Available: <http://www.who.int/publications/almaata_declaration_en.pdf> (3 Apr 2014).

World Health Organization, 1986. The Ottawa Charter for Health Promotion. First International Conference on Health Promotion, Ottawa, 21 November 1986. Online. Available: <http://www.who.int/healthpromotion/conferences/previous/ottawa/en/> (3 Apr 2014).

World Health Organization, 1997. Jakarta Declaration. Fourth International Conference on Health Promotion, Jakarta, July 1997.

World Health Organization, 2005. Bangkok Charter for Health Promotion. World Health Organization (WHO), Geneva.

World Health Organization, 2008. The WHO agenda: leadership priorities. Online. Available: <http://www.who.int/about/agenda/en/index.html> (3 Apr 2014).

World Health Organization, 2011. Global coordination mechanism. Online. Available: <http://www.who.int/global-coordination-mechanism/background/en/> (22 Apr 2015).

World Health Organization, 2012. WHO reforms: programmes and priority setting. WHO reforms: meeting of member states on programme and priority setting. Document 1, 20 February 2012. Online. Available: <http://www.who.int/dg/reform/consultation/WHO_Reform_1_en.pdf?ua=1&ua=1> (22 Apr 2015).

World Health Organization, 2013. The Helsinki Statement on Health in All Policies. 8th Global Conference on Health Promotion. World Health Organization (WHO), Geneva. Online. Available: <http://www.who.int/healthpromotion/conferences/8gchp/en/> (3 Apr 2014).

World Health Organization, 2014. WHO reform. Online. Available: <http://www.who.int/about/who_reform/en/> (5 Feb 2014).

World Health Organization Commission on Social Determinants of Health, 2005–2008. website. Online. Available: <http://www.who.int/social_determinants/thecommission/en/> (3 Apr 2014).

CHAPTER 2

History and development of public health

Mary Louise Fleming

Learning objectives

After reading this chapter, you should be able to:

- briefly describe the importance of public health history to contemporary public health

- discuss the major developments in the ancient history of public health

- outline the key periods and activities in the modern history of Western public health

- describe and understand the important roles of political, social, environmental and economic factors as they impact on health

- consider the major factors that have influenced contemporary public health in the past 50 years.

Introduction

This chapter and the others that follow have the study of population health as their focus, as opposed to a focus on individual care and treatment. Clearly, however, we are concerned with the way in which population health is influenced by biomedical theories and practices, and the way population health is funded and is influenced by the importance placed on therapeutic medicine. The discussions that follow include a brief overview of the ancient history of public health, and the modern history of Western public health dating from 1850. This date signifies the beginnings of a more organised, collective effort to protect the public's health. These discussions will help you further expand your definition of public health.

You will have an entertaining journey through public health achievements, and less successful outcomes, by examining the historical developments that have led us to a modern understanding of public health. The ancient Greeks and Romans, for example, had public health measures to ensure the safety and health of their populations, for a range of social and economic reasons. Convicts arrived in Australia with many health problems, and were put to work to satisfy the needs of a fledgling colony. It is important to understand the historical journey of public health and the way it is critically analysed, as it provides a looking-glass onto the present and the future.

The importance of the past in public health

Examining the historical evolution of public health is important because, as George Rosen said:

> There can be no real comprehension of the history of public health at any period without a thorough understanding of the political, economic and social history of that period in its relation to the contemporary public health situation. (Rosen 1953 p 430)

In a similar vein, Tosh (1984), in *The Pursuit of History*, commented that to know the past is to understand that things have not always been the same, and that they need not remain the same in the future.

History is also relevant because we need to be able to 'observe public health over a long period of time in order to be able to evaluate progress, or the lack of progress, in improving it' (Scally & Womack 2004 p 751). In an interesting article, Ogilvie and Hamlet (2005) present a dialogue between Socrates and Panacea, the goddess of healing, in the year 2055, about the history of the Western obesity epidemic. Socrates and Panacea discuss why information to the public about this issue had little or no impact on the community; they talk about the shortcomings of environmental changes, and the expectations of society regarding advancing economic development and access to healthy foods. At the conclusion of the article, Socrates asks Panacea why a discipline that was 'fond of phrases like "primary prevention" and "going upstream" never came up with a serious challenge to obesity' (Ogilvie & Hamlet 2005 p 1547): a sobering thought for us to contemplate in the second decade of the twenty-first century.

An understanding of how public health practitioners can influence the health of the population requires knowledge of how the discipline has evolved, and its successes and failures. Infectious diseases, which as a public health community we thought had mostly been eradicated, are once more threats to the population worldwide. For example, avian influenza A (H7N9), a subtype of influenza viruses, had not previously been seen in either animals or people until it emerged in March 2013 in China.

Historical awareness 'helps us to be alert to the resurgence of practice that has held sway in the past but been out of fashion in more recent times' (Scally & Womack 2004 p 752). It is important to be able to appreciate why particular approaches to public health are no longer used, and to determine the relevance of old approaches and their likely usefulness in thinking about contemporary approaches. For example, the rise of coronary heart disease and cancer in the period between the two world wars led to an emphasis on adult risk factors. In more recent years a return to a concept prevalent in the first half of the twentieth century—that of lifecourse epidemiology, where early life experiences influence adult mortality risk—has become more important.

Historical accounts of public health, up until the past 50 years, were strongly influenced by public health activity in the nineteenth century, and by the work of people such as Edwin Chadwick and John Snow. The Englishman John Snow, who had the handle from the Broad Street water pump removed, which led to a rapid decline in the number of cholera cases, demonstrated the early use of epidemiological analysis to pinpoint more extensive outbreaks of the disease. Edwin Chadwick's work on improving drinking water and sanitation actually marked the end of the era of social reform in public health in favour of advances in drainage systems and other more practical solutions (Berridge 2000). When we consider that, from the 1850s on, the links between poor sanitation and disease and the control of infectious diseases were the primary elements of public health, it is easy to argue that the foundations had been laid back through time, such as the Roman baths and aqueducts (Porter 1999). However, since the early 1960s a social history of public health has emerged where the focus is on 'economic, political, social and ideological responses to disease and the exploration of complex ways in which change both caused and was determined by the impact of epidemics' (Porter 1999 p 2).

Other more recent tensions evident in public health, such as the identification and classification of HIV/AIDS in the late 1980s, 'revived the historical study of stigma … and forcefully added to new debates about the social construction of everyday life' (Porter 1999 p 3). Placing current practice, organisational structures, and political and public health philosophies within a historical framework can increase our sense of identity and purpose (Scally & Womack 2004).

The history of public health provides a useful vehicle for teaching the principles of public health. It enriches our critical perspective of the 'social effects of initiatives undertaken in the name of public health, shows the shortcomings of public health interventions based on single factors and uses a wider time scope in the assessment of current problems' (Perdiguero et al. 2001 p 667). For example, there are similar issues between the story of opium at the end of the nineteenth century and its cultural and legal identification, and that of tobacco use at the end of the twentieth century (Berridge 2000). If you look at the website for the organisation Action on Smoking and Health (ASH website), there are key dates in the history of anti-tobacco campaigning in the United Kingdom.

It is interesting to note how many years passed between developments. It was not until the second half of the twentieth century that significant progress was made on a range of fronts; however, the power of the tobacco industry still remains a major stumbling block to achieving the overall objectives of the anti-smoking campaign. The ups and downs of this story are a message to today's practitioners to consider the timescale and effort entailed when dealing with vested interests (Scally & Womack 2004).

The following quote from Scally and Womack (2004) is worth including in full here, because it sums up why public health history is such an important aspect of our understanding of modern public health:

> An understanding of the rich and diverse history of public health cannot only support contemporary innovation but can help reduce the risk of public health practice being too narrowly focused on specific influences on the health of individuals rather than maintaining an overview of the full range of factors at work across a population. (Scally & Womack 2004 p 752)

Advancing population health—individual intervention or collective action?

One of the most prominent authors writing about changes to population health in nineteenth-century Europe was Thomas McKeown. He suggested that medical intervention, while playing a role in advancing health, was not responsible for the significant reduction in patterns of mortality and morbidity. He pointed out that diseases were declining prior to the advent of effective therapy (Lewis 2003). Szreter (2002), among others, has seriously challenged McKeown's thesis. Szreter (2002, 2003) has indicated that McKeown was right that material living standards, such as food availability, and therefore economics, were crucial to the health of the population. However, he also argued vigorously that McKeown was wrong in failing to 'foreground the importance of politics, ideologies, states, and institutions in producing the kind of societies that distribute their material wealth, food, and living standards in a health-enhancing way for all concerned' (Szreter 2002 p 724, 2003 p 427).

McKeown's critique of the medical establishment also found support in discourse emerging from the United States, Canada and the United Kingdom that focused on the importance of individual responsibility for health (we discuss these issues later in the chapter) (Colgrove 2002). However, Colgrove (2002) and Szreter (2002) have both suggested that McKeown had allowed his assumptions about the limited value of medical interventions, and the need for social reform, to predetermine his analytical categories and thus bias his interpretation of evidence.

What is clear in McKeown's argument is that nutrition and public health clearly have roles in the explanation, along, however, with living and working conditions, urbanisation, education, the aetiology of diseases, doctors and medical knowledge, mothers' attitudes, knowledge and behaviour, politics, reformers and climate (Lewis 2003).

However, McKeown's research has continued to hold a place in public health history because his research posed a fundamental question:

> Are public health ends better served by narrow interventions focused at the level of the individual or the community, or by broad measures to redistribute the social, political, economic resources that exert such a profound influence on health status at the population level? (Colgrove 2002 p 728)

In answering this question, Colgrove (2002) concluded that the choice of targeted interventions versus social change should not be viewed as dichotomous forces, but as complementary to each other. The challenge for health workers is to find ways to 'integrate technical preventive and curative measures with more broad based efforts to improve all of the conditions in which people live' (Colgrove 2002 p 729).

For the sake of the public's health?
The ancient history of public health

The ancient history of public health is permeated with examples of efforts to keep people healthy. However, it is unlikely that many of those efforts were designed to protect the public's health, but rather to enable other activity that would deliver a social or economic benefit to the State. In ancient societies, collective action to advance the health of populations was reserved for promoting the comfort of élites (Porter 1999).

Actions to protect the public's health are obvious throughout history, especially those activities relating to sanitary measures to ensure safe water and food supplies. For example, the earliest records of Chinese public health practice include providing drinking wells, building ditches around houses, protecting drinking water, and killing rats. Two centuries before the birth of Christ, the Chinese had invented rudimentary sewers, water spray carts and toilets. There was an emphasis on providing for personal hygiene and on preventive practices. In addition, herbal medicines, diagnostic procedures and preventive concepts—such as feeling the pulse and acupuncture—were in use.

In Egyptian and Babylonian societies, there were systems for sewage disposal and rainwater collection. Hygiene customs included personal cleanliness, frequent bathing, simple dressing, and the use of 'earth closets' (the forerunner of the modern-day toilet). The *Code of Hammurabi*, adopted by Babylonian society, guided the conduct of physicians and prescribed healthful practices. Temperance was recommended for all, at least 3000 years ago.

For Greek civilisation, the emphasis was placed on the individual. Consequently, the Greeks focused on the harmonious development of all faculties, where exercise and personal cleanliness were important. Little attention was afforded to environmental protection. The *Hippocratic Oath* (attributed to Hippocrates) still guides the ethical practice of medical practitioners. Hippocrates is also credited with a treatise on environment and health. Hippocrates in the fifth century BC, and Galen in the second century AD, described what were called the *four humours*: phlegm (phlegmatic), blood (sanguine), black bile (melancholy) and yellow bile (choleric) (Lawson & Bauman 2001). When in harmony, these four humours were believed to be responsible for health.

By contrast, in the Roman Empire, the State, not the individual, was considered more important. This meant that the regulation of building construction, sewage disposal and the destruction of decaying goods and buildings were of fundamental concern. Town planning, street and gutter paving, establishing drainage networks, and public bathing were very important aspects of Roman society, because they reinforced the philosophy of the importance of the State. Both the Greeks and the Romans protected the health of the wealthy, and their military, by providing fresh food, and water supply aqueducts, and enacting environmental protection laws.

Unlike the Greek and Roman eras, the Middle Ages marked a dark period in history. Throughout Europe there were major epidemics of infectious diseases. An emphasis on the spiritual aspects of life increased substantially, and if people were unwell they were often thought to have done something against the will of God. Islam rose to prominence during the sixth and seventh centuries, and a series of pilgrimages to Mecca saw several cholera epidemics emerge, while leprosy flourished in Egypt, Asia Minor and Europe.

Between 1096 and 1248, there were six great Crusades. These events all contributed to the spread of disease, as men were travelling together in large groups where diseases spread easily, and, with limited means to treat such outbreaks, large numbers of men were lost to disease rather than to war. In the period up to 1453, a number of pandemics and epidemics emerged. Diseases that flourished during the time included cholera, bubonic plague and pulmonary anthrax. A variety of factors contributed to the spread of epidemics and pandemics, including poor personal hygiene, inadequate nutrition, clustering of population groups, and increased contact through trade. Quarantine was used to prevent further spread of disease, because there was no scientific understanding of the cause and the nature of a disease, or how disease was spread.

During the Renaissance, the period from 1453 to 1600, the emergence of individual scientific endeavour led to a better understanding of the natural history of infectious disease. This increasing scientific knowledge enabled treatment activities to be put in place that were more closely linked with an understanding of disease processes. Although these processes were not at all sophisticated, their implementation marked the beginnings of scientific medicine and the development of a treatment focus, as opposed to a population health approach. The Renaissance was also a time of increasing social density, the expansion and further development of trade between countries, and general population movements, all of which encouraged the development and spread of disease.

Changing definitions of 'disease'

An understanding of the history of public health would not be complete without some consideration of the definitions of 'health' and 'disease'. The occurrence of death and disease can only rarely be described as a matter of chance. They are influenced by a number of determinants, including: the social and spatial organisation of a population; the individual's genetic endowment and exposure to a range of risk factors; the physical environment; patterns of relationships and mobility; and access to health services (Perdiguero et al. 2001, Scott 2004).

As the nineteenth century emerged, a number of disease theories formed the framework for the debate about causes of ill health. The germ (or contagion) theory held that for every disease there was a corresponding pathogen. It was only in the nineteenth century that this theory gained further prominence, when the theory of microorganisms could be substantiated with the aid of suitable medical apparatus, such as a rudimentary microscope. By contrast, the environmental theory supported the sanitary reforms that represented the first great revolution in public health. Unfortunately, that support was based on the incorrect belief that illness was a sign of dirty air, or, as it was known at the time, 'miasma'. While the theory of divine retribution suggested that a person's illness was a punishment for sinning, disease as a personal defect was another prominent theory on the cause of disease that suggested illness was attributable to an individual's social class or behaviour (Pickett & Hanlon 1990).

What becomes clear to us from the preceding discussion is the complexity related to defining health and disease. The germ theory supported the development of scientific medicine and treatment of the individual, although, with the recognition of contagious diseases, public health measures such as quarantine were introduced. The divine retribution and personal defect theories cited the cause of illness as either spiritual or the individual's class or behaviour. The personal defect theory had as its core the notion of individual responsibility for illness.

Edwin Chadwick supported the environmental theory of disease and pushed for sanitary reform; the culture of nineteenth-century Britain gave him the opportunity to write about the poor as the population group most often exposed to disease. They were 'less susceptible to moral influences, and the effects of education are more transient than with a healthy population; these adverse circumstances tend to produce an adult population short-lived, improvident, reckless and intemperate, and with habitual avidity to sexual gratification …' (Pickett & Hanlon 1990 p 28).

Only the environmental theory of disease can be clearly linked with sanitary reform measures; however, even though this strategy improved the health of the population, its use was initially based on incorrect assumptions about the cause of disease. As time passed, it became clear that changing patterns of mortality and morbidity, and significant decreases in the rate of death due to infectious diseases, were related to sanitary reforms. In addition, the militancy of the nineteenth-century working class resulted in improved wages and working conditions, and thus improved living standards and nutritional status, which significantly heightened people's resistance to microorganisms in the air, food and drinking water. The interrelationship between the two theories of disease is evident when one considers that clean water and proper sewerage are environmental changes that work, because they reduce or eliminate exposure to microbes (Fleming & Parker 2007).

In Chapter 1, we examined concepts of health and illness in contemporary society, and the diversity of perspectives that exist between, for example, professional and lay definitions. The ways in which professionals define health and illness are different from the ways in which other members of society conceive of them. Across time and cultures, depending on people's concerns, there have always been varied conceptions of health and illness (Waltner-Toews 2000).

The colonial era: colonisation and health

The colonial period extended from around 1600 to 1800. In the United Kingdom, for example, boards of health were established to examine prevalent health problems, and to protect the population from the spread of diseases caused by unsafe drinking water and tainted food supplies. Boards of health were the first employers of public health professionals. However, the ineffectiveness of the original boards of health in controlling infectious disease was partly due to the limited strategies they had at their disposal. Treatment options were minimal, and often dangerous to the patient, and prevention consisted primarily of quarantine. These quarantine measures were resented by the merchants, who understandably wanted to retain the flow of goods and customers. The religious orders also resented the boards and their powers to ban public congregations during an epidemic (Lewis 2003).

Improved understanding of the causes of ill health, and advances in the scientific basis of medicine, further increased the possibility that people might recover from an illness when treated with procedures that were based on increasing evidence. Community sanitation legislation was introduced in England in 1837 as a mechanism to ensure that at least fundamental public health activity was being pursued. Edwin Chadwick was the author of the *Report on the Sanitary Condition of the Labouring Population of Great Britain* (1842), and the initial driving force behind public health reform. In 1848, the *Public Health Act* came into being as a mechanism to remedy unsanitary conditions and provide adequate drainage and sanitation. This Act was primarily due to the efforts of Edwin Chadwick (Porter 1999). By 1872, a new public health Act required every statutory authority to appoint a medical officer of health.

In the colonial era, despite the improved understanding of the causes of disease, actions designed to protect the public's health often came *after* an epidemic had established itself in a population. Isolation and quarantine were still the major mechanisms to deal with outbreaks. Public health advances in the eighteenth century included developing rudimentary occupational hygiene practices, considering the health and safety of workers, introducing procedures to improve infant hygiene practices, and some attention to mental health issues (Lewis 2003).

Certainly, the public health movement was essential for the survival of the burgeoning cities created by nineteenth-century industrial capitalism (Susser 1981). Public health remained progressive, even though at times social and economic reforms were absent. The pursuit of community health at a population level was new, and the assumption of State responsibility for maintaining community health was equally so (aside from acute emergencies, such as plague or other epidemics). The originality of public health was to attack disease and poverty—in the community at large—at their perceived source in the environment.

Colonisation and health, and a maturing Australia

While Australia may have been a British colony, a somewhat different picture of public health emerged from that in nineteenth-century Europe, and the role of public health in the aftermath of the Industrial Revolution. The first phase of public health intervention in the fledgling colony, between settlement and the early 1800s, was marked by British administration of a colony fighting for its survival (O'Connor 1991).

BOX 2.1

DIFFERENCES BETWEEN THE BRITISH STATE AND THE AUSTRALIAN COLONY

- The force that was applied to control the convicts and the Indigenous people
- The degree of power vested in the military, a factor that permeated all aspects of the colony
- A complex range of factors contributed to rises and falls in patterns of mortality and morbidity in the colonial population:
  ○ the transmissibility of infections
  ○ increased population density
  ○ the creation of a permanent infectious disease 'pool'
- New diseases decimated segments of the Indigenous population, who were more susceptible to diseases to which their communities had not previously been exposed
- Resistance to infection among the colonists fluctuated, particularly with respect to infants and children (O'Connor 1991)

Lord Sydney, commenting on the establishment of the colony in New South Wales, claimed that there were two primary reasons for the settlement. These were the potential threat of escape of large numbers of prisoners from the overcrowded prisons in England, and the danger of the breakout of 'infectious distempers' (Historical Records of New South Wales 1892–1901 p 14). Other authors have commented on two further reasons for establishing a colony in New South Wales: first, the availability of materials useful to the navy in its activities in the Indian Ocean; and secondly, the colony being founded to promote trade with China (Fleming & Parker 2007).

The British State was not simply reconstructed in a colonial outpost. In addition, biology was not the direct determinant of the health of the colonial population; it was mediated by the colonial society's social organisation, its administration and economic development, and colonial beliefs about disease causation and the action needed to promote health (Fleming & Parker 2007). The colonial State departed from the British model in a number of ways. These differences are identified in Box 2.1.

There have been several important influences on the development of public health in Australia. These are similar to general themes identifiable in public health development overseas, but are modified by factors such as colonisation, federation, and federal and state relationships. Table 2.1 outlines these major influences.

A general history of public health: evolution and influences

The early developments that were designed to protect the health of the public can be charted by examining a number of important phases in public health history. Each of these phases is related to a particular time in history, and represents the prevailing thinking of the time about the causes of disease. What is important for us to remember is that the history of public health has benefited over the past five decades from scholars

TABLE 2.1 Six major influences on the development of public health in Australia

Major influence	Explanation
State promotion of national efficiency and national development	Efficiency was the application of expert or scientific knowledge to economic, social and political spheres of national life. The basis to this endeavour was the 'physical efficiency' of the population.
Bureaucratic ascendancy in Australian society	The growth of bureaucracy consequent on the expansion of State functions. In Australia, established in the colonial period where reliance was placed on bureaucrats for rule-making and arbitrative functions. This focus has continued, with bureaucrats both creating and administering policy in public health.
Federation and the constitutional division of powers between the Australian and the state governments	Following federation, the Commonwealth was obliged, under the Constitution, to give three-quarters of its revenue back to the states, thus greatly retarding its growth. Formal legal extension of Australian government functions, including health-related activities, were blocked. Some growth of functions, notably in health, scientific research and overseas marketing, took place in the 1920s via extra-constitutional and bureaucratic means. Further growth in federal responsibility for health occurred after World War 2.
Existence of a well-organised and politically sophisticated medical profession	Private practice of medicine and professional independence from the State, with the profession ready to sanction State intervention—both in the traditional public health sphere and in healthcare—if the intervention was on terms it found acceptable.

from a range of intellectual disciplines who have broadened the study of the economic, political and social relations of health and society. A history of public health is much more about the social, economic and political influences of the time and the interplay of these influences on health, disease and population health (Porter 1999). It is no longer only a narrative about individuals and their heroic contribution to improving health.

TABLE 2.1 Continued	
Major influence	Explanation
Reformist Labor Party	Labor Government focus on a policy of collective responsibility and equitable access in health matters, compared with conservative parties' emphasis on individual responsibility in a contributory insurance approach to health. Election of the Whitlam Labor Government (1972). Impacts include: changes to federal and state relationships; significant federal responsibility for public health, with the establishment of a community health scheme; introduction of Medibank and a Health Insurance Commission.
Advance of scientific knowledge in medicine and public health	Prominence of bacteriology shifted the focus of public health from the sanitary environment to identify infectious disease in the individual, and to control by isolation and later by mass vaccination. The emergence of modern laboratory-based medicine, the development of new diagnostic techniques, and the production of new therapeutic agents gave curative medicine unpredicted effectiveness. Technologically intensive medicine increased costs and focused on hospitals. Tension between state and federal responsibility for the health of the population compared with effective but expensive curative medicine resulting in State intervention to finance hospitals and the technological infrastructure needed for the new therapies. More recently tension between prevention and management of chronic diseases and re-emerging infectious diseases.

(Adapted from Baum 2008, Lewis 1989, Lin et al 2014, O'Connor 1991)

There are numerous ways to divide up the history of public health. Table 2.2 shows one of a number of different ways of conceptualising the periods that have been seen as important phases in the modern history of public health. The time periods mentioned are only a guide, and phases overlap and continue to have an influence over longer periods of time than might be suggested by this table. The major themes developed over time are influenced by shifting political imperatives, advancing

TABLE 2.2 Phases in the history of public health		
Historical phase	**Examples of major health issues**	**Measures to protect the population**
Miasma (1850–1880)—noxious odours caused disease	Malaria	Environmental reforms General cleanliness focus—*English Manual of Hygiene* as an example Emerging rudimentary influence of medicine
Bacteriological (1880–1910)	Specific organism, specific disease—plague, cholera, typhoid	Even before the isolation of specific agents, identifying certain modes of transmission of disease allowed limited public health measures to be put in place Development of rudimentary laboratory measures Quarantine still the major form of intervention
Health resources (1910–1960)	Infectious diseases early in this period; emergence of lifestyle diseases at end of period	Expansion of state health departments Improvements and development of hospitals as primary source of care for ill Expansion in the nature and role of health professionals Biomedical knowledge advances, and concentration on a medical focus Voluntary health agencies established and developed Major advances in laboratory measures
Social engineering (1960–1975)	Focus on individual health—lifestyle diseases	Treatment focus, and improvements in medical services Advances in medical technology, and increases in costs of care and treatment Recognition of social equity aspect of health through providing medical care for all Health education emerged to deal with individual lifestyle diseases

	TABLE 2.2 Continued	
Historical phase	Examples of major health issues	Measures to protect the population
Old public health (1975–mid-1980s)	Lifestyle diseases; some infectious diseases	Epidemiological studies identify determinants of health, and strategies focus on factors impacting on individual health Environmental health strategies are also considered important
New public health/health promotion (early 1980s to late 1990s)	Reduction in infectious diseases generally, but emergence of diseases that have no cure—HIV/AIDS; lifestyle diseases continue; emergence of chronic diseases as a major challenge	Health promotion World Health Organization (WHO) *Health for All by the Year 2000* (1981) Lalonde Report—Canada (1974) US Surgeon General's Report (2014) WHO *Ottawa Charter*, and elements of the charter to focus on population approach Old versus new public health—primary healthcare Continuation of tension between medical care strategies and promotion and prevention Equitable access to promotion, treatment and prevention services Recognition of, and strategies to deal with, influences of social, economic and political contributions to health and illness
Ecological public health (2000–)	Global warming; infectious diseases return; chronic diseases expand	Ecological and environmental sustainability strategies WHO *Health for All* 2010; 2020 Strategies to encourage wise use of resources, both human and material Multidisciplinary, multisectoral strategies to deal with complexity of health issues in twenty-first century

medical knowledge, economic perspectives, and social changes. Here, we take four themes in the development of public health to provide an overview of changes to organised efforts to promote, protect and restore population health. These four major themes include:

- environmental protection
- individualism and State involvement
- therapeutic era and medical dominance
- contemporary public health: 'ecological and sustainable' public health.

After we introduce you to each of the major themes, there is an activity for you to undertake to help you understand each of these developments. We ask you to think about these changes, and the impact on public health philosophy and strategies. Some of the changes were associated with increasing knowledge, some with mechanisms that worked to protect the public, even though at the time public health workers were not sure why they worked, and some brought about a shift in professional practice and a focus on the individual rather than on the population. Others recognise that social, political and economic issues mediate the ability of individuals to make changes to their health. In more recent times, the survival of the planet as we know it has challenged public health to engage in a consideration of ecological sustainability as the ultimate goal for our world.

Environment protection

The key public health activities throughout this phase ensured appropriate sanitary conditions, and laws to provide clean water, adequate food supplies and the safe disposal of personal and household waste. Diseases and illness were associated with overcrowding, poor hygiene, tainted water supplies, a failure of personal hygiene, and contaminated food supplies. There was a divide between those with the economic and social means to ensure basic sanitation, hygiene and adequate food supplies, and those with little economic or social opportunity (Consider Activity 2.1 and then read through Reflection 2.1).

Individualism and State involvement

This phase emerged after some of the most pressing environmental problems were brought under control, and scientific knowledge led to a greater understanding of the natural history of diseases. This greater understanding in turn led to a shifting focus on medical intervention, rather than prevention and promotion activities with populations and subpopulations. In addition, the State came to see its role far more clearly as the important player in developing public health. For example, the establishment of a federal health department in Australia and the notion of a division of responsibility between state and federal systems came into play early in the twentieth century (consider Activity 2.2 now then consider Reflection 2.2). Developments of school health education programs, nursing and family planning programs, and hospital services became more sophisticated and more clearly focused on the complexity of medical care and treatment.

In Chapter 3, we discuss the division of responsibility for public health between all levels of government. Have a look at this chapter to see how responsibility is divided.

Therapeutic era

This era heralded the incredible growth in the use of drug therapies to cure a wide range of diseases, or to at least enable people to continue to live with diseases that cannot be cured. Drugs such as insulin and penicillin were discovered, and new generations of drug therapies have emerged through the continued advancement of biomedical science.

The therapeutic era represented a time of attention to a medical model of public health, where the focus was on treating and curing health problems for the individual rather than at the population level. At the end of the nineteenth century, both the moral and the economic boundaries of public health were at issue, as public health agencies intruded into activities that the medical profession believed to be rightly its own. This conflict has long antecedents, but it was intensified by an historic convergence between medicine and public health (Starr 1982). This notion was discussed earlier in the chapter when we considered the changing historical trends in public health.

The impact of scientific development further intensified the conflict between medicine and public health. This meant that public health exponents increasingly came to rely on the techniques of medicine and personal hygiene (Starr 1982). As public health authorities gradually developed a more precise conception of the sources and models of the transmission of infectious diseases, and concentrated on combating particular pathogenic organisms, attention shifted further from the environment to the individual (Fleming & Parker 2007).

The road was open for action directed towards health that had as its central concern the personal behaviours of individuals and the contribution of a person's lifestyle to their health and wellbeing. These personal behaviours, and the ways in which the individual could modify them, became the subject of scientific judgements about the protection of the public's health (Reflect on Activity 2.3 and Reflection 2.3).

ACTIVITY 2.2 Population health programs at federal and local levels

Look up the website for the Australian Government Department of Health. In the top banner of that website, click on 'Programs & Campaigns'. Scroll down to 'Programs & Initiatives'. Click on the number 3 in the search list, 'Browse all programs and initiatives', which will reveal a large number of programs. Scroll down to number 6, 'A Healthy and Active Australia', and click on this link. Now consider the following activity.

- Select four of the 10 examples provided. Click on the visual for each of the four programs. For example, 'Get Set 4 Life—habits for healthy kids' might be one of your four choices.
- Draw up a table with a column for each of the four programs: one for the programs' purposes, one for the target groups for the programs, and one for the range of strategies for each program. Are the programs state, federal or shared initiatives?
- Think about an example in the press where there is an expressed tension between state/territory and Australian Government responsibility for a component of the health system. Why is this so? Do you think this tension is inevitable? Can you think of any solutions to this tension?
- Are there examples where state/territory and federal systems are working together? Does the website give you an idea about how that relationship works? What do you think would make it easier for state/territory and federal governments to work together in population health? In particular, look at the information on 'Healthy Spaces and Places'.

REFLECTION 2.2

In an example like the one presented above, you should be able to identify arrangements where there is a partnership between federal government and other agencies. What relationship is there between the federal health department and your state/territory health department? Look at your state/territory health department website and see if there are common programs listed. How do the programs at the federal level differ in terms of structure and outcomes from state/territory initiatives? You might expect that the federal department would have more of a policy and oversight role, with the state department having more of an implementation and evaluation role. Why do you think there might be tension between the two levels of government? Can you see, or do you know of, any programs that were well integrated between state and federal governments?

Contemporary notions: ecological public health

We now turn our attention to a discussion of a very recent iteration of the contemporary public health movements—'ecological public health'.

Recent approaches to public health provide an insight into the changing face of the politics of health. The 'new public health' prominent in the early twenty-first century emphasised the role of health promotion to advance population health, and focused on the elements of *The Ottawa Charter for Health Promotion* (World Health Organization 1986) (see also Chapter 14 for further detail on the 'new public health').

The 'ecological public health' approach emerged from the 'new public health', and it adds to health promotion by focusing on ecological sustainability. Figure 2.1 highlights the contributions of the 'old' and 'new' public health to this new approach.

ACTIVITY 2.3 Influences on individual health choices

- You have seen information on TV and in magazines about the importance of healthy nutrition and exercise, and their contribution to your health, so you decide to try to make some changes to your lifestyle. You join a fitness club and purchase some fresh fruit and vegetables. All is going well with your plan, except when you arrive at work you find that the only coffee shop there has no food to eat that fits in with your diet plan. Chips, hot dogs and greasy hamburgers are on offer. You are very hungry, have made good intentions and started the day well.

- You have also seen some information in the press about surgery to help you reduce weight. It has been very difficult for you to change your behaviour, and your environment is not helping because of limited healthy food choices in your workplace. Perhaps surgery might make it easier for you to lose weight?

- What do you do? How would you make a decision about your options?

REFLECTION 2.3

This scenario illustrates one of the dilemmas of the therapeutic model that focuses on individual responsibility for health choices. While it is important that individuals accept personal responsibility for their health, this is often not easy unless structures to assist individual decisions are also in place. On a broader scale, you need the economic resources to be able to purchase food (you can't eat without money); employment is a mechanism for supporting yourself, but the level of your education and whether you have a roof over your head and appropriate transport all impact on the decisions you will make. Access to adequate food and shelter, sufficient knowledge about healthy behaviours, health literacy and public health protection are considered to be widely available to the majority of the population. However, as Legge (1989 p 472) suggests, the individually focused therapeutic approach 'overlooks', or assumes as inevitable, the economic and social inequalities that affect health opportunities. We also need to consider the role of surgery for the individual as a mechanism for longer-term weight reduction and sustainability. Make a list of what you think are the advantages and disadvantages of surgery as a means to sustained weight reduction.

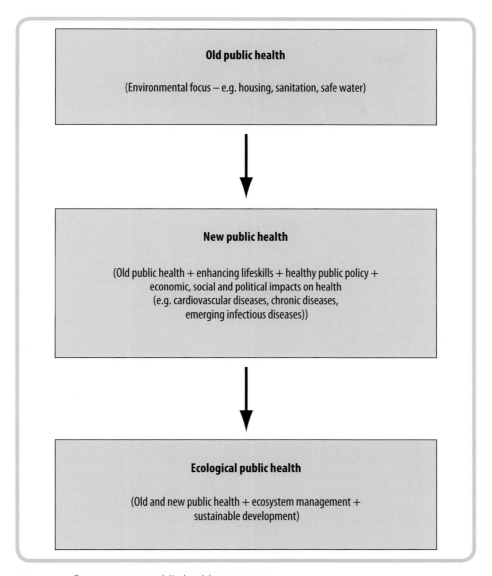

FIG. 2.1 Contemporary public health movement.

Sustaining the environment in which we live is central to our ongoing existence on this planet. This concept includes: making cities less polluted; becoming more energy-efficient; providing more social space and more trees; placing more emphasis on recycling and reducing waste; and becoming more self-sufficient in food production (Morris 2010).

This approach assumes that health results from a complex, dynamic, interconnected set of living systems existing in a delicate balance. It importantly considers equity, sustainability, consideration towards others, and preservation. Figure 2.2 succinctly demonstrates that our community needs to recognise that ecology sustains a society and its economic and political structures.

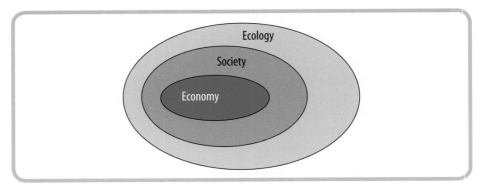

FIG. 2.2   The relationship between ecology, society and economy.

Ecological public health acknowledges that economic, environmental and social issues are interrelated, and recognises the sensitive interface between the natural and built environments. As a society, we clearly need to move away from polluting and wasteful behaviour, and towards protecting our natural, cultural, historical and human assets. We need to promote good environmental practices through collaboration and participation, and develop products and services that are environmentally friendly.

These challenges will not be easy; in fact, many political, economic and social factors act as barriers to ecological sustainability. Political commitment to the notion of ecological sustainability, while growing, is certainly not comprehensive, and in fact many of the emerging economies have found it hard to commit to such a concept and to associated targets to reduce carbon emissions.

Applying the models

Case Study 2.1 summarises the issues we have been discussing in the final section of this chapter. The questions provide you with an opportunity to think about how health professionals might address a series of key public health issues according to their philosophy of public health.

As a future practitioner, aside from deciding on strategies for action, it is most important that you think about why you have selected a particular strategy above

---

CASE STUDY 2.1

Alice, a homeless woman

Alice is an 18-year-old homeless woman who has been living on the streets for two months and does not want to go home. She has little money, is drinking a lot of alcohol with the money she does have, has the 'flu and few friends. Although Alice is living in a squat with some other street people, it is cold and inadequate. She is concerned about her 'flu getting worse, and is worried about money for food. Her money is running out. Alice left school at Year 11, but would like to finish school and get a job in a health-related area. She is not sure what the future holds for her, but she knows that she has to try to make a break from the life she has been living. How might Alice do this, and who might be able to help her?

another, and how that might improve Alice's life and possibly her health. Many would argue that strategies such as providing a safe home, adequate food and a source of income would be the essential first strategies for someone in Alice's position. Others might argue that the social and economic issues that make it difficult for Alice to make the necessary changes are the responsibility of governments, and so should be part of a range of government-managed strategies to assist Alice to find a safe environment, to provide medical care for her, and to support her to regain her self-confidence and self-respect.

A final word

What this chapter clearly shows us is that the past is a signpost for the present and the future. The ancient history of public health, briefly presented here, demonstrates to us that, even though efforts were in place at various times in history to protect the population's health, the purpose of that protection was often not for health reasons at all, but rather for social and political reasons. Throughout history, it is evident that the sanitary measures and environmental protections put in place in the early years of organised efforts to protect the health of the public worked to achieve these objectives. As we have seen in this chapter, the history of public health is a rich tapestry that has been impacted on by a wide range of social, economic and political factors that have shaped society's responses to health and diseases.

Removing environmental hazards and protecting the environment marked the first public health revolution. Environmental health today is still important to public health endeavours. Providing appropriate housing, safe water supplies, and nutritious food are fundamental to the health of the population.

What characterised the period up until the nineteenth century was the general lack of scientific evidence that could be brought to bear to explain disease, its transmission, and its human and social consequences. An increase in evidence about the cause of disease and its spread led to a focus on individual treatment and medical intervention. This development enabled the focus of public health to shift from the population to the individual, and reinforced the dominance of the medical profession and a biomedical model of health.

Accompanying the shift to medical dominance, and an individual focus on health and illness, was the role of the State in managing health services. Increasing costs of medical treatment, drug therapies and use of high-tech machinery to manage health conditions placed the State under extreme pressure to control health costs while providing a range of services. It also ensured that the gap between developing and

---

ACTIVITY 2.4 Public health interventions

- You have been appointed as a senior policy officer in a state or territory health department. In reflecting on Alice's predicament and issues (see Case Study 2.1), look at the public health models listed below and suggest one or two public health actions that could assist Alice for *each* of these models.

Public health model	Public health action to assist Alice
Environmental protection	
Individualism and medical intervention	
Therapeutic intervention	
Ecological sustainability	

REFLECTION 2.4

How different were the actions you suggested for Alice between the individual and medical intervention approaches and the ecological model of public health? There are a multitude of actions to assist Alice in this scenario. For example, in an individual model you may have thought that Alice needed to make personal changes to her lifestyle by finding a safe place to live and a job, and that Alice had to make this choice for herself. On the other hand, you may have felt that Alice's circumstances were created by multiple factors over which she had little or no control. How might you, as a senior policy officer, try to change the circumstances in which Alice finds herself?

developed countries, and the range of public health services available, would widen even further.

In the most recent past, public health has moved to a 'new public health' paradigm where there is a strong focus on prevention and health promotion, and on using public health policy to advance the case for a focus on population health, and subsequent funds to support such a focus.

Ecological public health marks contemporary public health efforts, and relies on the notion of an ecological contribution to public health that considers the environment in which we live and work, and in which our ecosystem functions, as the most important influences on population health.

In the chapter that follows, we examine contemporary public health policy, and the structure and function of the organisational systems that support public health.

REVIEW QUESTIONS

1 Jot down some ideas in bullet point form that explain the reasons behind changing definitions of 'public health'.

2 Write a paragraph or two on the work of McKeown and Szreter in describing the factors that contributed to major advances in the health of the population.

3 How did Australian public health develop, and what factors contributed to the nature of these developments?

4 Identify the main themes, and briefly describe the characteristics of each theme in the history of public health in Australia.

5 Describe the major themes and strategies for an 'ecological public health' approach.

6 Summarise how the history of public health can assist us in our understanding of contemporary public health.

References

Action on Smoking and Health (ASH) website. Facts and stats. Online. Available: <http://www.ash.org.uk/information/facts-and-stats> (9 Apr 2014).

Baum, F., 2008. The New Public Health, third ed. Oxford University Press, South Melbourne.

Berridge, V., 2000. History of public health: who needs it? Lancet 356, 923–925.

Colgrove, J., 2002. The McKeown thesis: a historical controversy and its enduring influence. American Journal of Public Health 92 (5), 725–729.

Fleming, M.L., Parker, E., 2007. Health Promotion: Principles and Practice in the Australian Context, third ed. Allen and Unwin, Crows Nest.

Historical Records of New South Wales, 1892–1901, Vol. 1, part 2, Phillip, 1783–1793, W. Britton, Government Printer, Sydney.

Lalonde, M., 1974. A New Perspective on the Health of Canadians: A Working Document. Government of Canada, Ottawa.

Lawson, J.S., Bauman, A.E., 2001. Public Health in Australia: An Introduction, second ed. McGraw-Hill, Sydney.

Legge, D., 1989. Towards a politics of health. In: Gardner, H. (Ed.), The Politics of Health: The Australian Experience. Churchill Livingstone, Melbourne.

Lewis, M.J. (Ed.), 1989. Health and Disease in Australia: A History. AGPS, Canberra.

Lewis, M.J., 2003. The People's Health: Public Health in Australia, 1950 to the Present, vol. 1 and 2. Praeger, Westport.

Lin, V., Smith, J., Fawkes, S., 2014. Public Health Practice in Australia: The Organised Effort, second ed. Allen and Unwin, Sydney.

Morris, G.P., 2010. Ecological public health and climate change policy. Perspectives in Public Health 130 (1), 34–40.

O'Connor, M., 1991. A Socio-Historical Study of Health and Medical Care in New South Wales from Settlement to 1850. Unpublished PhD thesis. University of Queensland, Brisbane.

Ogilvie, D., Hamlet, N., 2005. Obesity: the elephant in the corner. British Medical Journal 331, 1545–1548.

Perdiguero, E., Bernabeau, J., Huertas, R., et al., 2001. History of health, a valuable tool in public health. Journal of Epidemiology and Community Health 55, 667–673.

Pickett, G., Hanlon, J.J., 1990. Public Health: Administration and Practice, ninth ed. Times Mirror/Mosby College Publishing, St Louis.

Porter, D., 1999. Health, Civilization and the State: A History of Public Health from Ancient to Modern Times. Routledge, London.

Rosen, G., 1953. Economic and social policy in the development of public health: an essay in interpretation. Journal of History of Medicine and Allied Sciences 8, 430.

Scally, G., Womack, J., 2004. The importance of the past in public health. Journal of Epidemiology and Community Health 58, 751–755. doi:10.1136/jech.2003.014340.

Scott, W.G., 2004. Public policy failure in health care. Journal of American Academy of Business 5 (1&2), 88–94.

Starr, P., 1982. The Social Transformation of American Medicine. Basic Books, New York.

Susser, M., 1981. Ethical components in the definition of health. In: Caplan, A.L., Engelhardt, H.T., Jr., McCartney, J.J. (Eds.), Concepts of Health and Disease: Interdisciplinary Perspectives. Addison-Wesley, Reading, PA.

Szreter, S., 2002. Rethinking McKeown: the relationship between public health and social change. American Journal of Public Health 92 (5), 722–725.

Szreter, S., 2003. The population approach in historical perspective. American Journal of Public Health 93 (3), 421–431.

Tosh, J., 1984. The Pursuit of History. Longman, London.

US Surgeon General's Report, 2014. The Health Consequences of Smoking—50 Years of Progress: A Report of the Surgeon General. U.S Department of Health and Human Services, Rockville MD.

Waltner-Toews, D., 2000. The end of medicine: the beginning of health. Futures 32, 655–667.

World Health Organization, 1981. Global Strategy for Health for All by the Year 2000. Health For All Series No. 3. WHO, Geneva.

World Health Organization, 1986. The Ottawa Charter for Health Promotion. First International Conference on Health Promotion, Ottawa, 21 November 1986. Online. Available: <http://www.who.int/healthpromotion/conferences/previous/ottawa/en/> (20 May 2014).

CHAPTER 3

Contemporary public health policy

Elizabeth Parker

Learning objectives

After reading this chapter, you should be able to:

- identify the terms 'policy', 'public policy' and 'health policy', the stages of policy development, and the role that values and politics play in policymaking

- recognise contemporary international developments in public health, and their impact on national policymaking and the health of Australians

- describe the basic structure and financing of Australia's health system, and the role of public health within it

- identify Australia's national public health priorities, and be able to critique the development of health policies.

Introduction

This chapter builds on the definitions and history of public health in the previous two chapters, and provides an overview of contemporary health priorities. Understanding health policy is important for you as a health professional, whether as a nurse, paramedic, nutritionist/dietitian, podiatrist, public health/health promotion officer, occupational therapist, doctor or other health worker, as your practice will be influenced by changing health policies and priorities. For example, there are increasing roles for health professionals to play in preventing and managing chronic diseases and conditions, so understanding the relevant policies and programs will prepare you for your practice. We introduce you to definitions and types of policy, and the role of politics and values in public policymaking, and provide examples of these. We describe the role of the World Health Organization (WHO) in identifying global health trends, and how these impact on Australia's health policy.

What is 'policy'?

'Policy' has various definitions. For example, 'the process by which governments translate their political vision into programmes and actions to deliver "outcomes" … desired changes in the "real world" ' (Cabinet Office 1999). Policy can also be defined as a broad pattern or framework of collective action in a particular field (e.g. health policy), based on specific decisions that aim to realise the visions and goals of that field. Policy is usually about problem-solving, but it can also be about preventing or minimising problems. Policy can refer to a number of intentions and actions:

- a general statement of intentions and objectives (political leaders preface many speeches during election campaigns with 'our policy' statements)
- the past set of actions of government in a particular area, such as economic, refugee or health policies
- a specific statement of future intentions—for example, 'Our policy will allow people to opt out of Medicare in order to take up private health insurance'
- a set of standing rules intended as a guide to action or inaction, such as 'It is our policy not to interfere in those matters that are the responsibilities of the states' (Palmer & Short 2010).

The focus of policy is usually reform, establishing priority goals, and accomplishing policy objectives. Policy can thus be seen as the exercise of argument through the use of evidence, and an ability to juggle competing interests to achieve a collective purpose. Eva Cox (Cox n.d.) claims that 'public policy' also refers to the decisions taken at a government level to run, fund, support, regulate or ban certain services or activities. At its broadest, it is any intervention by the State in the community—encompassing the issues and ideas, the decision-making and the actions taken to implement those decisions (sometimes called the 'policy instruments').

Stages of the policy process

Ideally, the policy process consists of a number of stages (see Box 3.1). In reality, there are often no discernible stages and no rational sequence, because the policy process is changeable and influenced by many players. Determining policy goals is often not easy, as different stakeholders will have diverse interpretations of the problem and its solutions.

BOX 3.1

STAGES OF THE POLICY PROCESS

1 Hear about issues
2 Understand options
3 Learn of informed opinion
4 Make choices
5 Test decisions
6 Evaluate actions

(Source: Althaus et al. 2007 pp 1–2)

Policy can be seen as a framework for actions on specific public health issues. Policy development and implementation are also shaped by values and norms, which are often not explicit. For example, policies concerning Aboriginal and Torres Strait Islander Australians have reflected social and political values that have changed over time. Protectionism was the policy enacted in the first half of the twentieth century for Aboriginal and Torres Strait Islander peoples. However, a period of social change in the 1960s raised 'political and social consciousness among the general community and the plight of Aboriginal people constituted an urgent human rights issue' (Couzos & Murray 2003 p 5). Mobilisation actions by Aboriginal and Torres Strait Islander Australians led to the establishment of the first Aboriginal and Torres Strait Islander community-controlled health organisation in 1971, at Redfern in Sydney. Community self-determination was a key principle in establishing this health centre and all subsequent Aboriginal and Torres Strait Islander health organisations across Australia. See Chapter 16 for a comprehensive analysis of the health of Aboriginal and Torres Strait Islander peoples.

Policies, by their very nature, are not value-free. They underpin how governments distribute and redistribute resources, and how judgements are made in implementing policies (see Case Study 3.1).

CASE STUDY 3.1

Breast and cervical cancer screening

In the 1980s, Australian policymakers grappled with whether to introduce mammography screening for breast cancer. There was empirical evidence that mammography screening was an effective tool for early cancer detection for older women. The question was asked: 'How should we decide whether or not to introduce mammography screening?' The screening principles adopted by the WHO in 1968 (Wilson & Junger 1968) came into play by posing questions not only about the importance of the disease, but also about the acceptability of the screening test to the population. The values held by women about screening and its acceptability were taken into consideration; thus, the policy combines 'empirical criteria' (the evidence of the effectiveness of mammography screening) with 'value criteria' (the acceptability of the service to women) (in Lin & Gibson 2003). Established in 1988, the National Cervical Screening Program promotes Pap smear screening for women aged 18 to 69 years, to reduce morbidity and mortality from cervical cancer. Recall and reminder systems, adequate training of Pap-smear providers, and appropriate follow-up are integral to the program. The acceptability of services to women—that is, the 'value criteria' (Lin & Gibson 2003)—is particularly important in services for Aboriginal and Torres Strait Islander women, because of linguistic, cultural and geographical barriers.

CASE STUDY
3.2

Needle and syringe programs

In 1986, the first needle and syringe program (NSP) began in Sydney as a pilot project to address the high prevalence of needle-sharing among injecting drug users, and thus to reduce the spread of the human immunodeficiency virus (HIV). Other states, except for Tasmania, developed similar programs. Despite public controversies, particularly in the late 1990s, international and Australian research demonstrated that NSP programs were effective in maintaining low rates of needle-sharing-related HIV transmission. The value of harm minimisation and empirical research are linked under a policy framework of harm minimisation, through enabling individuals to exercise self-care and reduce harm, and through the coordinated efforts of public health workers, law enforcement workers and drug-user groups (adapted from Lin & Gibson 2003).

Drug and alcohol policies are often fraught with different and sometimes conflicting viewpoints. How should people who are users of illegal drugs be dealt with—through the criminal justice system or rehabilitation programs? Case Study 3.2, on harm minimisation[1] for injecting drug users, shows how empirical evidence together with values and a focus on the care of individuals were blended into a policy framework in establishing safe injecting facilities.

In this discussion of policy, the claim of the great nineteenth-century German pathologist Rudolph Virchow is pertinent: 'political action as well as rational science is necessary to initiate action to control public health problems' (Gunn et al. 2005 p 11). The case studies on breast cancer screening and needle and syringe programs illustrate how Virchow's statement is relevant to the complexities of public health policymaking in contemporary Australia.

The next section introduces various types of public policy.

Types of public policy

Various public policies affect the way communities live, their quality of life, and their access to services. Public policies may be categorised in different ways.

ACTIVITY 3.2 Values underpinning national public health policies

Choose one of the national public health policies of interest to you, from the Australian Government Department of Health, and analyse what, if any, values underpin the policy.

REFLECTION 3.2

Did the policy statement you chose identify any explicit values? For example, harm minimisation, universal access to prevention and treatment services, or equity? If you are doing this activity with other students and were not unanimous in your thinking, you can see how the policymaking process is complex and considers many viewpoints and values.

Distributive policies

These policies involve providing services or benefits to particular subpopulations. For example, pensions for people with a disability, pensioner health benefit cards, or youth allowances. They are relatively non-controversial and are implemented 'without any noticeable reduction in the benefits provided to other groups' (Palmer & Short 2010 p 24).

Regulatory policies

These are policies that restrict the behaviour of individuals and groups. For example, tobacco control policies are regulatory policies that restrict the sale of tobacco to minors and smoking in public places, and increase taxes on tobacco. Regulatory policies can also include the requirement that professionals be licensed before they can practise their profession (Palmer & Short 2010).

Self-regulatory policies

These policies are those often sought by organisations as a means of 'promoting their own interest' (Palmer & Short 2010 p 24). Some actions by self-regulatory boards can be seen in the establishment of the 'Australian Council on Healthcare Standards, which accredits hospital and nursing homes' (Palmer & Short 2010 p 24).

Redistributive policies

These policies are those that attempt to redistribute resources among the population. A classic health example is the universal health insurance scheme—Medicare—financed by compulsory income tax. For unemployed people and/or low-income earners, health insurance is subsidised by others. 'Universality' is an important public health principle, and there are other examples of such redistribution; for example, government-funded mass universal vaccination against childhood diseases (Palmer & Short 2010).

Hayes (2007) critiques these four policy typologies, claiming that they do not consider the influence of political dynamics on policies, particularly redistributive policies. The effect of politics on policy should be understood within the policymaking process in a democracy like Australia; especially as 'policy' is related to 'people and the needs of groups of people, be they patients, providers, communities or states' (Leeder 1999 p 74). So what are the influences of these types of policy on health outcomes?

Is there one type of policy that has a specific impact on public health? Navarro et al. (2006) analysed public health outcomes and policy developments in Organisation of Economic Cooperation and Development (OECD) countries with different political systems and various kinds of health insurance policy. They found that 'redistributive policies were positively associated with health outcomes', and that a long period of government with pro-redistributive policies is 'associated with low infant mortality' (Navarro et al. 2006 p 1035).

What is policy for?

The focus of policy in public health is to promote and restore the health of populations. Health policies are tools that can be used to identify, plan responses to, and act on prioritised health problems. Health policies and priorities must be periodically revised, according to changing patterns of morbidity and mortality, as the breast cancer and drug use examples demonstrate.

ACTIVITY 3.3 Types of public health policy

- Define 'distributive', 'redistributive', 'regulatory' and 'self-regulatory' policies, and list their advantages and disadvantages. How do these policy types impact on health policy? Are there community groups or health professions that are influential in making public health policy? How are their voices heard?

REFLECTION 3.3

Were there common themes in your list of advantages and disadvantages? Is it possible to use a mix of policy types to improve population health? Are physicians and nurses influential in the distribution of resources for public health policy?

John Last, a well-known epidemiologist, identified five essential ingredients for solving public health problems:

1   awareness that the problem exists
2   understanding of what causes it
3   having or developing the capability to deal with the problem, to solve or to reduce it, based on understanding its causes
4   a sense of values that it is worthwhile to deal with the problem
5   the political will to do what is necessary (Little 2010 pp 751–752).

These processes influenced the public health reforms of the nineteenth and twentieth centuries, and are still relevant to our discussion.

Politics and policy

Australia has a 'liberal-democratic' political system. Such a system of governance and a society ideally has numerous channels for participation in political parties and being involved in community organisations and special-interest groups, and the media is 'free'—meaning that freedom of expression is encouraged (Baum 2002). There is wide scope in such a society for public health professionals, individuals and communities to advocate to improve health opportunities and services. Kickbusch (2010 p 263) claims that 'politics in democracies is all about bargaining and compromise'; this is played out daily in liberal democracies. Current issues in Australian politics exemplify this, such as recognition of same-sex marriages, climate change, and the national education curricula (see Chapter 12 for an analysis of climate change, health, and policy developments). So while we may think that politics is only about politicians, 'politics' comes from the Greek *polis*, which referred to the city-state or its citizens, so politics can be seen in terms of governance of citizens and, in a liberal democracy, opportunities for participation in society.

As public health is about maximising the health of the population, it seems inevitable that the means to reach this public health goal would be challenged in an open society. Politics and policy is a recurring theme in public health in Australia and internationally (Baum 2002, Navarro et al. 2006, Palmer & Short 2010).

Health is political, because there is variation in access between groups; social determinants of health are amenable to political action, and the right to a standard of living adequate for health is an aspect of citizenship and a human right (Bambra et al. 2005). Health problems are also complex. Kickbusch (2010 p 261) argues that the visibility of health issues 'relate[s] to larger agendas such as the freedom of markets, the responsibility of individuals, the protection of vulnerable groups and the extent of state intervention—this makes any health issue inherently political'. The process of policy development in public health is, therefore, an intensely political one, which is aggravated by the different parties being in control of different governments or houses (the House of Representatives and the Senate), and the vested interest of those playing the political game.

Each political party in Australia designs policies on national issues based on that party's political ideology—what the party stands for. Review the websites of the various parties to ascertain party health policies and how they differ on particular issues. These policies are often released near an election, and have usually been debated at party conferences. Anyone can join a political party in Australia, and therefore participate in party committees and activities. In reality, there are often obstacles to enshrining party policy through the House of Representatives and the Senate, as different sections even within the same party may disagree regarding the proposed policy. For example, advocacy groups, such as groups of patients, powerful health professional groups, such as the Australian Medical Association, the registration boards of health professionals, and the media may have lobbied a Member with concerns about a policy.

'Social media—talkback radio and letters to the editor as well as blogs, social websites and microblogs, such as Twitter—provide constant qualitative and quantitative feedback on the issues of the day' (Baume 2011 p 1). Thus the principles and foundations of health policy and directions for its implementation can be shaped by numerous influences.

Political priorities in health are tempered not only by political realities, but also by economic realities and political promises.

Health economics

Governments and other healthcare organisations need to balance their own health policy priorities against political and economic realities within societies that have increasing demands for healthcare, 'and the costs of supplying healthcare services are rising' (Graves et al. 2009 p 81). Health economics can assist governments and departments within governments and other healthcare organisations to make decisions on the most effective economic investments to maximise health. Health economics can examine the cost-effectiveness and cost–benefit of different interventions, and provide economic evaluations 'aimed at examining alternative courses of action' (Hale 2000 p 341) to assist in making choices. Traditionally, health economists have focused on important research on the 'economics of the delivery of medical care services' (Halpin et al. 2009 p 276), but there is a need for 'economic analysis in public health interventions' (Ammerman et al. 2009 p 273) to decide how to allocate scarce public health resources.

Such economic analyses are being used increasingly in public health, as the following example demonstrates. An economic analysis of the impact of the National Tobacco Campaign, contained in the National Preventative Health Strategy, predicted that there would be 'a sustained 1.4% drop in prevalence [of smoking] observed in the first phase of the campaign that will prevent an estimated 55,000 premature deaths (in an investment of $9 million over only seven months), and will lower health care spending by at least $740 million on the four major diseases caused by smoking' (National Preventative Health Taskforce 2009 p 44). As a health professional, it is important that you understand the influence of politics on public health, what the government's priorities are, and how you can participate in shaping public health policy, and be aware of the increasing value of health economics as a tool to aid decision-makers in allocating scarce health resources. See Chapter 9 for the use of evidence in public health.

International developments and their impact on contemporary health policies

In Chapter 1 you were introduced to the WHO's six-point action plan (WHO 2008). Nearly 70 years have passed since the WHO was constituted, yet its relevance to public health policies and practice is still substantial, as it identifies world trends for public health action.

The WHO identifies several principles that underpin global and national health policies:

- 'The health of all peoples is fundamental to the attainment of peace and security and is dependent upon the fullest cooperation of individuals and States.

- The achievement of any State in the promotion and protection of health is of value to all.
- Unequal development in different countries in the promotion of health and control of disease, especially communicable disease, is a common danger.
- Healthy development of the child is of basic importance; the ability to live harmoniously in a changing total environment is essential to such development.
- The extension to all peoples of the benefits of medical, psychological and related knowledge is essential to the fullest attainment of health.
- Informed opinion and active cooperation on the part of the public are of the utmost importance in the improvement of the health of the people.
- Governments have a responsibility for the health of their peoples, which can be fulfilled only by the provision of adequate health and social measures.' (WHO 1948 p 2).

In the 1940s, representatives of 50 countries met to draw up the *United Nations Charter*. The United Nations (UN) officially came into existence on 24 October 1945, with broad aims to 'maintain international peace and security, to develop friendly relations among nations based on respect for the principle of equal rights and self-determination of peoples, [and] to solve international problems of an economic, social, cultural or humanitarian character' (United Nations (UN) 1945). On 10 December 1948, the General Assembly of the UN adopted and proclaimed the *Universal Declaration of Human Rights*. The declaration was seen as a common standard of achievement for all people and all nations, and, through teaching and education, would 'promote respect for these rights and freedoms'. Article 25(1) is relevant to our discussions of health policy, claiming:

> [e]veryone has the right to a standard of living adequate for the health and wellbeing of himself and of his family, including food, clothing, housing and medical care and necessary social services, and the right to security in the event of unemployment, sickness, disability, widowhood, old age or other lack of livelihood in circumstances beyond his control. (General Assembly of the United Nations 1948 p 5)

The WHO (2005) report *Preventing Chronic Disease: A Vital Investment* is a pivotal document that examines the rise of chronic disease. Contrary to the popular belief that chronic conditions (such as heart disease, diabetes and cancers) occur more frequently in developed countries, four out of five chronic disease deaths in the world now occur in low- and middle-income countries. In this report, the WHO assembled global data and made recommendations for future action, demonstrating their role in monitoring global health.

International health policy has traditionally been the domain of governments and non-government organisations (NGOs)—for example, World Vision. This field is altering rapidly with the entry of private philanthropists, and organisations comprising government and private industry partnerships (see Case Study 3.3).

As you can see, the dynamics and opportunities presented in the international health policy arena create potential for learning and translation into national policy developments in Australia, to assist us in creating health opportunities and services for all.

In the next section we introduce you to the Australian healthcare system and health policy.

CASE STUDY 3.3

The UN's Global Fund

The *Global Fund* was established in 2001 through the United Nations Secretary-General as an investment attempt to ensure that the *Millennium Development Goals* were met (see Chapter 1). The Global Fund, administered through the World Bank, is a different mechanism from previous development assistance agencies. It is a public–private partnership (PPP) 'tasked with administering and allocating funds provided by both governments and private sector donors to countries to combat HIV/AIDS, malaria and tuberculosis' (Feachem 2007). Other public–private partnerships have been established, including links between the Clinton Foundation, the Global Fund, the World Bank and UNICEF to assist with price reductions of AIDS drugs and diagnostics for disease identification. The Bill and Melinda Gates Foundation is a global health foundation that has funded health projects in over 100 countries, including the United States (see 'Useful websites' at the end of this chapter for more details of this enterprise).

ACTIVITY 3.4 The WHO and Australian public health policies

Write down the answers to the following questions:

- What is the relevance of the WHO for Australia's contemporary health policies?
- What is the significance of Article 25(1) for policy development in Australia, particularly the role of individual 'rights'?
- Can you think of examples in Australia where there is public–private investment in public health policy?

REFLECTION 3.4

There are many non-government organisations, such as the cancer councils, that contribute to health, and these are usually not-for-profit. Would private health insurers be considered private companies that contribute to health policy? If so, how?

Health policy and the Australian healthcare system

'Health policy' and 'healthcare policy' are terms that are used interchangeably. In political and media terms, healthcare policy can have a focus on 'illness care', with its nearly daily focus on the funding crises of hospitals, reduction of elective waiting lists, and workforce shortfalls in specific professions, particularly in rural and remote Australia. Health policy is simultaneously the goal, instrument and process by which systemic health-related decisions are made, implemented and evaluated. It is influenced by many factors, including public consciousness, political power and will, scientific understanding, and economic and environmental concerns.

Gardner and Barraclough (2002) claimed that 'health' in Australia includes medical and pharmaceutical services, institutions (e.g. hospitals, nursing homes and ambulance services), medical aids and appliances, non-institutional services (e.g. community services), and public health, dental services and health research. With this vast canvas illustrating how 'health' is used every day, health policy debates can range across a broad spectrum of issues and include many vested interests!

Health expenditure is a large sector of the economy, consuming around 9.5% of the gross domestic product[2] (Australian Institute of Health and Welfare (AIHW) 2013) and a 'significant proportion of both Commonwealth and state government outlays' (Duckett 2007 p 37). So financing the health system is always going to be a challenge, in terms

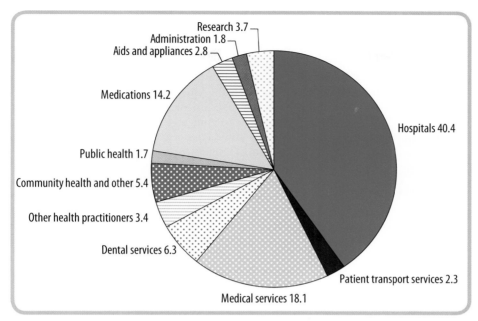

FIG. 3.1   Proportions of recurrent health expenditure, current prices, by area of expenditure, 2011–12, expressed as a percentage

Note: Components do not add to exactly 100% due to rounding.

(Source: Adapted from: Australian Institute of Health and Welfare, 2013. Health expenditure Australia 2011–12. Cat. No. HWE 59. AIHW, Canberra. Table A9: Proportions of recurrent health expenditure, current prices, by area of expenditure, 2001–02 to 2011–12 (per cent), p 77)

of rising consumer expectations, changing patterns of disease and illness, treatment options, and the competing interests of various health professions.

In 2011–12, Australia spent an estimated $140.2 billion (AIHW 2013) on health goods and services, an increase of $9.9 billion since 2010–11 (AIHW 2013). The largest increase from the period 2010–11 was for public hospital services, 'followed by spending on medical services' (AIHW 2013 p viii). However, 'funding of public health services *declined* [emphasis added] by 3.3% between the periods 2006–07 and 2011–12' (AIHW 2013 p 39). Figure 3.1 shows the recurrent expenditure by broad area of expenditure.

As a proportion of recurrent health spending, public health was at its highest in 2007–08 (2.3%), declining to 1.7% in 2011–12. Hospital spending and medications increased slightly over the same period, 39.3% up to 40.4%, and 14% up to 14.2%, respectively (AIHW 2013 Table A9, p 77).

Taylor et al. (2007) identify three distinct features of Australia's health system. The first is the complex relationships between the Australian Government and the states and territories. The federal government maintains a critical role in funding health-care for all Australians, and has played an increasing role in establishing a national agenda for health priorities and coordinated action.

The second feature is Medicare, introduced in 1984. Under Medicare, all Australians have equal access to care in a public hospital: 'out-of-hospital medical services at no, or minimal, cost to the service user due to benefits paid under Medicare and affordable pharmaceuticals through the Pharmaceutical Benefits Scheme (PBS)' (Taylor et al. 2007 p 48).

The third feature of Australia's healthcare system has been the growth of the 'private sector' in healthcare. In 1999, a 30% tax incentive was introduced to encourage people to take up private health insurance. In 2005, the rebate increased from 30% to 35% for Australians aged from 65 up to and including 69 years, and from 30% to 40% for Australians 70 years and over. From 2012, the government introduced income-testing for the rebate. Taylor et al. (2007) claim that this has meant individuals are paying more for their healthcare and are incurring more out-of-pocket payments for services.

Duckett claims that the argument that increasing private spending is advantageous becomes confused 'because advocates of increased private spending are usually from wealthier groups … this disguises a redistributive intent from the poor who are more reliant on tax-funded services' (2007 p 40). With these distinct features of the health system, what are the roles of the various levels of government, and how is healthcare funded? In the next section, we introduce aspects of the management of the healthcare system.

The Consumers' Health Forum of Australia (CHFA) provides community feedback to the government on health issues and initiatives, and represents patients, consumers and health professionals on policy initiatives. In 2010, the Forum described the government's MyHospitals website as 'contemporary, transparent and accountable information to help consumers make better health care choices' (CHFA 2010). MyHospitals is an open-access site that provides an overview of the performance of public and private hospitals provided through the National Health Performance Authority, an independent agency of the federal government.

ACTIVITY 3.5 Other important features of Australia's healthcare system

- Are there other important features of Australia's healthcare system that are not mentioned? What comments can you make about expenditure on public health? Research the role of consumers in current reforms to the Australian healthcare system. Are there plans for an increased consumer voice in policymaking?

REFLECTION 3.5

Think about the issues that encompass 'health' that Gardner and Barraclough (2002) identify, and examine the distribution of recurrent health expenditures in Figure 3.1. Should we increase the investment in public health? What arguments would you offer to make this case? Did you consider the influence of not-for-profit organisations, including church-based organisations such as Blue Care, Lifeline and the Salvation Army, which deliver health services?

Management and reform of healthcare

Each of the three tiers of government has a role to play in funding and delivering health to Australians. The Commonwealth government contributes to the main policy objectives, including health financing, as it has the power to raise revenue through the tax system and does that through a special Medicare levy (1.5%), and it sets the health agenda on national priorities, including public health. It contributes to the funding of major healthcare in the states and territories via a number of intergovernmental and constitutional definitions. The states deliver the services that are agreed upon (Barraclough & Gardner 2008), as well as fund some specific state priority programs. Local government monitors the physical environment for health and safety concerns, water quality, mosquito control, food safety, surveillance and education, and infection control. See Chapter 12 for more detail on local government and environmental health.

Five-year *Australian Health Care Agreements* outline the funding agreements between the state/territory governments and the Commonwealth, and the directions for priority spending and conditions. One of the drivers for national and intergovernmental reform is the Council of Australian Governments (COAG). Established in 1992, COAG comprises the prime minister, state premiers, territory chief ministers and the president of the Australian Local Government Association (ALGA). COAG is pivotal to health reform—when an issue reaches COAG for discussion, it is considered a priority. Between 2008 and 2012, the previous government initiated the National Health and Hospitals Reform Commission (2009) to develop a long-term health plan for Australia. A National Health and Hospitals Network (NHHN) for Australia's Future (Australian Government Department of Health 2010a) proposed altering the funding arrangements of public hospitals through local hospital networks, with the Commonwealth government being the majority (60%) funder of public hospitals. The NHHN was agreed to through COAG, and included equal funding of growth in costs, and the introduction of local hospital networks and 61 primary healthcare organisations (Medicare Locals). Medicare Locals replaced Divisions of General Practice, and were developed to integrate after-hours medical care, and importantly link hospitals with community-based services and with allied health professionals (e.g., dietitians, occupational therapists), and to address local health needs. The new government reviewed Medicare Locals in March 2014. The review found that patients experienced fragmented care, and that there was a need for an organisational 'linking' structure to improve health outcomes and efficiencies. From July 2015, Medicare Locals will be replaced by primary health networks. There will be fewer primary health networks than Medicare Locals, they will establish clinical councils with a significant general practice presence, and will establish a consumer advisory committee. Each primary health network will be contracted with the Department of Health to coordinate services to ensure improved patient outcomes within their jurisdiction, and be aligned with their respective local hospital network. Currently, there are 123 local hospital networks, so a primary health network may need to link with several local hospital networks. Medicare Locals and primary health networks are initiatives from different political parties in government (Medicare Locals—Labor; primary health networks—the Coalition). It is noteworthy that primary healthcare has remained a service delivery principle in both policy initiatives. (For further information about primary health networks, see the Department of Health website in 'Useful websites'.)

New 'super clinics' were developed in 2011; these provide patients with well-integrated multidisciplinary patient-centred care—that is, patients are able to consult several health professionals in the same visit. The Australian Government committed $650 million to build 60 general practitioner (GP) super clinics, in order to build a strong, integrated, multidisciplinary level of care for the management of chronic disease, disease prevention and health promotion. The GP super clinics can offer a potential range of multiple services besides a traditional medical practice, such as physiotherapy, dietary advice, health promotion and podiatry. These will be determined according to community healthcare needs. Around 425 general practices, primary care and community health services, and Aboriginal Medical Services will be upgraded (DoH 2013). GP super clinics provide direct services to patients. This is in contrast to the primary health networks, which

---

ACTIVITY 3.6 Super clinics

- Have you attended a GP super clinic near you? They are listed on the Department of Health website.
- What advantages can you see to attending a super clinic?
- Why is the Council on Australian Governments important for a unified health system?

REFLECTION 3.6

You can see the complexities of creating a unified private and public health system. Since 2010, different federal governments have attempted to integrate hospitals and primary healthcare services, the latter with a focus on a 'whole of care' approach, where a patient has a spectrum of health professionals to attend to their health needs, and there is potential scope for community input into service design and delivery.

are coordinators of primary healthcare services that link to the local hospital networks.

Despite the inherent complexities, there are strengths in having a unified approach to health issues. The Australian Government has played a pivotal role in setting a national public health policy agenda that began in the late 1980s, with many subsequent initiatives to drive a 'health for all' agenda across numerous health areas.

National public health priorities— an evolving agenda

The introduction of national public health policies in the 'new era of public health' began with the development of national goals and targets in the 1990s. This work built on the Better Health Commission (1986), which for the first time in Australia utilised policy analysis of the current health status of Australians, identified priority health issues, and proposed recommendations to address health problems. *Health for all Australians* (Australian Health Ministers' Advisory Council (AHMAC) 1988) was published in 1988. AHMAC, which meets three times a year, comprises the heads of each state and territory health department. It advises the Australian Health Ministers' Conference.

The national public health policy agenda has had a number of iterations. In 1993, a report entitled *Goals and Targets for Australia's Health in the Year 2000 and Beyond* was launched (Fleming & Parker 2007 p 71). In 1996, the federal and state governments endorsed four *National Health Priority Areas* (NHPAs)—cardiovascular health, cancer control, injury prevention and control, and mental health. Diabetes mellitus was added in 1997, asthma in 1999, arthritis and musculoskeletal disorders in 2002, obesity in 2008, and dementia in 2012. The specific actions required in the priority areas are:

- monitor health outcomes and progress towards set targets
- identify the most appropriate and cost-effective points of intervention
- identify the most appropriate role for government and non-government organisations in fostering the adoption of best practice
- investigate some of the basic determinants of health, such as education, employment and socioeconomic status (National Health Priority Action Council (NHPAC) 2002 p 8).

The *National Chronic Disease Strategy* was developed in 2006. The National Preventative Health Taskforce (NPHT), established in 2008, developed a strategy aimed at preventing 'hundreds of thousands of Australians dying prematurely, or falling ill and suffering, between now [2008] and 2020' (NPHT 2009 p 8). The strategy comprises seven strategic directions:

- Shared responsibility—developing strategic partnerships at all levels of government, industry, business, unions, the non-government sector, research institutions and communities
- Act early and throughout life—working with individuals, families and communities
- Engage communities by working with people where they live, work and play
- Influence markets and develop coherent policies through taxation, responsible regulation and through coherent and connected policies

- Reduce inequity through targeting disadvantage
- Contribute to 'Close the Gap'[3] for Indigenous Australians
- Refocus primary healthcare towards prevention (NPHT 2009 p 6).

The strategy concentrated on three main risk factors: overweight and obesity, smoking, and harmful consumption of alcohol. In 2012, an Australian National Preventative Health Agency (ANPHA) was established to: advise COAG, through the Australian health ministers, on national preventative health priorities; be a national clearing house for the evaluation and monitoring of policies and programs; and develop and implement comprehensive social marketing campaigns around obesity, tobacco and alcohol. The ANPHA was a key element of the COAG-agreed National Partnership Agreement on Preventive Health (NPAPH), but was closed in 2014.

Current national public health policies build on previous public health policy successes, where coordinated action in developing and implementing policies through consultation, coordination and financial investments have seen changes in health outcomes. They are founded on national health priorities, established through coordinated federal and state policy development and agreements. Many of these public health policies were initiated in the 1980s, and include the *National Drug Strategy*, the *National Aboriginal Health Strategy*, the *National HIV/AIDS Strategy*, *BreastScreen Australia*, and the *National Cervical Screening Program*.

> **ACTIVITY 3.7 Unified approaches to health policy**
>
> - What are the strengths and limitations of national public health policy approaches to contemporary health problems?
> - What are the limitations of a unified approach?
> - What are the implications if a state or territory government has a different view on implementing these policies?
> - Is there a role for consumers in national public health policy development?
> - Provide two examples of how nurses, physicians, dietitians or other health professionals have contributed to changing health policy.
>
> **REFLECTION 3.7**
>
> Were there more strengths than limitations in having a national approach to major health issues? Would it mean that, without such an approach, people in different states might receive different services? Do you think there are enough avenues for consumers to have a voice about public health priorities and services? If not, what changes would you suggest?

The National HIV/AIDS Strategy

To explore the role of national public health policies further, we draw attention to two of these policies. The first is the National HIV/AIDS Strategy. From the endorsement of the first National HIV/AIDS Strategy in 1989 through to the Sixth National HIV Strategy 2010–2013 (Australian Government Department of Health 2010b), Australia has recognised the need for a coordinated response to HIV. Furthermore, HIV/AIDS is still an important health issue in the Oceanic region. In December 2013, the new government pledged $200 million over three years to support the Global Fund to Fight AIDS, Tuberculosis and Malaria. The Global Fund is the world's largest multilateral funder of health programs in over 140 countries. It is a key partner with Australia in combating these three diseases in the Indo-Pacific region (Department of Foreign Affairs and Trade 2013).

While the HIV epidemic in Oceania is small, the number of people living with HIV in this region more than doubled between 2001 and 2009, from around 28,000 to approximately 57,000 (UN AIDS Report 2010), and then declined to 51,000 in 2012 (UNAIDS Report 2013 p A12). The number of people newly infected with HIV has begun to decline from about 4700 in 2001 to 2100 in 2012 (UNAIDS Report 2013 p A24). Analysis of available data from Papua New Guinea shows that the epidemic there is starting to level off. The national adult HIV prevalence in 2009 was estimated at around 0.9%, with about 34,000 people living with HIV (UNAIDS Report 2010), and in 2012 the national adult HIV prevalence was 0.5%, and there were 25,000 living with HIV (UNAIDS Report 2013).

The National HIV/AIDS Strategy was drafted to operate as a flexible framework for responding to the challenges it identified that emerged during its five-year term. Policy development and implementation can seem mysterious, and something that governments and sections of the health sector 'do', but what is illustrative in the policy success of the HIV/AIDS policy, in particular, is the active roles of those community groups affected by the virus. Moreover, if we return to our original discussions about the role of values in public policymaking, the strategies and services had to be suitable and accessible for those affected by the virus. A unique approach was adopted in Australia, with the input of sex workers, 'men who have sex with men', physicians, politicians and well-known spokespeople in policy development. The policy outcomes saw the opening of the first needle-exchange program in Sydney. It is the involvement of such diverse stakeholders that has contributed to its success. We alluded to the political dynamics in policymaking at the beginning of the chapter, and this case demonstrates how skilful the key policymakers in government were in harnessing various lobbyists and advocates and implementing an agreed national policy. It must be remembered that the context for policymaking was a difficult one.[4]

The National Chronic Disease Strategy

Nine public health priorities were introduced in our previous discussion of the NHPAs. We mentioned the National Chronic Disease Strategy (NHPAC 2006). This landmark Australian policy document provided direction for the prevention and care of chronic disease, and focused particularly on asthma, cancer, cardiovascular disease, diabetes, and musculoskeletal conditions—arthritis and osteoporosis. Importantly, the strategy provided a series of National Service Improvement Frameworks to fund programs and services to improve the prevention and care of chronic disease in each state. The programs and services are coordinated through each state health department.

So what is chronic disease, and why do health professionals need to understand its dimensions? The AIHW (2010) reiterates claims that most premature deaths are due to chronic disease. 'Chronic disease has complex and multiple causes with a gradual onset, becomes more prevalent with older age, can compromise quality of life through physical limitations and disability, is long-term and persistent, leading to a gradual deterioration of health, and [is] the most common leading cause of premature mortality' (NHPAC 2006 p 1). For example, 'diabetes prevalence has more than doubled over the past two decades affecting over one million Australians. Type 2 diabetes is expected to have the largest increase of chronic disease by 2020' (NHPAC 2006 p 1). The prevalence and increase in chronic disease has implications for health professionals. For example, podiatrists will probably see more patients with

---

ACTIVITY 3.8 Priorities and issues of interest

- Are there lessons that can be drawn from the HIV/AIDS health policy discussions? What role did social and cultural approaches to this issue have in developing improvements in health? What was the role of a range of stakeholders in policy development? Choose a health priority or health issue of interest. Could you apply the same process of engagement with consumers, private industry, researchers, non-government health agencies, and federal and state governments to address your issue? What are the barriers to such a process, and what ideas have you for overcoming these?

diabetic foot problems; nurses and occupational therapists will need to understand self-care management techniques for patients in cardiac rehabilitation; paramedics will need to know how to care for a patient in diabetic shock; public health nutritionists will be planning community-based healthy food programs in schools; and health promotion professionals may collaborate across education, local councils and sport and recreation facilities to implement physical activity programs and services.

New challenges confront Australians' health, and public health practitioners respond through policy and service initiatives based on compelling evidence and opportunities. Under the 'chronic disease' umbrella, obesity has received national and international attention. To many, obesity may have emerged as a new priority in 2003, yet the NHMRC reported on this issue in 1997 (NHMRC 1997). Lin and Robinson (2005 p 3) claim that, despite national cooperation on promoting the importance of physical activity and nutrition, the public and political imaginations were not captured until the issues were recast as 'obesity'. The authors claim that the Commonwealth strategy is 'relatively weak on intersectoral policy and regulatory measures' (Lin & Robinson 2005 p 3). And that on this national policy the Commonwealth 'apparently chose not to consider how it might exercise its relevant taxation or legislative powers' despite the evidence that public policies beyond the health system can have an impact on health (Lin & Robinson 2005 p 3). An example is the attempts to limit food advertising to children during scheduled children's program time, as occurs in Sweden, and imposing higher costs on soft drinks. Again, does this speak to a policy landscape with different interests, values and, therefore, actions?

However, overweight and obesity in the Australian population continues to rise. The Australian Health Survey 2011–12 reported that the prevalence of overweight and obesity in Australian adults aged 18 years and over has continued to rise, to 63.4% in 2011–12 from 61.2% in 2007–09, and 56.3% in 1995 (Australian Bureau of Statistics (ABS) 2013); in other words, there has been a increase in overweight and obesity in Australian adults of 7.1% in 16 years. Of concern is the increasing overweight and obesity of children, making them more likely to remain obese in adulthood, with increased risks of short- and long-term health problems, such as type 2 diabetes and cardiovascular disease. In 2011–12, approximately 25% of Australian children 5–17 years were obese or overweight. In 2011–12, 7% of boys 5–12 years were obese; and for girls aged 13–17 years, 18% were overweight (ABS 2013).

We explore briefly another public health issue that does not receive as much attention as it should—oral health—and we present a policy initiative that has been controversial for many years in Australia. Oral health does not feature in the list of national public health priorities, yet dental health accounted for 6.3% of the total expenditure on health goods and services (AIHW 2013). Most of the expenditure on chronic diseases partly reflects the use of hospitals and general practitioners, and for oral health, out-of-hospital services, mainly dental services.

From survey data in 2010, more than a quarter of people aged five or older (28%) avoided or delayed going to a dentist due to cost. From 1994 to 2010, there was a noted rise in the proportion of adults avoiding dental visits from 25% to 30% (AIHW 2014).

In Chapter 7, we discuss the link between regional and rural locations, type of neighbourhood and health. This link is true for oral health, with the proportion of

---

REFLECTION 3.8

Did your lessons contain any insights that could be applied to other health issues nationally? Did engaging stakeholders play a part in ensuring a positive implementation? Were there lessons to be learned from being attuned to social and cultural approaches, and from policymakers 'listening' to these? What views do you have regarding Australia's commitment to the Oceanic region to deal with the HIV/AIDS issue?

CASE STUDY
3.4

Oral health in Queensland

Queenslanders have the highest levels of tooth decay and the lowest level of access to water fluoridation in Australia. Levels of tooth decay for Queensland children are much higher than those in other states and territories, and 67% of Queensland children have experienced tooth decay by eight years of age. In 2007, 'Queensland had the highest mean number of teeth with untreated decay per child (0.69), and the greatest mean DMFT [permanent decayed, missing (due to decay) and filled teeth] score per child (1.32)' (Mejia et al. 2012 p 17). However, Townsville children aged 5 to 12 years have 45% less tooth decay than Brisbane children.

Townsville fluoridated its water in 1965 (Queensland Government water fluoridation website). The oral health program—as a public health priority that provides universal access to fluoridated water supplies—was to be implemented to cover 90% of Queenslanders by 2012 (Bligh 2007). With the change to a Liberal National state government in Queensland, in 2012 local councils were given back the responsibility of deciding whether their water supplies were to be fluoridated (Government News 2014). At least seven councils have decided against fluoridation, some because of pressure from anti-fluoride lobby groups, and others for budgetary reasons (Government News 2014). This is at odds with the recommendation of the National Advisory Committee on Oral Health (2004 p viii) to 'extend fluoridation of public water supplies to communities across Australia with populations of 1000 or more'.

people with untreated tooth decay greater in remote/very remote areas (38%) than in major cities (24%) and for people with lower household income (AIHW 2014).

The NHMRC completed a systematic review of the efficacy and safety of different forms of fluoridation (NHMRC 2007). In December 2007, the Queensland Government acted to improve the oral health of Queenslanders through fluoridating Queensland's water supplies. Case Study 3.4 profiles the poor dental health of many children, and the implementation of a new public health policy to improve their dental health outcomes through a universal public health approach.

We conclude this chapter by introducing the Australian Institute of Health and Welfare.

The role of the Australian Institute of Health and Welfare

The development of national public policies is not possible without robust data on which to make policy decisions on public health priorities. The Australian Institute of Health and Welfare (AIHW) is an independent government agency established to develop, collect and disseminate reliable, timely facts on the health of Australians, and on health and community services. National agreements commit all of the nine governments, the AIHW and the ABS to work together to further this endeavour. The data are freely available on the AIHW website.

A final word

This chapter presented definitions and types of health and public policy, and stages of policy development. The role of values and politics within a liberal-democratic society, and their influence on health policy, were outlined. COAG as a mediator between state and federal interests was described, with examples. International health policy developments, including the roles of the WHO and the UN, were discussed, as was the changing architecture of international policy developments with the advent of public–private partnerships and health investments by philanthropic trusts. The structure and financing of Australia's health system was touched on briefly.

Australia has a tradition of the federal government taking a lead in public health policy developments, and some of the history of this tradition and its current public health priorities were introduced. Four case studies were presented: breast cancer screening, needle and syringe programs, the UN's Global Fund, and oral health. The role of the AIHW was outlined.

In summary, health and public policies are intended to improve the quality and wellbeing of people's lives (Bessant et al. 2006 in Taylor et al. 2007). These aims are positioned against a backdrop where, in an adaptation of the words of Virchow (in the seventeenth century) and Walt (2004), one cannot separate policy from politics.

REVIEW QUESTIONS

1 What do you understand by the terms 'policy', 'public policy' and 'health policy'?

2 What are the stages of policymaking?

3 What role do values and politics play in health policymaking?

4 What is the relationship between the Australian Government and state governments, and what are the agreements that are important in funding the health system?

5 How are international organisations such as the WHO relevant for Australia's health policy directions?

6 Why is there more policy action on some issues and not on others?

7 Explore the roles for health professionals in primary healthcare settings such as super clinics and the new primary health networks. Do you see yourself working in such settings?

8 Obesity is a national priority within the National Chronic Disease Strategy. Research what role you will play within your health profession in addressing this growing risk factor for chronic disease.

9 Research current initiatives to improve the oral health of Australians, and describe the link between poor dental health and chronic disease.

10 Should the Medicare levy be increased to pay for the additional demands on the healthcare system? What are implications of such an increase for consumers?

Endnotes

1 'Harm minimisation links the ethical consideration of expanding the autonomy of the drug user with the utilitarian principle of aiming to achieve net benefit for the individual and the community.' (Lin & Gibson 2003 p 308).

2 Gross domestic product: 'The GDP of Australia is the total market value of all goods and services produced within Australia in a given period of time.'

Parliament of Australia Parliamentary Library. Available: http://www.aph.gov.au/About_Parliament/Parliamentary_Departments/Parliamentary_Library/pubs/MSB/feature/FeatureGDP 7 Apr 2014.

3   The Close the Gap campaign 'calls on federal, state and territory governments to commit to closing the life expectancy gap between Indigenous and non-Indigenous Australians within a generation.' Available: https://www.oxfam.org.au/explore/indigenous-australia/close-the-gap/ 8 Apr 2014.

4   In 2007 the Australian Broadcasting Commission (ABC) produced a documentary called *Rampant* that traces the Australian AIDS story.

Useful websites

- Australian Broadcasting Commission: www.abc.net.au
- Australian Government Department of Health: www.health.gov.au
- Australian Government Department of Health, Primary Health Networks: http://www.health.gov.au/internet/main/publishing.nsf/Content/primary_Health_Networks
- Australian Institute of Health and Welfare: http://www.aihw.gov.au
- Australian Institute of Health and Welfare (NHPA): http://www.aihw.gov.au/nhpa/
- Bill and Melinda Gates Foundation: http://www.gatesfoundation.org
- Council of Australian Governments: http://www.coag.gov.au
- MyHospitals website: http://www.myhospitals.gov.au/
- Public Health Association of Australia: http://www.phaa.net.au
- The Clinton Foundation: www.clintonfoundation.org
- The Consumers' Health Forum of Australia: http://www.chf.org.au
- The Global Fund: www.theglobalfund.org
- United Nations Children's Fund (formerly United Nations International Children's Emergency Fund): http://www.unicef.org
- World Bank: http://www.worldbank.org

References

Althaus, C., Bridgman, P., Davis, G., 2007. The Australian Policy Handbook. Allen and Unwin, Crows Nest.

Ammerman, A., Farrelly, M., Cavallo, D., et al., 2009. Health economics in public health. American Journal of Preventive Medicine 36 (3), 273–275.

Australian Bureau of Statistics, 2013. 4125.0—Gender indicators, Australia, Jan 2013. Overweight/obesity. Online. Available: <http://www.abs.gov.au/ausstats/abs@.nsf/Lookup/4125.0main+features3330Jan%202013> (11 Apr 2014).

Australian Government Department of Health, 2010a. A national health and hospitals network for Australia's future—delivering better health and better hospitals. Online. Available: <http://www0.health.nsw.gov.au/resources/Initiatives/healthreform/pdf/NHHN_report3_RedBook.pdf> (11 Apr 2014).

Australian Government Department of Health, 2010b. Sixth National HIV Strategy 2010–2013. Online. Available: <http://www.health.gov.au/internet/main/publishing.nsf/Content/ohp-national-strategies-2010-hiv/$File/hiv.pdf> (18 Feb 2014).

Australian Health Ministers' Advisory Council Health Targets and Implementation (Health For All) Committee, 1988. Health For All Australians. Report to the Australian Health Ministers' Advisory Council and the Australian Health Ministers' Conference. Australian Government Publishing Service, Canberra.

Australian Institute of Health and Welfare, 2010. Premature mortality from chronic disease. Bulletin No. 84. Cat. No. AUS 133. AIHW, Canberra.

Australian Institute of Health and Welfare, 2013. Health expenditure Australia 2011–12 Cat. No. HWE 59. AIHW, Canberra. Online. Available: <http://www.aihw.gov.au/WorkArea/ DownloadAsset.aspx?id=60129544656> (17 Feb 2014).

Australian Institute of Health and Welfare, 2014. Oral health varies by wealth and location. Online. Available: <http://www.aihw.gov.au/media-release-detail/?id=60129546485> (11 Apr 2014).

Australian Institute of Health and Welfare, 2015. National health priority areas. Online. Available: <http://www.aihw.gov.au/national-health-priority-areas/> (22 Apr 2015).

Bambra, C., Fox, D., Scott-Samuel, A., 2005. Towards a politics of health. Health Promotion International 20 (2), 187–193.

Barraclough, S., Gardner, H. (Eds.), 2008. Analysing Health Policy: A Problem-oriented Approach. Elsevier, Marrickville.

Baum, F., 2002. The New Public Health, second ed. Oxford University Press, South Melbourne.

Baume, P., 2011. Forget focus groups, the answer's in the ether. The Australian, 7 March 2011. Online. Available: <http://www.theaustralian.com.au/business/media/forget-focus-groups -the-answers-in-the-ether/story-e6frg996-1226016759509> (8 Apr 2014).

Bessant, J., Watts, R., Dalton, T., et al., 2006. Talking policy: how social policy is made. In: Taylor, S., Foster, K.Fleming, J. (Eds.), Health Care Practice in Australia: Policy, Context and Innovations. Oxford University Press, South Melbourne, p. 2007.

Better Health Commission, 1986. Looking Forward to Better Health: Report of the Better Health Commission. Australian Government Publishing Service, Canberra.

Bligh, A., 2007. Fluoridated to deliver better oral health for Queenslanders. Queensland Government. Press release. December 2007.

Cabinet Office, 1999. Modernising Government White Paper. Cm 4310. HMSO, London.

Consumers' Health Forum of Australia, 2010. MyHospitals website a good start. Media release, 10 Dec 2010. Online. Available: <https://www.chf.org.au/pdfs/med/med-my-hospitals -10Dec2010.pdf> (7 Feb 2014).

Couzos, S., Murray, R., 2003. Aboriginal Primary Health Care: An Evidence-based Approach, second ed. Oxford University Press, Melbourne.

Cox, E., n.d. What is policy? The Centre for Policy Development, Sydney. Online. Available: <http://youthscape.vibewire.org/wp-content/uploads/2010/07/whatispolicy.pdf> (8 Apr 2014).

Department of Foreign Affairs and Trade, 2013. Australia supports fight against AIDS, tuberculosis and malaria. Online. Available: <http://aid.dfat.gov.au/LatestNews/ Pages/australia-supports-fight-against-aids-tuberculosis-and-malaria.aspx> (8 Apr 2014).

Department of Health, 2013. About the GP Super Clinics Program. Online. Available: <http://www.commcarelink.health.gov.au/internet/main/publishing.nsf/Content/pacd -gpsuperclinic-about> (8 Feb 2014).

Duckett, S., 2007. The Australian Health Care System. Oxford University Press, Melbourne.

Feachem, R., 2007. New ways of funding development assistance. Speech given at the Lowy Institute, 16 May 2007. Online. Available: <http://www.lowyinstitute.org/news-and-media/ audio/new-ways-funding-development-assistance> (9 May 2014).

Fleming, M.L., Parker, E., 2007. Health Promotion: Principles and Practice in the Australian Context, third ed. Allen and Unwin, Crows Nest.

Gardner, H., Barraclough, S., 2002. Health Policy in Australia. Oxford University Press, Melbourne.

Government News, 2014. Dentists drill councils over water fluoridation decay. Online. Available: <http://www.governmentnews.com.au/2014/01/dentists-drill-councils-over-water-fluoridation-decay/> (11 Apr 2014).

Graves, N., Halton, K.A., Paterson, D., et al., 2009. The economic rationale for infection control in Australian hospitals. Healthcare Infection 14 (3), 81–88.

Gunn, S.W.A., Mansourian, P., Davies, A., et al., 2005. Understanding the Global Dimensions of Health. Springer, New York.

Hale, J., 2000. What contribution can health economics make to health promotion? Health Promotion International 15 (4), 341–348.

Halpin, H.A., Hankins, S.W., Scutchfield, D., 2009. Broadening the role of the health economist to include public health research: a commentary. American Journal of Preventive Medicine 36 (3), 276–277.

Hayes, M.T., 2007. Policy characteristics, patterns of politics, and the minimum wage: toward a typology of redistributive policies. Policy Studies Journal 35 (3), 465–480.

Joint United Nations Programme on HIV/AIDS (UN AIDS), 2013. Global report: UNAIDS report on the global AIDS epidemic 2013. Online. Available: <http://www.unaids.org/en/media/unaids/contentassets/documents/epidemiology/2013/gr2013/UNAIDS_Global_Report_2013_en.pdf> (17 Feb 2014).

Kickbusch, I., 2010. Health in all policies. Editorial. Health Promotion International 25 (3), 261–264.

Leeder, S., 1999. Healthy Medicine: Challenges Facing Australia's Health Services. Allen and Unwin, Melbourne.

Lin, V., Gibson, B., 2003. Evidence-based Health Policy: Problems and Possibilities. Oxford University Press, Melbourne.

Lin, V., Robinson, P., 2005. Australian public health policy in 2003–2004. Australia and New Zealand Health Policy 2 (1), 7.

Little, J., 2010. A conversation with John Last. Epidemiology (Cambridge, Mass.) 21 (5), 748–752.

Mejia, G.C., Amarasena, N., Ha, D.H., et al., 2012. Child Dental Health Survey Australia 2007: 30-year trends in child oral health. Cat. No. DEN 217. AIHW, Canberra. Online. Available: <http://www.aihw.gov.au/WorkArea/DownloadAsset.aspx?id=10737421871> (20 Apr 2014).

National Advisory Committee on Oral Health, 2004. Australia's National Oral Health Plan 2004–2013. National Advisory Committee on Oral Health—a committee established by the Australian Health Ministers' Conference. Online. Available: <https://www.adelaide.edu.au/oral-health-promotion/resources/public/pdf_files/oralhealthplan.pdf> (11 Apr 2014).

National Health and Hospitals Reform Commission, 2009. A healthier future for all Australians: final report, June 2009. Online. Available: <http://www.health.gov.au/internet/nhhrc/publishing.nsf/Content/1AFDEAF1FB76A1D8CA257600000B5BE2/$File/Final_Report_of_the%20nhhrc_June_2009.pdf> (7 Apr 2014).

National Health and Medical Research Council (NHMRC), 1997. Acting on Australia's weight: strategic plan for the prevention of overweight and obesity. Online. Available: <http://www.nhmrc.gov.au/publications/synopses/n21syn.htm> (11 Apr 2014) *This publication was rescinded on 22 September 2006. Rescinded publications are publications that no longer represent the council's position on the matters contained therein. This means that the council no longer endorses, supports or approves these rescinded publications.*

National Health and Medical Research Council (NHMRC), 2007. Public statement: the efficacy and safety of fluoridation 2007. Adapted from: Water fluoridation information for health professionals. Queensland Health 2005, State of Queensland.

National Health Priority Action Council, 2006. National Chronic Disease Strategy. Australian Government Department of Health and Ageing, Canberra. Online. Available: <http://www.health.gov.au/internet/main/publishing.nsf/Content/pq-ncds> (11 Apr 2014).

National Preventative Health Taskforce, 2009. Australia: the healthiest country by 2020: National Preventative Health Strategy—Overview. Online. Available: <http://www.health.gov.au/internet/preventativehealth/publishing.nsf/Content/AEC223A781D64FF0CA2575FD00075DD0/$File/nphs-overview.pdf> (7 Feb 2014).

Navarro, V., Muntane, C., Borrell, C., et al., 2006. Politics and health outcomes. Lancet 368, 1033–1037.

Palmer, G., Short, S., 2010. Health Care and Public Policy, fourth ed. Palgrave Macmillan, Melbourne.

Queensland Government water fluoridation website. Online. Available: <http://www.health.qld.gov.au/fluoride/> (11 Apr 2014).

Taylor, S., Foster, K., Fleming, J., 2007. Health Care Practice in Australia: Policy, Context and Innovations. Oxford University Press, Melbourne.

UN AIDS, 2010. Report on the global AIDS epidemic. Online. Available: <http://www.unaids.org/globalreport/> (8 Apr 2014).

United Nations, 1945. Charter of the United Nations. Online. Available: <http://www.un.org/en/documents/charter> (8 Apr 2014).

United Nations General Assembly, 1948. The Universal Declaration of Human Rights. Adopted and proclaimed by General Assembly resolution 217 A (III) of 10 December 1948. Online. Available: <http://www.un.org/Overview/rights.html> (7 Feb 2014).

Walt, G., 2004. Health Policy: An Introduction to Process and Power. Zed Books, London.

Wilson, J.M.G., Junger, G., 1968. The Principles and Practice of Screening for Disease. World Health Organization, Geneva.

World Health Organization, 1948. The Constitution was adopted by the International Health Conference held in New York from 19 Jun to 22 Jul 1946, signed on 22 Jul 1946 by the representatives of 61 States, and entered into force on 7 Apr 1948. Constitution of the World Health Organization. WHO, Geneva.

World Health Organization, 2005. Preventing chronic diseases—a vital investment: WHO global report. Online. Available: <http://www.who.int/chp/chronic_disease_report/> (8 Feb 2014).

World Health Organization, 2008. The WHO agenda: leadership priorities. Online. Available: <http://www.who.int/about/agenda/en/index.html> (3 Apr 2014).

There are numerous books on the structure of the Australian health system, and a comprehensive text is Palmer and Short (2010). Other useful resources are the websites of: the Australian Institute of Health and Welfare (http://www.aihw.gov.au), which publishes an annual Health Expenditure Australia series and a profile of the health of Australians in its bi-annual reports; and the Australian Government Department of Health (http://www.health.gov.au), which presents the structure and priorities for attention to improve health and healthcare for Australians.

CHAPTER 4

Public health and social policy

Greg Marston

Learning objectives

After reading this chapter, you should be able to:

- understand how trends in the welfare state are impacting on the funding and delivery of public health

- briefly describe the history of universal health in Australia, and how it compares with that in other countries

- understand what is meant by the term 'neo-liberalism', and how it influences the design of health services and ideas about risk

- understand how other areas of social policy, such as employment, income support and housing, impact on population health and wellbeing

- identify the difference between a health and welfare system that has a high degree of commodification and targeted programs (market-based provision), and a health and welfare system that has a high degree of direct government provision and universal-based health services

- discuss the potential benefits of the National Disability Insurance Scheme.

Introduction

This chapter places public health in the broad context of social policy and how social problems like growing income inequality, unemployment or insecure housing can impact on health and wellbeing. The previous chapter provided a range of definitions of policy and the policy process, emphasising the importance of action and values in framing what is considered a public or collective responsibility. Value debates are constantly played out in the field of social policy. The term 'social policy' is often used to refer to all areas of government, private and community activity that contribute to health, education, employment and related welfare outcomes. Health policy is somewhat unique compared with other areas of social policy, in that there is a seemingly limitless demand for more and different services, and issues of life and death are tied up with questions about rationing public resources for healthcare (Lewis 2010). Health policy analysis, like other fields of social policy, is often concerned with who gets what, when and how, in terms of the distribution of public goods and services. Health policy is also about advocating across the policy sectors of housing, urban design, income support and education to improve access to good-quality healthcare, as well as improving community health and creating quality of life.

As Chapter 2 illustrated, the notion of healthcare as a public good is something that has evolved over time. This idea became institutionalised with the advent of the post-World War 2 welfare state. Central to all definitions of 'the welfare state' is a notion of government as either the direct provider or a regulator of private and non-profit health, education and social welfare services. In Australia, the welfare state includes public schools and hospitals, income support payments (e.g. unemployment benefits, the aged pension), community services (e.g. counselling and homelessness services), and various forms of occupational welfare (e.g. superannuation and fringe benefits).

The justification for the welfare state grew out of nineteenth- and twentieth-century ideas about the appropriate role for government, which changed due to the processes of urbanisation, industrialisation and global conflict; all of which demanded a greater role for governments in regulating not only private property and guarantees of basic political freedoms, but also an expanded notion of citizenship in terms of social rights and reward for sacrifices made by all citizens during World War 2 (1939–1945). Some examples include the introduction of widow's, sickness and unemployment benefits in 1945. While there is strong public support for aged and veterans' pensions, unemployment benefits continue to be controversial. The able-bodied unemployed have always been seen as less 'deserving' of public support in the Australian welfare system, echoing a longstanding moral distinction in Western countries between the 'deserving' and 'undeserving' poor (see Activity 4.1 and Reflection 4.1).

The other difference between unemployment benefits and healthcare is that unemployment benefits are 'targeted' to people who meet certain eligibility

---

Activity 4.1 Unemployment

Write down your answers to the following questions:

- How important do you think the 'work ethic' is to shaping attitudes to unemployment and the unemployed in Australia?
- Which groups in society are typically thought to be deserving of government support, and which are generally seen as less deserving?
- What are some of the derogatory terms that are used to describe someone who is long-term unemployed in Australia?

REFLECTION 4.1

Did you find it easy to come up with descriptions of the long-term unemployed? How similar do you think these descriptions are to how citizens and governments in other wealthy countries talk about unemployment? Certain labels for social problems minimise the economic dimensions; for example, talking about unemployment as the problem of the unemployed individual means giving less attention to systemic factors. These include the shortage of paid jobs in the Australian economy, as well as the role of workplace discrimination in making it more difficult for some groups to get paid work, particularly women, older workers and people from culturally and linguistically diverse backgrounds.

requirements, whereas access to healthcare in Australia is provided on a more universal footing, which is why it receives wider public and political support (Denmark et al. 2007). This chapter focuses on policy principles and health service delivery, with a particular focus on the relationship between the government and citizens, and key social policy principles of access, equity and social justice. There are different philosophical definitions of 'social justice', ranging from a notion of justice as the equal distribution of a nation's wealth and resources (a social contract between all citizens and government) to minimal state intervention to redress social inequalities, which is the idea of justice as just deserts (those who work harder deserve more, and those who show little effort deserve less). The chapter also focuses on the interconnection between social needs and public health outcomes, emphasising that what happens in other fields of social policy, such as housing and unemployment, is important in terms of people's standard of living and quality of life.

Health policy: a key foundation of the welfare state

Health services became a central component of the post-World War 2 welfare state. In the United Kingdom the twentieth-century economist and social reformer William Beveridge proclaimed that the aim of government investment in welfare services would be as a reward for the sacrifices made by everyone during the war, to attack the five 'giant evils' in society: 'squalor, want, ignorance, idleness and disease' (Abel-Smith 1992 p 5). This rallying cry became the basis of the modern welfare state, which saw governments getting involved to an unprecedented degree in the provision of housing, creating employment opportunities and providing an income support system as a 'safety net' for the unemployed. Some elements of the post-war welfare state were highly targeted, such as unemployment benefits, while others were provided more universally, such as healthcare and, initially, public housing. The assumption at the time was that not everyone would experience unemployment, but everyone gets sick and needs shelter, therefore all citizens should be provided with a basic level of healthcare and access to housing. Initially, public housing in Britain and Australia in the 1940s was targeted towards returning soldiers and their families at a time of chronic housing shortages, but, as more housing was built, public housing was opened up to a wider range of citizens. However, as demand for public housing has grown, access has again become much more restricted. By comparison, public healthcare has continued to be provided on a more or less universal basis.

Universal health initiatives (e.g. immunisation and sanitation) underpin the improvement in key indicators of public health over the past 50 years, such as increased life expectancy and reduced rates of infant mortality in Western Europe and Australia. However, these positive overall trends in health and wellbeing outcomes disguise continuing health inequalities. Health gains have not been equally shared across all sections of the population, and four significant factors continue to exacerbate this trend. These are: an ageing population; the growing burden of chronic disease (we are living longer but not necessarily any healthier); growing levels of income inequality within wealthy nations; and the organisation of funding and delivery of health services, which means that healthcare is treated in contradictory terms in policy, as both a commodity and a basic human right. As discussed in Chapters 2 and 3, and in more detail in Chapter 7, inequalities in health are of growing policy concern.

The notion of a right to healthcare establishes the grounds for the State to provide a social and physical environment conducive to citizens' health, and services designed to maintain and enhance their health (Jamrozik 2009). Expectations about standards of health have also increased in line with advances in health technology, and as a result of policy activism on the part of citizens to demand more affordable medicines and timely healthcare. It was these demands that led to the introduction of the Pharmaceutical Benefits Schemes in the 1940s and 1950s; and the introduction of Medibank and Medicare in the 1970s and 1980s in Australia. These schemes have been informed by principles of social justice; that is, the fair distribution of national resources and opportunities, which reflects an egalitarian philosophy of social justice, and ensuring that all citizens have access to decent healthcare, regardless of their capacity to pay.

Health policy, social justice and risk

Discussions of justice within health have often concentrated on questions of how public health priorities should be set, particularly in a fiscal climate of scarcity. Should more resources be spent on infant and prenatal health as opposed to aged care? Should additional resources be directed towards regional and remote areas to help overcome locational disadvantage? Questions of justice are both particular and universal. They are universal in the sense that the principle of redistributing resources towards the groups with the greatest need can form a basis of policymaking irrespective of context; however, the particular requirements for achieving justice will change over time and across different spaces.

There are competing conversations about wellbeing and contested representations of health policy problems and solutions in Australian social policy. How we define 'health' and 'illness' influences health policy and its legitimate concerns. Moreover, conceptions about health and wellbeing vary both within and between societies and cultures. For social scientists, the terms 'health' and 'illness' are not only defined in terms of anatomy, physiology and genetic makeup, but also in terms of the experience of sickness, disability and pain (Fox & Ward 2006, cited in Pietsch et al. 2010). These experiences are often mediated by class, gender, age and ethnicity, which in turn can affect people's capacity to achieve a level of economic security. In contrast to a biomedical view of the diseased individual body, a social model of health directs the focus from individuals who are ill to social groups with high illness rates; the aim is to find the causes of inequality and, if they include aspects of people's living and working conditions, to use public policy to change them (Burdess 2011). In examining public policy, the aim is to see whether the balance is right between funds being directed to biomedical-orientated solutions, and public health initiatives that seek to address the social aspects of health, such as occupational health and safety and working conditions. The basic point of a sociological approach is that in order to understand health you need to know more than what is going on inside people's bodies—you need to know about the social system in which they live (Burdess 2011) (see Activity 4.2 and Reflection 4.2).

This means using social and economic statistics, first-hand accounts and reports to develop community profiles in areas where public health workers operate. This information can then be used to tailor public health campaigns and related initiatives. More broadly, taking the social model seriously means addressing inequalities and injustices. Achieving system-level change is more difficult and takes longer than simply focusing on individual health problems; thus, different disciplines need to collaborate on complex issues. Public health and social work have long shared a mission to protect and enhance community wellbeing and to promote social justice. In hospitals, schools, government agencies, and local community-based settings, public health social workers forge the connection between prevention and intervention, from the individual to entire populations. It is these kinds of coalitions between professionals, and between professionals and their clients, which put the social model of health into action.

A social perspective of health may look at how the profit motive can affect the delivery of healthcare, or how people from lower socioeconomic groups suffer higher levels of poor health and stress (Pietsch et al. 2010). In Australia there has been an expanding research and policy agenda around the social determinants of health, emphasising the social and economic conditions that influence individual and group differences in health status. These social factors also include public policies and politics. As the World Health Organization (WHO 2008 p 1) argues:

> The unequal distribution of health-damaging experiences is not in any sense a 'natural' phenomenon but is the result of a toxic combination of poor social policies, unfair economic arrangements and bad politics.

Health systems are coming under pressure due to the increasing demand and rising costs of health infrastructure and technology. Contemporary media reports in Australia about healthcare and health services often represent the system as being in crisis (Lewis 2010). The 2014 Federal Budget announcements, which include a proposed $7 co-payment for every GP visit, also present the health system as being in a state of crisis and being unsustainable. A mix of moral and economic arguments is used by the government to justify the co-payment. Attempts to increase user-charges for primary healthcare to assist with rising costs have been met by resistance from citizens.

Demographic and technological changes will be major factors behind increases in health costs in coming decades. Between 2010 and 2050, health spending is expected to increase sevenfold on those 65 and over, and twelvefold on those 85 and over (Australian Treasury 2010). As Chapter 3 has shown, health services constitute one of the largest components of government expenditure. High levels of expenditure are in line with community expectations about access to health services being a right in modern societies. Increasingly, rights are being tied to responsibilities, and the collective pooling of risk through a welfare state is being challenged on both moral and economic grounds (Marston & McDonald 2013). The attempted introduction of co-payments for general practitioner (GP) visits, increased education charges for university students, and periods of non-payment for unemployment benefits in the 2014 federal budget are examples of where both economic and moral arguments are being used to justify proposed policy changes.

Health inequalities are likely to intensify as a result of policy measures that seek to individualise risk. In recent decades, welfare states have been struggling to meet both old and new lifecycle risks. The old risks are those that the market was generally unable to provide for during the industrial era, such as unemployment, old age and disability. These risks were a key justification for the twentieth-century welfare states. New risks are those generated by post-industrial changes to the labour market, where there has been a decline in full-time work and changing family and household dynamics, an ageing population and chronic diseases. Ironically, some of these new risks have been generated by the success of the welfare state in increasing life expectancy and expanding consumption. These risks result in a larger claim being made on governments, which has governments worried about the sustainability of health and welfare measures. Thus governments are increasingly asking citizens to bear more of the responsibility for life risks, either informally or through the market. For example: asking workers to delay and self-fund their retirement; prioritising private rental subsidies rather than building public housing; and encouraging middle- to high-income earners to use private health providers. In short, the government is reducing its role in the direct provision of social services and support. The US political scientist Jacob Hacker (2006) refers to this change in government role as 'the great risk shift' to highlight the institutional transformation that is taking place in health and social policy more generally.

The guiding assumptions in the post-war period about the role of governments in regulating risk came under attack in the mid-1970s as a result of rising unemployment and inflation, and the subsequent loss of faith in Keynesian economic prescriptions for economic and social security. Keynesian economics came to prominence in the post-war period as an approach to economic outputs that emphasised government spending to increase aggregate demand (total spending in the economy); therefore, government spending could help to minimise the effects of an economic recession. Since the 1970s, economic policy started to turn away from Keynesian demand-side job creation and welfare state expansion. Subsequently, in Australia and other advanced economies, mass unemployment started to be accepted as inevitable, as 'fighting inflation first' became the mantra of economic governance. Significantly, governments started to position themselves as risk managers of last resort, with a preference for non-State actors, particularly market providers, filling the gap left by the withdrawal of government services. The current Australian Federal Government's general objective of increasing individual and family responsibility for community services is characteristic of this trend. Criticism of privatisation centres on concern that the needs of disadvantaged groups in the community may not be met by the process, and that the financial gains enjoyed by some as a result of privatisation may well result in socioeconomic disadvantage for others.

In practice, the privatisation process transformation is uneven. Some social policy fields, such as employment assistance, have been essentially fully privatised with a range of for-profit and non-profit providers, such as Salvation Army Employment Plus, providing all employment and training services to the unemployed. Other fields, like education and health, maintain a mixed economy of welfare, although even here individuals are encouraged through a range of government-funded rebates and incentives to opt out of the public system and into private forms of provision. This process of institutional transformation has been legitimated through a neo-liberal economic orthodoxy. Common to all neo-liberalism variants is a belief that market mechanisms of exchange are morally and economically superior to government-provided schemes, which are represented as inefficient and as responsible for creating 'welfare-dependent' citizens (Fraser 1997, Peck 2010).

While neo-liberalism undoubtedly changed the politics and character of health and welfare provision during the 1990s, it did not lead to an overall decline in social expenditure, as was predicted. Figure 4.1 shows how, even during periods of fiscal restraint and an ideology of a 'small state', funding for social welfare actually increased. This reinforces the point that neo-liberalism does not necessarily mean the end of State regulation and spending, it simply changes the means and ends of government spending and activity.

A continuing rise in expenditure during the 1990s and early 2000s led social policy researcher Frank Castles (2004) to proclaim that Australia has a 'steady, steady welfare

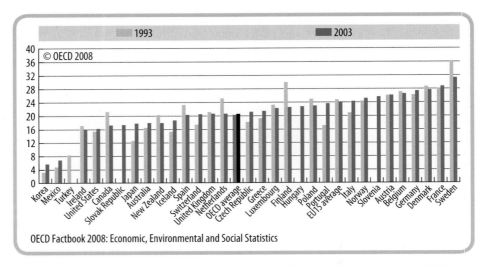

FIG. 4.1   Public social expenditure as a percentage of gross domestic product (GDP).
(Source: OECD 2008)

state', meaning that, despite the talk about welfare state retrenchment, the welfare state is proving more resilient than crisis theorists had predicted. Whether the amount of spending is adequate, or it produces new inequalities, depends on how the expenditure is being distributed and which groups are being targeted. Measures such as tax rebates and concessions may disproportionally benefit middle- and upper-income earners, and are therefore likely to exacerbate inequalities. For example, superannuation tax concessions and negative gearing of investment properties favour high-income earners. Neoliberalism's emphasis on market solutions and individual responsibility can lead to a health and welfare system where people's capacity to pay has a large bearing on whether they receive high-quality healthcare. This development works against greater health equality and principles of equity and justice.

While Australia is spending about the average on healthcare compared with other OECD countries, overall social expenditure is towards the lower end of the spectrum. Australia is similar to nations such as the United States, the United Kingdom, New Zealand and Canada. This group of countries is referred to as 'liberal welfare states' (Esping-Andersen 1990); that is, they favour market-based solutions (commodification) to meet social needs (e.g. private rental housing, private health insurance) compared with social democratic countries, such as Sweden and Norway, which preference universal health and welfare coverage. The 'social democratic welfare states' are at the high end of public expenditure, because they have wider universal coverage of the population (de-commodification) in terms of healthcare, dental care, education, childcare and paid parental leave, largely funded by higher rates of direct and indirect taxation. The social democratic welfare states have lower rates of income inequality, and the way they structure social relations is arguably more conducive to a healthier population.

As discussed in more detail in Chapter 7, Wilkinson and Pickett's landmark study (2009, 2010) on social inequality and the impact on health outcomes claimed that for many health and social problems—such as drug abuse, crime, obesity, diminished trust and community life, violence and teenage pregnancies—outcomes are significantly worse in more unequal countries. The design of welfare states and their equalising

CASE STUDY
4.1

Joined-up problems need joined-up solutions

Joan is a single parent living in private rental in outer Western Sydney. She has three children, aged 9, 12 and 15. Joan has her name down on the public housing waiting list, but has been told by the state housing department that it could be three years before she gets a place. The two-bedroom flat she is living in has rising damp, and is difficult to keep cool in summer and warm in the winter. Her nine-year-old son has asthma, and Joan has noticed that it has been getting worse since they moved into the flat, which she did after separating from the children's father. Joan wants a permanent part-time job to fit in around the school hours, but all she can get is casual work at the local supermarket during school hours. The extra income supplements her unemployment benefit, which is less than the single parent's pension, which she received until her youngest child turned eight. Her casual job makes it difficult for her to predict what her income will be each fortnight, and so reporting her income to Centrelink is a challenge. Joan finds they have very little money left over after paying the rent and the bills. She feels a lot of shame about her situation, and guilty that she can't buy the kids the things they need, like new shoes for school. Although Joan manages to put food on the table for the kids, she sometimes goes without. She feels stressed and tired a lot of the time, and wishes she had more time and money.

capacity therefore plays a significant role in population health outcomes. If someone has to work three jobs to make ends meet, while constantly living under the threat of eviction, then their physical and mental health is likely to be poorer than someone with stable employment and housing. Furthermore, precarious paid employment can actually be worse for someone's mental health than no job at all (Butterworth et al. 2011). Thus, what is happening in other fields of social policy has an important bearing on public health outcomes (see Case Study 4.1, and Activity 4.3 and Reflection 4.3).

Different systems of government, and overall policy governance across countries, also play an important role in the effectiveness of health systems and outcomes for citizens. The United States, for example, spends more on health services per capita than Australia, and yet it has poorer outcomes. The costs of drugs, medical technology and a complex profit-orientated private-sector model of health insurance continue to drive costs upward in the United States. Sweden, with a healthcare budget that is about half that of the United States, has a higher life expectancy, and an infant mortality rate that is about 40% of the US rate (Blau 2007). The United States and Australia have federal systems of governance, where the different levels of government have different

ACTIVITY 4.3 Interconnected problems

- List the problems Joan faces, and explain how they are interconnected.
- How does Joan's precarious employment impact on her health?
- How do you think Joan's feelings of stress might impact on her health and her children's health?
- Who should Joan speak to, to get something done about her poor-quality housing?

REFLECTION 4.3

Did you identify any common themes in the problems Joan is facing? There is a lot of uncertainty in Joan's life, and it sometimes easy to forget how important having economic security is to being able to develop one's full potential in all areas of life, not just paid work.

responsibilities in terms of funding, regulation and provision; whereas Sweden has a unitary system of government, making it easier to stipulate and implement national standards of healthcare. Joint responsibility for health between levels of government does not necessarily lead to cooperative and effective outcomes. Funding inadequacies and poor services tend to be explained by buck-passing in federal systems of government (Jamrozik 2009).

The structural explanation for this competitive federalism is what economists call 'vertical fiscal imbalance', which means that the national government raises most of the revenue while the state and territory governments are largely responsible for policy implementation and service delivery. Moreover, state and territory governments argue that they are closer to the needs, and should therefore have greater autonomy over how funds are spent, while the national level of government argues the case for consistency of service quality, regardless of which state and territory a citizen resides in. Furthermore, industry and health professionals also have competing interests. The recent controversy in Australia over a voluntary star-rating system to be applied to processed foods illustrates this point. Government and industry had worked on the development of the system over many months, but, despite agreement between state and federal ministers to proceed with the star-rating website, the website was taken down the day it was launched in February 2014. The federal Assistant Health Minister Fiona Nash said the website was pulled because it was a draft; and also indicated that the CEO of the Australian Food and Grocery Council expressed his opposition to the scheme (ABC News 27 February 2014). Clearly, as food processing is now Australia's largest manufacturing sector, it has a significant lobbying presence (see Activity 4.4 and Reflection 4.4).

One of the common features in many health systems around the world is the division between public and private interests. These competing interests are intensified by the considerable amount of funding involved in the area of health policy and programs, which makes health funding vulnerable during times of fiscal constraint. In the United States, these differences were recently revealed when the US government, led by President Obama, sought to introduce Medicaid. Republican politicians, supported by private health funds, labelled the scheme 'socialist'. The Health Care Reform Bill, passed in the United States in 2010, essentially did three things: (1) restricted the freedoms of private insurance companies, forcing them to provide coverage for pre-existing conditions, among other things; (2) increased regulation of these private insurance companies, forcing them to compete in healthcare exchanges in an effort to lower costs; and (3) mandated that individuals purchase health insurance. None of these actions transferred ownership of the health insurance industry from private firms to the federal government, so there was no new 'mixed economy' and therefore no new 'socialism' (Knoll 2012). This resistance by US private health insurers to health reform highlights the difficulties of health policy development.

ACTIVITY 4.4 Influence of lobbies

Go to the Australian Food and Grocery Council website (http://www.afgc.org.au/) and do a keyword search for 'star rating'.

- What is their policy position regarding the proposed labelling scheme?
- Do you see any contradictions in what they are advocating on this issue, particularly in relation to other policy positions they are advocating?
- How much say do you think this industry body should have on public health policy?
- Whose interests should take priority in cases like this?

REFLECTION 4.4

Did you consider whether the influence of professional lobbyists is limiting the role of ordinary consumers in these policy debates? How much government regulation of food packaging should there be? Can we have too much regulation in this field?

International comparisons are one way to understand Australia's health system; another is by looking at continuities and discontinuities over time. As Chapter 2 illustrated, history is important for public health policy, particularly as it can demonstrate how contingent and fragile policy agreement can be. The next section considers changes to Medicare since its inception, and the health outcomes for different groups in Australian society, to illustrate what is changing about health and social policy in Australia since the 'golden age' of the post-World War 2 welfare state. This discussion further develops the theme introduced in Chapter 2 on health policy and the Australian healthcare system by examining ideational and institutional change to conceptions of health and wellbeing.

History of Australian health policy—policy design and funding arrangements

As discussed in Chapter 2, compared with most other Western countries, with the exception of the United States, Australia was late in developing a national health insurance scheme (Lewis 2010). Various failed attempts were pursued through the 1940s. Subsidised voluntary health insurance was progressively introduced from 1950 to 1953. This included a national pharmaceutical scheme, a means-tested medical benefits scheme with heavy involvement from the friendly societies, and hospital benefits with co-payments from users. Each was fought over and finally resolved (Lewis 2010 p 200). Australia continued with a residual health insurance system until the 1970s, when the Whitlam Government was elected on a platform of social justice and equity, and established a national health scheme named Medibank. Its aim was to provide public insurance for the whole population, which was important, given that in the early 1970s around 20% of the adult population, most of whom were on low incomes, did not have private health insurance.

The original Medibank program proposed a 1.35% levy (with low-income exemptions) to fund the scheme. These Bills were however rejected by the Senate, so Medibank was originally funded from general revenue. The Medibank scheme was partially dismantled by the Fraser Government, elected in 1975. Medibank was then restored, in a slightly different form, by the Hawke Labor Government in 1983. Renamed Medicare in 1984, it provides a fixed subsidy for different types of medical service and procedure, with patients responsible for paying any charges levied by providers above this subsidy out of their own pockets. The Medicare program, now nominally funded by an income tax surcharge, is currently set at 1.5%, with a higher levy for high-income earners.

Universal access to primary healthcare has been a political football since it was first introduced in the 1970s. This backwards and forwards policy movement led academic Frank Castles (1985 p 30) to conclude that Australia has the world's 'most reversible' welfare state. This form of policy development has been particularly acute in relation to the public versus private health insurance debate in Australia. Private health insurance declined significantly following the introduction of Medicare (Colombo & Tapay 2003). The Howard Government, elected in 1996, introduced various measures to reverse the decline in private health insurance. These included a substantial subsidy in the form of a non-means-tested 30% rebate to residents on the purchase of private health insurance (Duckett 2005, Hurley et al. 2002), a tax rebate for residents who bought private health insurance, and a range of financial penalties on those who did not take out private health insurance (Butler 2002). Consequently, membership of private health insurance rose from around 30% in 1998 to 46% in 2001 (Australian

Institute of Health and Welfare (AIHW) 2008, Hurley et al. 2002, Walker et al. 2006) and has settled at around 43% ever since (AIHW 2010).

The expansion of government support for private health insurance was framed in terms of supporting a *universal public health insurance system*. Critics say that the private health insurance rebate is an unfair subsidy to those who can afford health insurance (Lewis 2010), and that the money would be better spent on public hospitals where it would benefit everyone. Supporters of the tax subsidy say people must be encouraged into the private healthcare system, claiming that the public system is not universally sustainable for the future. Even after the introduction of the rebate, private health insurance organisations have raised their premiums most years, which negates the rebate somewhat. Segal (2004) argues that policies to boost private health insurance membership have undermined the efficiency and equity of the Australian healthcare system, and have not reduced waiting lists in public hospitals. Walker et al. (2006) argue that a boost to private health insurance through the rebate has provided substantial public subsidies to the wealthiest quintile of Australians, the group most likely to purchase private health insurance, while the impact of the reforms for the poorest 40% has been minimal.

A 2005 study found that only 24% of Australians who live in households with incomes below $25,000 per year were covered by private health insurance, while 69% of those in households with incomes over $100,000 had private health cover (Denniss 2005). As Chapter 3 illustrated, high income and personal wealth play a key role in people's private health insurance status.

The Australian Government's reliance on private health insurance as a tool of public policy is delivering a disproportionate benefit to high-income earners. Some areas of surgery are now performed predominantly in the private sector, and the 55% of Australians without private health insurance must wait, often for months, for elective surgery in the public system. Reforms to private health insurance have increased access to obstetricians in private practice, but primarily for high-income women. The out-of-pocket fees for private obstetric services are often substantial, and Australia has one of the highest rates of per-capita out-of-pocket expenditures (Van Gool et al. 2009).

Private health insurance allows women the choice of a private obstetrician, and generally offers continuity of care throughout pregnancy and childbirth, longer post-partum hospital stays if desired, and often superior hospital accommodation. However, current health policy in Australia makes access to these advantages inequitable. Policy channels public funds to private obstetric services (Van Gool et al. 2009), thus perpetuating the dominance of medicine and decreasing the efficiency of the maternity sector by utilising highly trained obstetricians as primary birth attendants for women regardless of their obstetric risk. Australian women giving birth in the public healthcare system have fewer opportunities for choice of maternity care provider, and little possibility of receiving continuity of care during the childbearing period. Within the maternity workforce, obstetricians have been the main beneficiaries of government policies promoting private health insurance, and the numbers of specialists qualified in obstetrics and gynaecology have grown substantially.

Dental health is another area where those who rely on the state-based system must wait longer for basic dental health services than those who can access privately provided dental care. Adults in the highest income quartile were more likely to have visited a dentist in the past 12 months than those in the lowest income quartile (76.9% compared with 55.1%). Those in the highest income quartile were also less likely to receive an extraction than those in the lowest income quartile (3.7% compared with 13.5%) (Spencer & Harford 2007). Dental health is excluded from the Medicare scheme, although universal dental healthcare gained some traction when the Labor Government

(2007–2013) made a commitment to expanding public dental health coverage. The dental profession argued against the inclusion of dentistry in any universal health insurance scheme, concerned that it would act as a price-control system (Matthew 2007). Despite these objections, new investment in dental care was one of the main conditions on which the Greens political party pledged their support for Labor in forming a minority government in 2010. A proposal, debated in the Federal Parliament in 2012, was to implement a six-year package, including $2.7 billion for children aged 2 to 18, $1.3 billion for adults on low incomes, and $225 million for non-metropolitan areas. The Coalition Government, elected in 2013, has indicated its support for the Child Dental Benefits Scheme, but not whether it will support other components of the six-year package.

The current situation is inequitable, in that timely access to healthcare in Australia can still be based on the ability to pay rather than the degree of need. Additionally, despite the expansion of the private health subsidy and the continuation of Medicare, the costs of healthcare for individuals continue to rise. The largest component of non-government funding for healthcare came from out-of-pocket payments by individuals, equating to 17.5% of total funding. When low-income status intersects with disability or ethnicity, it can create an even more dramatic profile of health inequalities, as the next section demonstrates.

Disability, Indigenous health and equity considerations

As discussed earlier, a social model of health is concerned with the health status of different groups in society, in terms of characteristics such as income, ethnicity, place, gender, disability and age. While many fields of social policy, particularly income support and public housing, have been tightening eligibility criteria, disability policy in Australia has been subject to major reforms, to increase choice and autonomy and relax eligibility criteria to provide higher levels of support and services for a greater number of Australians with a disability. This is the National Disability Insurance Scheme (NDIS), currently being trialled in most states and territories, with a view to being fully operational in 2019–20; it will provide support to around 460,000 Australians at a cost of $22 billion per year (Cullen 2013). The NDIS, which will be administered through a national fund, with money contributed at federal and state levels, is being touted as the most significant reform in health since the introduction of Medicare.

The NDIS is a national no-fault insurance scheme that guarantees a level of financial support to people with a disability. Currently, people with similar levels of functionality get access to quite different levels of support, depending on their location and the timing or origin of their disability. The NDIS will have individualised funding packages based on a client's level of need. The person with the disability, together with their family and carers, will be able to choose where they spend their entitlement, meaning that disability and some health service providers will no longer receive block funding from the Government but will instead compete for a client's funds. Theoretically, this should increase efficiency and give the client choice. Support and assistance associated with the implementation of the NDIS aim to increase opportunities for people with disability by tackling such things as inadequate housing, the need for personal care, and assistance in participating in the community. A lot will depend on the detail in determining whether this new social policy will meet the intended aims.

Another area of social policy where the outcome has not always matched initial expectations and hopes is Indigenous health. As discussed in detail in Chapter 16, there are major differences between the health status of Aboriginal and Torres Strait Islander Australians and non-Indigenous Australians, representing a chronic failure of health policy in Australia.

Indigenous children and young people are far more likely to be disadvantaged across a range of health and socioeconomic indicators: 2–3 times as likely to die, be of low birth weight or have dental cavities; 8–9 times as likely to be in the child protection system; and 24 times as likely to be in juvenile justice supervision. Such statistics are partly a legacy of colonisation and the disadvantaged socioeconomic position of Indigenous Australians, but they also reflect a clash of paradigms between Western medicine and Indigenous knowledge systems. The Australia Medical Association (AMA) recommends that 'a holistic, culturally appropriate approach informs all areas of government policy development, which supersedes the current disease-based and fragmented policy and funding strategies' (AMA 2005 p 4).

There is limited evidence that these principles are being widely incorporated into public health promotion and primary healthcare in Australia. There are some exceptions—for example, the hub-and-spoke model of service delivery provided by the Katherine West Health Board (KWHB). An Aboriginal community-controlled health organisation in the Northern Territory, the KWHB is governed by an 18-member board of Aboriginal representatives, who provide advice about the health concerns and priorities of their communities. The KWHB owns and operates a health centre in Katherine, and health centres in seven communities in the region, which are staffed by GPs, nurses, qualified and trainee Aboriginal health workers, administrative staff, and visiting specialists. The KWHB produces health outcomes that are better than average on nearly all of the key health performance indicators used in the Northern Territory (AMA 2011).

The Rudd Labor Government, elected in 2007, pledged that it would close the gap between the health outcomes of Indigenous and non-Indigenous Australians. The timeframes for the Closing the Gap targets recognise that comprehensive strategies and policies will need to be sustained for a long time. The Australian Government committed itself to releasing an annual report on how much progress it has made towards these goals. While important in tracking progress, these reports say little about service delivery models, particularly the crucial issues of ownership and control; and the report is still underpinned by a biomedical and disease approach to health, rather than one that focuses on the social environment, economic context and culture. For further analysis on Closing the Gap, see Chapter 16.

In the next section I will expand on the importance of context by considering the synergy between the social determinants of health perspective and the characteristics of class, ethnicity and gender. This discussion will highlight the competing discourses about health and the connections with wider debates about welfare and wellbeing in Australia.

Social determinants of health and environmental health discourses

This chapter has emphasised the importance of context, culture and other structural factors in making sense of health inequalities and in explaining the class, gender and ethnicity differential when it comes to assessing who benefits from good-quality healthcare. This framework is consistent with the social determinants of health perspective. It is also evident that environmental factors are important, and that the major determinants of health or ill health are inextricably linked to the social and economic context (Marmot & Wilkinson 2001). Factors such as housing, income, employment, geography—indeed, many of the issues that dominate political life—are key determinants of population health and wellbeing. Environmental health impacts, for example, tend to disproportionately affect population groups that have limited choices about where they live and work, and what they eat. A shift-worker living alongside a major freeway and in poor-quality or overcrowded housing is likely to have poorer health outcomes than does the individual who has a good job and lives in appropriate housing located close to public amenities. Yet this analysis is missing when the social policy problem is constructed in terms of behavioural explanations, where individuals are held responsible for making 'sensible choices' (Habibis & Walter 2009 p 232).

The definition of health that has conventionally been operationalised under Western capitalism has two interrelated aspects to it: health is considered both as the absence of disease (biomedical definition) and as a commodity (economic definition). These both focus on individuals, as opposed to society, as the basis of health: health is seen predominately as a product of individual factors such as genetic heritage and lifestyle choices, and as a commodity that individuals can access via either the market or the health system. Inequalities in the distribution of health are therefore either a result of the failings of individuals through their lifestyle choices, or a result of the way in which healthcare products are produced, distributed and delivered.

Since the beginning of the last century, there has been a dramatic decrease in the mortality rates of babies and children in Australia. However, children's life expectancy and quality of life is now threatened by an array of modern conditions. In what is described as 'modernity's paradox', many Australian children are not as healthy as were children of earlier generations. Children and young people today live in an environment that is vastly different from that of only a generation ago. Technological advances, new industrial processes, changes in food production, increased mobility, intensified urbanism, global warming, new individualised work practices, and increased consumption of media, processed foods and drinks and alcohol have radically changed the quality and patterns of life for children and young people (Wyn 2009).

Furthermore, these changes have been linked with a range of 'new childhood morbidities' (Baur 2002 p 525). These include: low birth weight; rising rates of obesity and diabetes; childhood asthma and increasing allergies; developmental disorders; autism; dental decay; congenital malformations; and mental health problems. There is an increase in learning disabilities, aggressive behaviour and violence. Such problems are likely to become more prevalent as these children become adults and parents of their own children. In Australia, the prevalence rates of asthma are high by international levels, and are a major cause of hospitalisation of children (Australian Centre for Asthma Monitoring 2011). Studies show that both outdoor (Barnett et al. 2005, Hinwood et al. 2006) and indoor pollutants contribute to increased respiratory symptoms in children (Nitschke et al. 2006, Ponsonby et al. 1999, Zhang & Smith 2007). In addition, exposure to ozone increases the severity of respiratory symptoms in children under the age of five years (Rodriguez et al. 2007).

The WHO acknowledges that 'only a small fraction of all childhood cancers are associated with heredity, genetics, infections, and viruses; instead environmental pollutants appear to play a major role and air pollution alone is associated with up to half of all childhood cancers' (WHO 2005 p 144). Generally, it is recognised that children suffer a disproportionate share of the environmental health burden (Prüss-Üstün & Corvalán 2006). The Australian Government has made it clear that children's and young people's health and wellbeing is a priority, recognising that the environment plays a critical role in their wellbeing (Council of Australian Governments (COAG) 2009). The vision for Australian children put forward by successive Australian Governments is clear: '[B]y 2020 all children have the best start in life to create a better future for themselves and for the nation' (COAG 2009 p 18). Despite this acknowledgement of the importance of children's health and a lifecycle approach to healthcare, federal or state governments do not appear to be moving away from traditional biomedical concerns towards more societal- and environmental-based approaches to health policy (Lewis 2010).

Australia could follow the lead of Britain, where there has been a paradigm shift since the early 2000s in terms of linking healthcare reforms with wider public-sector reforms to address the determinants of health inequalities (Lewis 2010). However, cutbacks to public-sector expenditure in the United Kingdom since 2010, following the Global Financial Crisis, are likely to undo some of these achievements. Preventative health requires a long-term approach to achieving the policy goals of improving access and equity, and is therefore always vulnerable to budget cuts and short-term electoral cycles. The contribution of social determinants and environmental approaches to public health are further developed in Chapters 6 and 7.

A final word

Social justice is essential, as it affects the way people live, their consequent chance of illness, and their risk of premature death. We watch in wonder as life expectancy and good health continue to increase in some parts of the world, and in alarm as they fail to improve in others. A girl born today can expect to live for more than 80 years if she is born in some countries—but less than 45 years if she is born in others (Commission on Social Determinants of Health 2008 p 3).

This assessment of the social distribution of health and wellbeing is not only relevant to developing economies. As this chapter has discussed, there are significant and growing inequalities within countries that mean some groups are doing better than others when it comes to health and wellbeing. Sociological understandings of health help to highlight the social inequalities in health and the impact of social location on the body, while political economy helps us to identify the private interests that seek to marginalise a universally-orientated public health system. Comparative evidence from OECD countries suggests that Australia's mixed public–private health system does a good job in ensuring high-quality access to doctor, hospital and dental care services. However, as in other OECD countries, Australians on higher incomes are more likely to consult a specialist, while those on lower incomes are more likely to consult a GP. The unequal distribution of private health insurance coverage by income contributes to the phenomenon that the 'better off' and the 'less well off' do not receive the same mix of services, nor have the same level of access.

As this chapter has shown, the entitlement to free medical care in Australia is not sufficient to ensure equitable access to timely and good-quality healthcare. Geographical location and demographic factors continue to have an important bearing on access to health services (AIHW 2013). Financial barriers to health service could be removed through policies that re-emphasise the universal nature of Medicare, by encouraging bulk billing for patients and by abolishing the private health insurance rebate (Lewis 2010). Abolishing the rebate would lower health costs overall, and reduce the inflationary pressures within the dual insurance system. Health budgets, however, are only part of the picture. Spreading the benefits of good-quality healthcare and addressing entrenched health inequalities will also require going beyond an individualised discourse of what good health means.

REVIEW QUESTIONS

1 How does the broader context of social policy and the history of the welfare state shape public health policy?

2 How do contemporary notions of risk and responsibility inform social policy decisions?

3 What role do private sector interests, such as health insurers and food-processing manufacturers, play in public health?

4 Why did a public health insurance scheme take longer to develop in Australia than in the United Kingdom?

5 What is the difference between a biomedical and a social model of health?

6 How does the National Disability Insurance Scheme differ from how services to people with a disability have traditionally been provided?

7 What is meant by the term 'neo-liberalism', and how does it influence the delivery of health services?

8 In terms of health and social policy, what are the main differences between 'liberal welfare states' and 'social democratic welfare states'?

9 What is meant by the phrase 'modernity's paradox' with regard to children's health?

10 What is meant by the 'great risk shift' with regard to health and social policy?

Useful websites

- Australian Institute of Health and Welfare: www.aihw.gov.au
- Australian Policy Online: www.apo.org.au
- Social Policy Research Centre: www.sprc.unsw.edu.au

References

Abel-Smith, B., 1992. The Beveridge report: its origins and outcomes. International Social Security Review 45 (1–2), 5–16.

Australian Centre for Asthma Monitoring, 2011. Asthma in Australia 2011: With a Focus Chapter on Chronic Obstructive Pulmonary Disease. Cat. No. ACM 22. Australian Institute of Health and Welfare, Canberra.

Australian Institute of Health and Welfare, 2008. Australia's Health 2008. AIHW Cat. No. AUS 99. AIHW, Canberra.

Australian Institute of Health and Welfare, 2010. Australia's Health 2010. AIHW Cat. No. AUS 122. AIHW, Canberra.

Australian Institute of Health and Welfare, 2013. Australia's Welfare 2013. AIHW Cat. No. AUS 174. AIHW, Canberra.

Australian Medical Association, 2005. Aboriginal and Torres Strait Islander health 2005. Online. Available: <https://ama.com.au/position-statement/aboriginal-and-torres-strait -islander-health-2005> (10 Apr 2014).

Australian Medical Association, 2011. 2010–11 AMA Indigenous health report card—'best practice in primary health care for Aboriginal peoples and Torres Strait Islanders'. Online. Available: <https://ama.com.au/article/2010-11-ama-indigenous-health-report-card-best -practice-primary-health-care-aboriginal> (23 Apr 2015).

Australian Treasury, 2010. Australia to 2050: The 2010 Intergenerational Report. Commonwealth of Australia, Canberra.

Barnett, R., Schwartz, J., Neller, A., et al., 2005. Air pollution and child respiratory health: a case-crossover study in Australia and New Zealand. American Journal of Respiratory and Critical Care Medicine 1 (171), 1272–1278.

Baur, L.A., 2002. Child and adolescent obesity in the 21st century: an Australian perspective. Asia Pacific Journal of Clinical Nutrition 11 (3), 524–528.

Blau, J., 2007. The Dynamics of Social Welfare Policy, second ed. Oxford University Press, Oxford.

Burdess, N., 2011. The social basis of health and illness. In: Germov, J., Poole, M. (Eds.), Public Sociology: An Introduction to Australian Sociology. Allen and Unwin, Sydney, pp. 330–348.

Butler, J., 2002. Policy change and private health insurance. Australian Health Review 25 (6), 1–12.

Butterworth, P., Leach, L., Strasdins, L., et al., 2011. The psychosocial quality of work determines whether employment has benefits for mental health: results from a longitudinal national household panel survey. Occupational Health and Medicine 68 (11), 806–812.

Castles, F., 1985. The Working Class and Welfare. Allen and Unwin, Sydney.

Castles, F., 2004. The Future of the Welfare State: Crisis Myths and Crisis Realities. Oxford University Press, Oxford.

Colombo, F., Tapay, N., 2003. Private Health Insurance in Australia. OECD Working Papers No. 8. Directorate for Employment, Labour and Social Affairs (DELSA).

Commission on Social Determinants of Health (CSDH), 2008. Closing the Gap in a Generation: Health Equity Through Action on the Social Determinants of Health. Final Report of the Commission on Social Determinants of Health. World Health Organization, Geneva.

Council of Australian Governments, 2009. Investing in the Early Years—A National Early Childhood Development Strategy: An Initiative of the Council of Australian Governments. COAG, Canberra.

Cullen, S., 2013. Early figures show cost of NDIS blowing out by 30 per cent. ABC News. Online. Available: <http://www.abc.net.au/news/2013-11-20/early-figures-show-ndis -scheme-cost-blowout/5105304> (2 May 2014).

Denmark, D., Meagher, G., Wilson, S., et al., 2007. Australian Social Attitudes 2: Citizenship, Work and Aspirations. University of New South Wales (UNSW) Press, Sydney.

Denniss, R., 2005. Who Benefits from Private Health Insurance in Australia? The Australia Institute, Canberra.

Duckett, S., 2005. Private care and public waiting. Australian Health Review 29, 87–93.

Esping-Andersen, G., 1990. Three Worlds of Welfare Capitalism. Princeton University Press, Princeton.

Fox, N., Ward, K., 2006. Health identities: from expert patient to resisting consumer. Health (London) 10, 461. doi:10.1177/1363459306067314.

Fraser, N., 1997. Justice Interruptus: Critical Reflections on the Post-Socialist Condition. Routledge, New York.

Habibis, D., Walter, M., 2009. Social Inequality in Australia: Discourses, Realities and Futures. Oxford University Press, Melbourne.

Hacker, J., 2006. The Great Risk Shift: The Assault on American Jobs, Families, Health Care and Retirement and How You Can Fight Back. Oxford University Press, Oxford.

Hinwood, A., De Klerk, N., Rodriguez, C., et al., 2006. The relationship between changes in daily air pollution and hospitalizations in Perth, Australia 1992–1998: a case-crossover study. International Journal of Environmental Health Research 16 (1), 27–46.

Hurley, J., Vaithianathan, R., Crossley, T., et al., 2002. Parallel Private Health Insurance in Australia: A Cautionary Tale and Lessons for Canada. Discussion Paper No. 448. Centre for Economic Policy, Australian National University, Canberra.

Jamrozik, A., 2009. Social Policy in the Post-Welfare State: Australian Society in the 21st Century, second ed. Pearson Education, Sydney.

Knoll, B., 2012. President Obama, the Democratic Party, and socialism: a political science perspective. Huffington Post. Online. Available: <http://www.huffingtonpost.com/benjamin-knoll/obama-romney-economy_b_1615862.html> (10 Apr 2014).

Lewis, J., 2010. Recent changes in health policy: stepping back and looking forward. In: McClelland, A., Smyth, P. (Eds.), Social Policy in Action: Understanding for Action, second ed. Oxford University Press, Melbourne.

Marmot, M., Wilkinson, R., 2001. Psychosocial and material pathways in the relation between income and wealth: a response to Lynch et al. British Medical Journal 322, 1233–1236.

Marston, G., McDonald, C., 2013. The Australian Welfare State: Who Benefits Now? Palgrave MacMillan, London.

Matthew, J., 2007. EPC Scheme developments. Australian Dental Association News Bulletin 357: 22–24 at p 26.

Nitschke, M., Pilotto, L., Attewell, R., 2006. A cohort study of indoor nitrogen dioxide and house dust mite exposure in asthmatic children. Journal of Occupational and Environmental Medicine 48 (5), 462–469.

OECD Factbook 2008: Economic, environmental and social statistics. Online. Available: <http://dx.doi.org/10.1787/factbook-2008-en> (25 Mar 2014).

Peck, J., 2010. Constructions of Neo-Liberal Reason. Oxford University Press, Oxford.

Pietsch, J., Graetz, B., McAllister, I., 2010. Dimensions of Australian Society, third ed. Palgrave Macmillan, Melbourne.

Ponsonby, A., Couper, D., Dwyer, T., et al., 1999. Relationship between early life respiratory illness, family size over time, and the development of asthma and hay fever: a seven year follow up study. Thorax 54 (8), 664–669.

Prüss-Üstün, A., Corvalán, C., 2006. Preventing disease through healthy environments: towards an estimate of the environmental burden of disease. World Health Organization, Geneva. Online. Available: <http://cdrwww.who.int/quantifying_ehimpacts/publications/preventingdiseasebegin.pdf> (14 Jan 2014).

Rodriguez, C., Tonkin, R., Heyworth, J., et al., 2007. The relationship between outdoor air quality and respiratory illness in children. International Journal of Environmental Health Research 17 (5), 351–360.

Segal, L., 2004. Why it is time to review the role of private health insurance in Australia? Australian Health Review 27 (1), 3–15.

Spencer, J., Harford, J., 2007. Inequality in oral health in Australia. Australian Review of Public Affairs. Online. Available: <http://www.australianreview.net/digest/2007/election/spencer_harford.html> (14 Apr 14).

Van Gool, K., Savage, E., Viney, R., et al., 2009. Who's getting caught? An analysis of the Australian Medicare safety net. Australian Economic Review 42 (2), 143–154.

Walker, A., Percival, R., Thurecht, L., et al., 2006. Distributional impact of recent changes in private health insurance policies. Australian Health Review 29, 467–473.

Wilkinson, R., Pickett, K., 2009. The Spirit Level: Why More Equal Societies Almost Always Do Better. Allen Lane, London.

Wilkinson, R., Pickett, K., 2010. Why Equality is Better for Everyone. Penguin Books, London.

World Health Organization, 2005. The World Health Report 2005: making every mother and child count. Online. Available: <www.who.int/whr/2005/en/> (10 Apr 2014).

World Health Organization, 2008. Closing the gap in a generation: health equity through action on the social determinants of health. Online. Available: <http://www.who.int/social_determinants/thecommission/finalreport/en/> (5 Jun 2014).

Wyn, J., 2009. Young people's wellbeing: contradictions in managing the healthy self. ACHPER Australia Healthy Lifestyles Journal 56 (1), 5–9.

Zhang, J., Smith, K., 2007. Household air pollution from coal and biomass fuels in China: measurements, health impacts, and interventions. Environmental Health Perspectives 115 (6), 848–855.

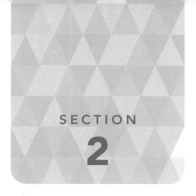

DETERMINANTS OF HEALTH

Introduction

- **An examination of** the nature and range of determinants that might impact on health and illness is the focus for Section 2.
- **The health of individuals** and populations is influenced and determined by many factors acting in various combinations. The dominant view is that health is *multicausal*—healthiness, disease, disability and, ultimately, death are seen as the result of the interaction of human biology, lifestyle and environmental (e.g. social) factors, modified by health interventions and other measures (Marmot & Wilkinson 2006). As Labonte (2012) commented when discussing global action on social determinants, we also need to consider global action that spreads far beyond a focus on health:

  > … there are three major crises confronting global health: ongoing financial crises; deepening ecological crises; and rapidly escalating income and wealth inequalities … (Labonte 2012, p 139).

  This adds a level of complexity to the conversation that we will return to in the last chapter of this book.

- **Health determinants** can be described as those factors that raise or lower the level of health in a population or individual (Australian Institute of Health and Welfare (AIHW) 2012). Determinants help explain and predict trends in health, and explain why some groups have better or worse health than others. They are the key to preventing disease, illness and injury (AIHW 2012).
- **Determinants may have** positive or negative effects. Factors such as tobacco smoking or low socioeconomic status increase the risk of ill health and are commonly termed *risk factors*. Positive influences, such as a high intake of fruit and vegetables, are known as *protective factors*. Unlike behaviour, some determinants such as age, sex and genetics cannot be altered. Some of these factors are the subject of

Chapter 5; while Chapters 6 and 7 discuss the biological, environmental, social and economic factors that influence health.

- **For almost all factors** that impact on health, the associated effect is not 'all or nothing'. For risk factors, rather than there being one point at which risk begins, there is an increasing effect as the exposure increases. For example, a person may be physically active but not in a way that increases heart rate on a regular basis each week, and therefore, in association with inappropriate food consumption, that person has an increased risk of ill health. Although the increasing risk often starts at relatively low levels, the usual practice is to monitor a risk factor by reporting the proportion at the riskier end of the spectrum (AIHW 2012).

- **Determinants can vary** in the extent to which they represent *relative risk* and *absolute risk* of developing disease. The concept of 'relative risk' is defined and discussed in more detail in Chapter 5. If, for example, a food product provided to a small group of people was contaminated with *Salmonella*, there would be a high relative risk of food poisoning among the group. However, as the product was only provided to a small group, there would be a relatively low absolute risk of poisoning from the food product in the population as a whole.

- **In addition to influencing** the occurrence of new cases of disease or injury, determinants can affect the continuation and prognosis of chronic diseases and their complications (AIHW 2012). The use of healthcare interventions can also be regarded as a determinant in that context. Determinants can also influence how individuals function, in terms of their activities and participation in society. Aspects of the physical environment can either facilitate functioning or act as a barrier to it, as can the availability of assistance from other people or functional support such as aids and appliances (WHO 2007).

- **Chapter 5 covers** the important role of epidemiology in determining the factors that influence patterns of mortality and morbidity. Epidemiology is the study of factors affecting the health and illness of populations, and serves as the foundation and logic for interventions made in the interests of public health and preventive medicine. It is considered a cornerstone methodology of public health research. Many authors (Buettner & Muller 2011, Gordis 2014, Last et al. 2000) have described the role of the epidemiologist as investigating the occurrence of disease or other health-related conditions or events in defined populations. The control of disease in populations is often also considered to be a task for the epidemiologist. Epidemiology has three main aims:
  - to describe disease patterns in human populations
  - to identify the causes of diseases (also known as *aetiology*)

- to provide data essential for managing, evaluating and planning services for preventing, controlling and treating disease (Australasian Epidemiology Association website 2010).

The chapter provides you with an introduction to epidemiology and its component parts, and gives you an idea of how useful the study of epidemiology is to public health as a fundamental discipline underpinning the subject.

- **Chapters 6 and 7** examine the multidimensional nature of the determinants of health. In recent years, the social determinants of health have taken centre stage—strongly supported by the work of the World Health Organization (2010; 2011)—in an attempt to place social determinants of health and health inequalities into the global health arena (Friel & Marmot 2011, Labonte 2012).

- **Determinants are not just** social in nature, as a range of factors impact on the health and wellbeing of the population, and Chapters 6 and 7 address these issues. There is a growing acknowledgement of the importance of a range of factors impacting on exposure to health hazards and risk conditions in the population. Some groups in society have a much poorer chance of achieving their full health potential as a result of their life circumstances—including political, social, economic and environmental conditions, as illustrated above. These factors interact with genetic and biological factors to impact on the health and wellbeing of the population in a wide variety of ways.

- **Chapter 6 concentrates on** the biological and environmental determinants of health. It discusses the contribution of genetic and biological factors that impact on the health of the population and subpopulations. The environment interacts with genetic and biological factors to influence health and wellbeing. Most health problems are multicausal and are influenced by a range of factors.

- **Social and economic factors** are known to be powerful determinants of population health in modern societies. There is acknowledged scientific justification for isolating different aspects of social and economic life as the primary determinants of a population's health. Chapter 7 addresses the issue of social determinants of health, and also considers the importance of emotional determinants—issues too often neglected in political and policy deliberations about health and wellbeing.

References

Australasian Epidemiology Association, 2010. What is epidemiology? Online. Available: <http://www.aea.asn.au/about-us/what-is-epidemiology> (28 Apr 2014).

Australian Institute of Health and Welfare, 2012. Australia's health 2012. AIHW Cat. No. AUS 156. AIHW, Canberra.

Buettner, P., Muller, R., 2011. Epidemiology. Oxford University Press, South Melbourne.

Friel, S., Marmot, M.G., 2011. Action on the social determinants of health and health inequalities goes global. Annual Review of Public Health 32, 225–236.

Gordis, L., 2014. Epidemiology. Elsevier Saunders, Philadelphia, PA.

Labonte, R., 2012. Global action of social determinants of health. Journal of Public Health Policy 33, 139–147.

Last, J., Spasoff, R., Harris, S., 2000. A Dictionary of Epidemiology. Oxford University Press, New York.

Marmot, M., Wilkinson, R.G., 2006. Social Determinants of Health. Oxford University Press, Oxford.

World Health Organization, 2007. Determinants of health. Online. Available: <http://www.who.int/social_determinants/en/> (6 May 2014).

World Health Organization, 2010. Equity Social Determinants and Public Health Programmes. WHO, Geneva.

World Health Organization, 2011. Closing the Gap: Policy into Practice on Social Determinants of Health. Discussion Paper. WHO, Geneva.

Epidemiology

CHAPTER 5

Catherine M. Bennett

Learning objectives

After reading this chapter, you should be able to:

- appreciate the role of epidemiology in public health

- understand exposure and outcome measures

- identify the main types of epidemiological study design

- report and interpret measures of association between exposures and health outcomes

- discuss the concepts of chance, bias and confounding.

Introduction

This chapter will provide you with a basic understanding of epidemiology, and introduce you to some of the epidemiological concepts and methods used by researchers and practitioners working in public health. Epidemiologists, often described as 'disease detectives', play a key role in identifying and presenting the evidence that underpins policy and practice in both the clinical and the public health settings. The ultimate goal of epidemiology is to contribute to the prevention of disease and disability and to delay mortality.

Epidemiology is fundamental to evidence-based medicine and to public health policy and practice. Rather than examine health and illness on an individual level, as clinicians do, epidemiologists focus on communities and populations where important information and insights can be gained regarding the health of populations, the distribution of disease and injury, and the determinants of these conditions, as well as the effectiveness of health interventions.

But why do we need epidemiology and this population-level understanding of health? Our health, risk of disease, and chance of having an injury are all determined by a complex interaction between multiple factors related to our family history, where we live, and how we live. These factors can be difficult to tease apart unless we have a systematic way of studying them and determining real causal associations. Only then can we determine the best ways to treat or prevent poor health outcomes. Epidemiology is a structured, logical framework for thinking, unravelling complex problems, and piecing together the best evidence available. Epidemiology therefore provides the basis for evidence-based clinical practice, strategic planning, prioritising health issues, and evaluating health services.

This example of an association between an exposure of interest and a health outcome will help you understand how epidemiology works, and how it is useful in public health. Australia has the highest incidence of asthma in the world; it is commonly found that people who own cats are less likely to have asthma. Does this mean that owning a cat protects you from developing asthma? Or that people with asthma tend to not own cats as it exacerbates their asthma? Or is it possibly a bit of both? Should doctors tell women with a family history of asthma to get rid of their cat, if they are planning to get pregnant; or get a cat if they are thinking of getting pregnant, to reduce the chances of their child having asthma? We will come back to this example at different times in the chapter to illustrate different aspects of epidemiological concepts and methods.

Defining epidemiology

Epidemiology can be defined as:

> The study of the *distribution* and *determinants* of *health*-related states or events in specified *populations*, and the application of this study to *control of health problems* [emphasis added]. (Last 1995 p 55)

This definition succeeds in capturing the scope of epidemiology in a clear and concise manner. Look carefully at each of the italicised words in the above definition of epidemiology.

Distribution refers to the pattern or frequency of health events by person (who gets affected), place (where it happens) and time (when it happens). We will expand on this when we consider 'person, place and time' in more detail, together with the ways we capture and measure health outcomes. *Determinant* refers to both the causes of, and risk factors for, health events. These can include any aspect of the environment we live in (e.g. biological, physical, cultural, social), including living organisms (e.g. viruses and bacteria), physical entities (e.g. radiation, pollution and dangerous machinery), lifestyle (e.g. stress and diet), social factors (e.g. poverty), and genetic factors (e.g. inherited or changed genes that cause genetic diseases). We will revisit health determinants when we consider how we might measure these exposures when trying to understand the patterns of disease that we see in populations.

The World Health Organization (WHO) defines *health* as 'a state of complete physical, mental, and social wellbeing and not merely the absence of disease or infirmity' (WHO 1948). Health could include a specific disease state, the absence of a disease state, a quality of life rating, life expectancy, or the incidence of mental illness or physical injury. *Population* refers to a group of people with definable commonalities—for example, the people who reside in a certain city or country, a school community, or a certain age, occupational or ethnic group. *Control of health problems* refers to reducing the burden of a health problem in a population. Epidemiology quantifies the burden of disease, the strength of the association between exposures and health states, the magnitude of risk at the population level, and the potential benefit of interventions, thus driving evidence-based health policy and practice.

Objectives of epidemiological studies

Epidemiological studies can fulfil three primary roles: description, analysis and intervention. Depending on the study design, the descriptive information may then be used to look for relationships between possible causal factors and health outcomes, through statistical analysis. This can help determine whether a certain population or individual factors seem to be associated with certain health outcomes (e.g. the inverse relationship between asthma and cat ownership). Finally, the outcomes of analytical studies can be used to develop and justify the implementation of further analytical studies to explore these associations (e.g. clarifying what is cause and what is effect), or there may be sufficient information to drive interventions, such as health promotion programs. Epidemiological approaches are also integral to the evaluation of the effectiveness of interventions.

> **ACTIVITY 5.1 Application of epidemiology to public health issues**
>
> - Think of a public health issue relevant to your area of interest. Write a paragraph to explain how epidemiology could contribute to identifying or quantifying the issue at the population level.

> **REFLECTION 5.1**
>
> This activity requires you to apply your understanding of epidemiology and its objectives. What resources will you use to identify the public health issue? Try using the definition of 'epidemiology' above to help you.

Measuring the occurrence of exposures of interest and of health outcomes

Measuring the health of populations can help to answer some fairly simple yet crucial questions. For example, how much disease is present? How quickly are new cases occurring? How long do people remain ill? How does the rate of disease or death differ over time within this population, or compared with another? Who does the disease affect? Where and when are they getting sick? What strategies are effective at reducing the occurrence of a certain disease or condition? *Health indicators* are measurable characteristics of a person, population or environment that are indicative of one or more aspects of a population's health (e.g. infant mortality rate).

Case definitions are fundamental in epidemiology; they must be unambiguous and consistently applied across populations and time in order to allow reliable reporting and comparison of health data. This is equally true of health outcome data, as well as exposures of interest.

CASE STUDY 5.1

Measuring exposure and outcome

Asthma data can be collected in a variety of ways. Asthma may be self-reported from symptoms (Have you ever had a persistent wheezing cough?), from a doctor's diagnosis of asthma (Have you ever been diagnosed by a doctor as having asthma?), from medication typically associated with asthma (Have you ever used a preventer or reliever puffer?), or directly from medical records. You can see that these measures might have varying degrees of reliability, and you would not want to compare the frequency of asthma based on different measures between groups. If the exposure of interest is 'cats', we must be equally careful to define whether this includes any cat ownership, or whether only 'indoor cats' will be counted. The timing of exposure is also important, and so you also need to know the timing of the cat exposure (Did you own a cat before you developed asthma?).

Epidemiologists can *count* disease events or, more usually, calculate rates and proportions, so comparisons of health status can be made between populations and over time. Several measures of disease frequency are employed. The simplest quantitative measure is a count—the number of people in a certain health state, or who die or become ill from a specified cause. These data have limited value without information about the population size or the number of people at risk.

CASE STUDY 5.2

Counting and reporting cases

We might count 20 influenza-related deaths; however, unless we know how many flu cases there were—that is, the number of people at risk of dying of flu—we cannot assess the mortality rate associated with this particular flu strain. Were there 20 deaths out of 100,000 cases, or 20 out of 200 cases? The implications are very different for managing this flu outbreak. For a count to be descriptive of a population, it needs to be reported as a *proportion* relative to the size of that population.

A *ratio* describes the magnitude of one group relative to another. For example, if, of the 20 people who died of influenza, 16 were men and 4 were women, then the sex ratio would be 4:1 male to female. Another commonly used measure is a *rate*, which is a measure of the frequency of occurrence of an event. A rate differs from a proportion in that it involves units of time in its calculation (e.g. the number of influenza cases in a given year).

Two of the most widely used measures of *risk* calculated from the frequency of a health outcome (e.g. asthma) or exposure (e.g. cat ownership) are prevalence and incidence.

Prevalence refers to the number of people in a defined population who have a specific disease, condition or exposure at a certain point in time (e.g. at the time the data were collected in a health survey). Measuring prevalence involves counting cases and dividing the count by the total number of people in the population from which the cases arose (e.g. the number of people who completed the survey).

Prevalence can either refer directly to a specific point in time (point prevalence) or to a period of time (period prevalence). For example, we might count the number of motor vehicle accidents occurring on 31 December, or the number of accidents that occurred between 1 January and 31 December.

Prevalence is calculated using the following equation:

$$\text{Prevalence} = \frac{\text{Number of people with the disease/condition at a specific time}}{\text{Number of people in the population at risk at the specified time}} \times 10^n$$

Multiplying by 10^n allows you to adjust the reporting units so that prevalence is expressed in the same standard units for comparison across populations or time. It also allows you to report very low prevalence as cases per 100,000 (e.g. 13 cases of meningococcal disease per 100,000).

Calculating prevalence

EXAMPLE   5.1

DURING a lecture we ask all students (in a class of 200) with a headache to put up their hands in order to calculate the prevalence of headaches. If 8 students put up their hands, the prevalence of headaches is 8 out of 200 students at that point in time = 4% of the class (or 40 cases per 1000 students)—this is *point prevalence*.

If we ask students in the same class to put up their hands if they had experienced a headache at any time during the past week, this would be *period prevalence*. If 15 students reported that they had experienced a headache during the past week, the period prevalence is 15 cases out of 200 students over a one-week period = 7.5% of the class per week (or 75 per 1000 students per week).

Note that period prevalence will include those with the condition at the start of the specified time period, and also all the new cases (incident cases) that develop the condition over that specified time period.

Incidence refers to the number of new cases of disease, injury or death in a population during a specified time period. For chronic diseases that are not that common and can last a lifetime (e.g. tuberculosis), there may be a large difference between incidence and prevalence, as there are few new, or incident, cases but many persistent cases. However, for acute diseases where all cases are incident cases (e.g. influenza), there will be little difference between incidence and prevalence estimates.

Unlike prevalence, incidence is a true rate, as it always specifies a unit of time in its calculation. There are two major measures of incidence: incidence rate and cumulative incidence. *Incidence rate* is a more precise measure that describes the rate at which new cases occur in a population over a specified period of time. *Cumulative incidence* is a simpler measure of the occurrence of disease or death, and tells us the proportion of a population at risk that develops a disease during a specified time period. As with prevalence, cumulative incidence can be expressed as a proportion, a percentage, or as the number of cases per population.

Incidence rate and cumulative incidence are calculated using the following equations:

$$\text{Incidence rate} = \frac{\text{Number of new people with the disease or condition in specified period}}{\text{Total 'person-time' at risk during specified period}} \times 10^n$$

Note: 'person-time' represents the sum of each participant's individual time at risk (i.e. duration of follow-up) and can be expressed in any time unit, depending on the context—for example, person years, person months or person days.

$$\text{Cumulative incidence} = \frac{\text{Number of new people with the disease or condition in specified period}}{\text{Number of people in the population at risk during specified period}} \times 10^n$$

(For further information on the concept of person-time, see Webb et al. 2011 pp 41–45).

CASE STUDY 5.3

When to use incidence rate

Many epidemiological studies follow people over time to see who develops certain health outcomes in a population deemed to be 'at risk'. Not everyone will be followed for the full study period (some drop out of the study, die from other causes, etc.), and we need to take this into account so that we do not underestimate disease incidence relative to time at risk. For example, say in a group of 100 people who have had a coronary artery bypass graft, 24 have had a myocardial infarction (MI) after 2 years. This gives a 2-year incidence risk of 24%. This could also be expressed as a risk of *12 MIs per 100 person-years*. However, that assumes that everyone was followed up for the full 2 years. If, instead, you find that the follow-up time was actually only 18 months, then this should then be reported as 12 MIs per 150 person-years (which is the same as saying *16 MIs per 100 person-years*). So you can see that we may underestimate the disease incidence, or disease risk, if we do not take into account the variation in the individual follow-up periods (Example 5.2).

EXAMPLE 5.2

Incidence of hearing loss among workers in heavy industry

Imagine you are studying the incidence of hearing loss in 16,000 workers in heavy industry in Victoria, Australia. There are 750 new cases of hearing loss over a 10-year period. During those 10 years, the employees worked a total of 116,000 years of work (calculated by adding up all the years of employment during the specified 10-year period for all the 16,000 workers). The average employment was 7.25 years over that 10-year period.

What was the incidence rate of hearing loss in workers in heavy industry in Victoria over the 10-year period (expressed in 1000 person-years)?

$$\text{Total person-years exposed} = \frac{750}{116,000}$$
$$= 6.47 \text{ per } 1000 \text{ person-years}$$

This figure can be compared with the incidence of hearing loss in people working in light industry (1.22 per 1000 person-years). Hearing loss among workers in heavy industry occurs more frequently than in workers in light industry.

What is the cumulative incidence of hearing loss in these workers?

$$\text{Cumulative incidence} = \text{Number of new cases in Victoria over 10 years}$$

$$\text{Total number of people at risk during 10 years} = \frac{750}{16000}$$
$$= 0.047 \text{ over 10 years}$$

You conclude that, among workers exposed to noise in heavy industry over a 10-year period, 4.7% developed hearing loss. This can be further interpreted as a risk statement: if workers are exposed to noise in heavy industry, they have a 4.7% chance of developing hearing loss in a 10-year period. However, it is more correct to report these findings in person-years (6.47 per 1000 person-years), as the risk is actually higher when you take into account the fact that not all workers were exposed for a full 10-year period.

Mortality rates and life expectancy are important health indicators. In Australia, a major public health effort is focused on Closing the Gap, to reduce inequalities between Indigenous and non-Indigenous Australians. However, progress is slow, and the discrepancy in the average age at death in 2014 of about a decade remains an important policy driver. Mortality patterns can be described using crude rates, age-specific rates, sex-specific rates and cause-specific rates (deaths attributed to a certain disease). Crude mortality rates (CMRs) are derived from the equation:

$$\text{CMR} = \frac{\text{Number of deaths in a specified time period}}{\text{Total population}} \times 10^n$$

CASE STUDY 5.4

When comparative mortality rates can be misleading

Crude mortality rates (CMRs) are affected by a number of population characteristics, particularly age structure. For example, in 1990, Sweden's annual death rate was 11 per 1000. This rate was higher than that of Guatemala (8 per 1000), even though life expectancy in Sweden (78 years) was greater than in Guatemala (63 years). The difference in crude mortality rates between the two countries was mainly due to differences in age structure: 18% of Sweden's population was aged over 65 years, compared with only 3% of Guatemala's population. The differences in the age structure of a population, together with the fact that risk of mortality varies with age, can cause misleading conclusions about comparative health status.

A range of approaches are used to take age structure into account when comparing populations:

- *Age-specific mortality rates* (ASMR): Calculated as for CMR, but both cases and the population denominator are restricted to a specific age group—for example, infant mortality rates (IMR) (birth to one year of age).

- *Direct age-standardised rates*: Adjusts for age differences between comparison populations. The age-specific rates from the two populations are applied to one standard population of known age structure to allow the overall adjusted mortality rates to be compared independently of age structure.
- *Indirect age-standardised rates*: Used when age-specific rates are not available for the populations being compared: the total observed death rate in each of the populations of interest is compared with the deaths expected from applying age-specific rates from a reference population to the given age structure of each population being compared. If the observed deaths in one population are higher than the other, then one or more of the age-specific rates in that population must also be higher, but in this case you do not know which age band(s) are involved without further study.

(If you are interested in reading further about these measures, see Gordis 2004).

Epidemiological study design

Different types of epidemiological study design are used to answer different research questions. Each has advantages and disadvantages in terms of the costs involved in carrying out the study, the quality of data the study generates, and the strength of the conclusions that can be drawn. (Table 5.1 summarises these advantages and disadvantages.) The research questions are usually based on existing hypotheses built on a biological understanding of the natural history of the disease of interest, and/or observations made by clinicians or public health practitioners from individual cases (case series), or observational studies that seem to suggest a possible association. The research questions must be biologically plausible.

Studies can be classified as either observational or experimental, and the distinction is an important one. Observational studies allow Nature to take its course, and the investigator simply observes events in different populations/groups. The investigator then seeks information about the patterns of diseases and potential risk factors, or exposures of interest. In contrast, in experimental (intervention) studies the investigator actively manipulates an exposure to judge its effect on a health outcome. This is a powerful study design for isolating the effects of an exposure and making causal inferences about the relationship between the exposure under study and the health outcome of interest.

Studies can also be classified as descriptive or analytical, but can be both. Descriptive studies are used to describe and measure health indicators or the burden of disease within a population, whereas analytical studies are performed to evaluate the association between one or more exposures and the development of a particular disease or health state, or a number of health outcomes.

Study designs differ with respect to the number of observations made, whether data are collected prospectively or retrospectively, the data collection procedures used, whether individuals or groups are studied, and the availability of participants or existing data. Epidemiologists use a range of study designs (see Figure 5.1).

Observational epidemiology

For ethical reasons, many factors thought to influence disease, or protect against it, cannot be imposed on a study population. Instead, researchers make use of naturally occurring situations, and observe and measure exposures and patterns of health in naturally occurring groups. The investigator does not intervene.

TABLE 5.1 Epidemiological study designs: advantages and disadvantages

Study type	Study design	Timeframe	Basis for recruitment	Basic design	Strengths	Practical challenges	Inference
• Observational	• Ecological	• Information on exposures and outcomes is collected at the population level, and may be collected independently and at different time points	• No recruitment as such; uses existing population-level data collected for other purposes	• Data on exposures and outcomes of interest collected in the same population to see if there is an association between the prevalence of exposures and outcomes	• Can include the whole population or the subset for whom data are available • Low cost relative to efficiency	• Making sure that data from different sources are comparable in population coverage, and are concurrent	• A useful way to see whether there is an association between a certain exposure and outcome at the population level. However, even if an association is observed, you cannot confirm that it holds true at the person level—i.e. were those individuals with the outcome the same people who also reported higher exposure?

TABLE 5.1 Continued

Study type	Study design	Timeframe	Basis for recruitment	Basic design	Strengths	Practical challenges	Inference
• Observational	• Cross-sectional	• Information on case status and history of exposure is collected at a single point in time	• Approach often used in large-scale surveys, so entire populations or a random subsample may be targeted	• One-time data collection, often via a survey or questionnaire if large-scale	• Can reach thousands of people through large-scale surveys • Cheap compared with other forms of data collection, low cost relative to efficiency • Allows examination of multiple exposures, including personal and social characteristics where demographic information is also collected	• Difficult to tease out the timing and sequence of exposures and outcomes • There is a risk of bias if people's exposure history is altered by the occurrence of the disease • People with long-term disease might be overrepresented compared with those with disease of short duration	• **Descriptive studies** (prevalence surveys, etc.) involve simple presentation of facts • As not selecting participants on either exposure or outcome, the prevalence of both exposures and outcomes can be measured • **Analytic studies** set inferences about associations that can be explored statistically. Where studies are prone to bias and confounding, associations observed between the presence of exposures and outcomes cannot be interpreted as evidence of causation

TABLE 5.1 Continued

Study type	Study design	Timeframe	Basis for recruitment	Basic design	Strengths	Practical challenges	Inference
• Observational	• Case-control	• Cases are recruited on the basis of their disease status, and then information on their exposure history is collected retrospectively • A group of controls selected at the same time, usually from the same population, is also asked about their exposure history	• Disease or health outcome: the study sample comprises people with the disease/ outcome (cases) and a comparison group at the same risk, but who do not have the disease (controls)	• Allows estimation of the odds of having been exposed to specific risk factor(s) given current disease/case status	• Useful for rare diseases • Can examine multiple risk factors at once • Low cost relative to efficiency	• Analyses are restricted to the outcome that cases were selected on • Finding a suitable group of controls who must be like the cases in every way and have the same potential opportunity for the outcome • Recall error— inaccurate information may be reported about exposures occurring some time ago • Recall bias—where someone's memory of their exposure history is distorted by the fact that they have developed the outcome • Identifying and measuring confounders that you may have to adjust for	• As for cross-sectional studies, with a particular risk of recall bias for cases who are selected on the presence of the disease outcome, and who may have an altered or distorted memory of their own exposure driven by their understanding of the possible causes of their own disease

TABLE 5.1 Continued

Study type	Study design	Timeframe	Basis for recruitment	Basic design	Strengths	Practical challenges	Inference
• Observational	• Cohort	• Sampled on exposure status and outcome information collected prospectively • You may see retrospective cohort studies using existing data (e.g. medical records) to determine past exposures and the subsequent incidence of outcomes	• People are recruited on the basis of their potential for exposure (e.g. asbestos workers) and/ or may be population-based (a particular birth-cohort followed over time)	• Allows estimation of the risk of disease in those exposed to specific risk factor(s) compared with those who are not	• Exposure status ascertained before the outcome appears • Incidence rates can be computed and compared for people with and without exposure	• Requires follow-up to monitor for disease development, expensive and difficult to prevent loss to follow-up • Need to measure all possible confounders, so can adjust statistically	• As for other observational studies; however, for prospective cohort studies there is less risk of bias, as exposure information is recorded before disease outcomes present

TABLE 5.1 Continued

Study type	Study design	Timeframe	Basis for recruitment	Basic design	Strengths	Practical challenges	Inference
• Experimental	• Clinical trials	• Prospective, with exposure allocated and follow-up to determine outcomes	• Recruitment is aimed at including people who would be exposed to that intervention/ treatment if rolled out in real life • Some clinical trials can have very restrictive inclusion and exclusion criteria to minimise adverse outcomes	• As for cohort studies; only here the exposure is allocated randomly to balance the presence of possible confounders between the different study arms so that they do not interfere with the estimation of the effect of the exposure under study	• If well designed and conducted, can minimise all forms of bias and confounding, allowing the researcher to isolate the true impact of the intervention under study	• Expensive to run and difficult to protect against various forms of selection and information bias, especially where the participants and researchers cannot be blinded to the arm of the study they are in • Can only study the exposure that was randomised • Participants studied may not be representative of the general population—need to look at both inclusion and exclusion criteria to ascertain potential selection bias	• This is the only study design where there is the potential to make direct inference about causation • If there has been selection bias, even if just by chance alone in smaller trials, then care must be taken to adjust for the impact this might have on effect size

TABLE 5.1 Continued

Study type	Study design	Timeframe	Basis for recruitment	Basic design	Strengths	Practical challenges	Inference
	• Community intervention	• Prospective with exposure allocated, and follow up to determine outcomes	• Unlike standard trials where the intervention is applied at the individual level, here a whole subpopulation (district or school, for example) is randomised to receive an intervention or not	• As for other trials, only here the exposure is allocated randomly at subpopulation level to balance the presence of possible confounders between the different groups across study arms	• Allows the trialling of community-based interventions and, as the whole local population is allocated together into the one study arm, it removes the risk of cross-contamination where people not allocated an intervention might learn about it from those who were, which may allow them to adopt some of the changes, thereby reducing their validity as a control arm member	• There are often relatively fewer population groups than there are individuals in regular trials; therefore, it is harder for the randomisation process alone to ensure that each arm contains similar populations. Analysis can also be quite complicated in these trials	• The outcomes measured are at population level, just as the intervention was allocated at this level; therefore, causation should strictly be inferred at the population level. For example, an education program may be shown to lift vaccine uptake in one population compared with another control population where there was no education campaign. Individual data on whether a person who was vaccinated had actually been exposed to the intervention itself may not be known

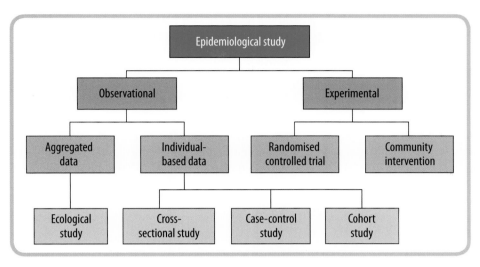

FIG. 5.1 Main types of epidemiological study design.

Ecological studies

Studies built on an ecological design are quick and cheap to run, and are usually based on the examination of existing data. In some cases, you can design a study that uses different data sets to extract information on exposures and disease outcomes. For example, there was some concern that mobile phone use might increase the risk of brain cancer. The first step in investigating this was to carry out an ecological study to compare mobile phone usage data at the population level with routinely collected cancer data for the same population. If there was a strong association at the population level, then it would be important to investigate further to determine whether the excess cases of cancer actually occurred in mobile phone users. As there are no data on individuals, care must be taken not to over-interpret any associations found.

Cross-sectional studies

Cross-sectional (prevalence) studies are one of the most common study designs used in descriptive epidemiology. Many health surveys in which people are interviewed are cross-sectional—that is, they collect data about both exposure and outcomes from an individual at one point in time.

The study group is chosen to be a cross-section of the population, and is usually selected in a way that makes them arguably representative of the whole population. For example, a questionnaire is going to provide more generalisable data if it is completed by a sample of 1000 people, based on randomly selected phone numbers, rather than 10 people visiting a particular shopping centre. This design is particularly

> **ACTIVITY 5.2 Inconsistencies between studies**
>
> If you search the literature, you will find that there have been around 30 cross-sectional studies focused on cat ownership and asthma. The results have been inconsistent; some studies found that cat ownership was positively associated with asthma prevalence, while some found the reverse.
>
> • Could these inconsistent results for cat ownership and asthma mean that the associations are different in the various populations studied around the world? Or could there be other study design factors that might explain these inconsistencies?

REFLECTION 5.2

Think about the range of exposure and outcome definitions that might be used in these studies, and also the way the information on cat ownership and asthma history is collected in a cross-sectional study. Might this lead to some of the differences in study outcomes we see?

useful for studies investigating the impact of multiple exposures on health, including personal characteristics such as socioeconomic status, country of birth, and age.

A good example of an Australian cross-sectional study is that of the Queensland Ambulance Service (Clark et al. 1999), which involved every patient ($n = 11,408$) who presented at Ipswich Hospital in a four-month period. Data were collected on demographic characteristics (e.g. sex, date of birth, marital status, country of origin), presentation details (e.g. arrival method, arrival date, complaint) and departure details (e.g. date of departure). This study provided a snapshot of ambulance service users at that time, and their reasons for calling an ambulance, which then guided the planning of future services and resource allocation.

Case-control studies

Case-control studies are increasingly being used to investigate the causes of diseases. This is a particularly useful study design when the disease or health outcome of interest is rare. Like cross-sectional studies, the information on case status and history of exposure is collected at a single point in time, so these studies can be quite economical to run and can yield results quite quickly. This is often an important consideration in public health practice, particularly in rapidly evolving disease outbreaks.

The case-control study design recruits a group of people with the disease/outcome (cases) and a comparison group who do not have the disease (controls). If we are interested in a disease that is found in only 1 per 1000 of the population, we would have to survey 1000 people just to find 1 case if we were conducting a cross-sectional study. The case-control design allows us to selectively recruit cases (e.g. identified through a disease register, a doctor, or laboratory diagnosis). The challenge is often in finding a suitable group of controls, who must be like the cases in every way but without the disease in question.

Case-control studies determine the proportion of cases that were exposed to the exposure(s) of interest, and compare this with the proportion of cases that were not exposed. The proportions of the controls that were or were not exposed to the same exposure(s) are also determined. The objective is to see whether there are differences in the odds of exposure between the two groups of people—that is, the ratio of the probability that the event will happen to the probability that the event will not happen. We anticipate that if the exposure (e.g. cat ownership) is related to a disease outcome (e.g. asthma), then the prevalence of a history of exposure will be significantly different in cases compared with controls: either greater if the exposure increases risk of disease, or less if the exposure is protective.

Like cross-sectional studies, case-control studies are asking about past exposures, so again the direction of enquiry is retrospective and is susceptible to errors in recall, thus making the data less reliable. Moreover, there is an additional challenge with case-control studies—ensuring the appropriateness of the control group. The control group should be drawn from the same population with the same potential for exposures as the case group, otherwise there is a risk that any differences observed are simply differences between the two different populations that were sampled for the cases and the controls.

CASE STUDY
5.5

Recall error and bias

A case-control study conducted between January 1996 and January 1997 in Brisbane investigated potential risk factors for *Campylobacter* infection in infants and young children (Tenkate & Stafford 2001). In this study, ownership of pet puppies and pet chickens, as well as mayonnaise consumption, were found to be strongly associated with *Campylobacter* infection. Can you think of reasons why these associations might have occurred? Do you think that everyone in the study would have remembered their exposure accurately? If not, what impact might that have had on the results?

Cohort studies

Cohort studies are generally considered to be the most robust of the observational designs. In this type of study design, we investigate groups of people who have no apparent symptoms of the disease under study at recruitment. A critical feature of a cohort study is that the study population is observed over a period of time so that the

CASE STUDY
5.6

A longitudinal cohort study

A well-known current Australian cohort study is the Tasmanian Longitudinal Health Study (TAHS), as described below in excerpts from the *Medical Journal of Australia*.

How do childhood factors affect adult-onset asthma? How do issues around the time of puberty influence the risk of breast cancer? When a disease 'runs in the family', is it because of environmental or genetic reasons? Today, the Tasmanian Longitudinal Health Study (TAHS) is attempting to answer these questions and more. The baseline study in 1968 surveyed all 8500 schoolchildren (probands) in Tasmania who were born in 1961 and were then 7 years old. The probands' brothers, sisters and parents were also surveyed, taking the total number of participants in the original survey to 45,900. Follow-up studies were conducted in 1974, 1979, 1992 and 1996. The aim of the current and next phases of the study is to investigate the total original cohort of 45,900.

The TAHS is unique internationally because it is the world's largest and longest running respiratory health study. However, because of the population-complete nature of the cohort, the length of follow-up and the opportunities for a general health study, research is now extending to other areas such as breast cancer, eye disease and social science. (Gregory et al. 2008).

Major findings to date include:

1 only 1 in 4 probands who had asthma in childhood continued to have asthma at age 32, and 1 in 10 probands who didn't have asthma as a child developed it later on (Jenkins et al. 1994).

2 for girls, being overweight at 7 years of age triples the risk of developing adult-onset asthma (Burgess et al. 2007)

3 early aggressive treatment of eczema and allergic rhinitis and reduced passive smoking exposure may facilitate asthma remission (Burgess et al. 2011).

What types of observational study designs are the following studies, designed to investigate the effect of raspberry leaf tea on length of labour?

- *Design 1*: A survey of women after they have delivered at the local maternity hospital, asking them about their use of raspberry leaf tea and other herbal supplements in the preceding year. Data on length of labour are collected from existing hospital medical charts upon discharge.

- *Design 2*: A study of 226 women giving birth and classified by length of labour (usual labour versus long labour), and then asked whether or not they used raspberry leaf tea during their pregnancy.

- *Design 3*: A group of 457 pregnant women, followed up from first antenatal visit to delivery, with questionnaires addressing current complementary medicine usage at each time/visit. Women will be classified according to whether or not they used raspberry leaf tea at all, and their length of labour compared once they have delivered.

REFLECTION 5.3

Did you consider whether the data were collected at one point in time or if the study required participant follow-up? Did any of the studies compare cases and controls?

rate of disease occurrence among people exposed to a suspected causal agent can be compared with that among unexposed people. Importantly, the measures of exposure and outcome are usually measured prospectively through time, so there is less chance of recall error. However, cohort studies are often large and expensive, because the participants have to be followed up over time, often years, to allow sufficient time for the disease outcomes of interest to present.

Experimental epidemiology

Experimental designs are used in clinical epidemiology where medical interventions are evaluated, and increasingly to evaluate the health impacts of population health interventions. The essence of experimental designs is comparing outcomes among exposed and non-exposed groups where the exposure is under the control of the investigator, therefore isolating the effects of the exposure of interest. This is the only study design that is considered to provide direct evidence of causation.

There are also limitations to consider in experimental design and conduct. They are often very expensive to run (given the control required for the exposure under examination, they may have to run for a long time if the disease development or prevention runs a slow course), and they can focus on only one or a few exposures and outcomes, and only those that are designed into the study in the first place.

Randomised controlled trials

Randomised controlled trials (RCTs) are a type of experimental study in which the participants are individually randomly assigned to either experimental or treatment groups, or a control group (sometimes more than one intervention is tested in the one trial). The experimental groups receive the treatment/intervention and the control group receives either no treatment/intervention or, preferably, a placebo treatment/intervention (something that appears similar to the real treatment, but is not active, such as a pill of same colour, size and shape but with no active ingredients).

Randomisation ensures that each participant has the same chance of receiving an intervention or entering the control group as the next person, which helps to ensure that the study groups (intervention and control) are the same from the start, so that any differences between the groups may be attributed to the intervention. RCTs are, therefore, thought to give the best quality of evidence out of all of the epidemiological study designs. An RCT has five important elements:

1 The investigator controls the exposure for each group of people to study the effect on an outcome.

2 The investigator has control over all elements of the research, including selecting the participants or subjects, measuring the exposure and the

outcome, and setting the conditions within which the experiment is conducted.

3   Participants are randomly allocated to intervention or control groups.

4   Effects of the intervention (exposure) are measured by comparing the outcome in the experimental group with that in a control group.

5   The investigators and the participants should ideally be unaware of the group to which they are allocated ('double-blind' describes where both investigators and participants are unaware).

ACTIVITY 5.4 Randomised controlled trials

• Could an randomised controlled trial (RCT) be designed to answer our questions about cat ownership and asthma? Would it be ethical to remove a pet cat or to impose cat ownership on families? If we restricted the RCT to only those who currently did not own a cat but would be willing to do so if assigned to the intervention group, would these participants be representative of the wider population?

CASE STUDY 5.7

RCT challenges

A randomised controlled trial (RCT) conducted in Izmir, Turkey, assessed the efficacy of honey as a wound dressing compared with a standard topical antibacterial cream in treating patients with pressure ulcers (Gunes & Eser 2007). After five weeks of treatment, results showed that patients receiving honey dressings healed approximately four times faster than patients receiving standard dressings. In this study, participants were aware of which treatment group they were in. Do you think this might have influenced the results? Imagine if half the participants who received standard dressings left the study before its completion. How might this change the results?

Community trials

Community trials, or field trials, are conducted at a population level rather than at an individual level. A good example of a community trial is the *10,000 Steps Rockhampton* study in Queensland, which assessed the effectiveness of a whole-of-community approach in improving levels of physical activity in the population (Brown et al. 2006). In this study, instead of selecting individual participants the researchers implemented multiple strategies across the whole Rockhampton community to improve population levels of physical activity.

Measures of association

Most epidemiological studies look for associations between different exposures and a particular health outcome. Measuring the occurrence of disease in a population (e.g. prevalence or incidence) describes the health of the population, but it does not tell us anything about possible causes of disease. The frequencies of disease or exposures in each group can

ACTIVITY 5.5 Study designs

Each study design in epidemiology has advantages and disadvantages. For the following research questions, which study design do you think would be the most appropriate?

• *Design 1*: What was the relationship in Australia between suicide and unemployment between 1950 and 2003?

• *Design 2*: Is green tea consumption associated with prostate cancer?

• *Design 3*: Does a daily dose of vitamin C prevent the onset of the common cold among élite athletes?

• *Design 4*: Is there an association between depression and physical abuse by partners of women attending general practice?

• *Design 5*: What are the health effects of long-term exposure to heavy metals among miners in Australia?

REFLECTION 5.5

The choice of study design (see Activity 5.5) will be dictated by the question asked and the particular outcome and exposures under study. Other practical factors, such as feasibility, finances, ethics and time, also need to be considered. All study designs, if well conducted, will provide useful information to the researcher, although some are better at providing evidence for causality. For this activity, it is important for you to be able to recognise the basic types of study design, and identify which are best for different types of research question. Consider whether the 'gold standard' RCT is an appropriate study design before considering the observational designs.

be compared in a *measure of the association* between an exposure and the risk of developing the disease.

The two-by-two table is a simple way of presenting data, and can be helpful to start looking for patterns in disease incidence or risk (Table 5.2). It consists of two columns, each representing the presence or absence of disease, and two rows, each representing the presence or absence of exposure. This orientation is important, and it is the standard way to present data.

Relative risk

In RCTs and cohort studies, the objective is to determine whether there is an increased or a reduced risk of a particular health outcome associated with a particular exposure. In other words, whether there is an association between a specific risk factor and the disease. This allows researchers to calculate and then compare the incidence rates in the exposed and unexposed groups. This is called the relative risk, and is calculated by dividing the incidence of disease in the group of exposed people by the incidence of disease in a group of people who are not exposed to the same factor.

$$\text{Relative risk (RR)} = \frac{\text{Incidence in exposed}}{\text{Incidence in unexposed}}$$

Or alternatively, using the two-by-two table:

$$\text{RR} = \frac{a/(a+b)}{c/(c+d)}$$

TABLE 5.2 Two-by-two table

		Disease		
		Yes	No	Total
Exposure	Yes	a	b	a + b
	No	c	d	c + d
Total		a + c	b + d	a + b + c + d

Note: The cells containing a, b, c and d each represent the number of individuals with a particular combination of disease and exposure:
a = Number of people who are exposed and who have the disease
b = Number of people who are exposed and who do not have the disease
c = Number of people who are not exposed and who have the disease
d = Number of people who are not exposed and who do not have the disease

Relative risks range in value from 0 to infinity. To interpret the relative risk (RR):
- if RR is near to or equals 1, there is no or little association (risk in exposed equals risk in non-exposed)
- if RR >1, there is a positive association (risk in exposed greater than risk in non-exposed)
- if RR <1, there is a negative or inverse association (risk in exposed less than risk in non-exposed).

Remember, relative risk values close to 1 may also be unimportant from a public health perspective. Well-designed studies will state up-front the degree of association considered to be clinically important or of public health significance. Measures of association must always be interpreted in the context of the study question and the potential application of the findings:
- A relative risk of 1.2 means that there is a 20% higher risk of developing the health outcome in the exposed group than the unexposed group; however, if the disease is very rare, this might not be important.
- A relative risk of 2.0 means that the exposed group is twice as likely, or 100% more likely, than the unexposed group to develop the health outcome. If the health outcome is positive (e.g. weight loss), then this may be sufficient evidence to justify expensive interventions being put in place. If the health outcome being measured is negative (increased likelihood of disease), then this is evidence against the intervention.
- A relative risk of 0.5 means that the exposed group is half as likely to develop the outcome as the unexposed group, and if the outcome is a disease, then we say that the intervention is protective.

Consider a comparison of death from coronary heart disease (outcome) between males and females (sex = exposure). One thousand women and 1000 men were recruited into a cohort study and followed over one year. Sixteen of the women and 20 of the men died from coronary heart disease within that year. The rate of death from coronary heart disease among females was 16 per 1000 person-years of observation, and the rate among males was 20 per 1000 person-years of observation. A two-by-two table for this scenario is shown in Table 5.3.

To calculate the relative risk in this example:

$$RR = \frac{a/(a+b)}{c/(c+d)}$$
$$= \frac{20/(20+980)}{16/(16+984)}$$
$$= 1.25$$

TABLE 5.3 The relative risk for coronary heart disease (CHD) mortality

| | | Death from CHD | | |
		Yes	No	Total
Sex	M	20	980	1000
	F	16	984	1000
Total		36	1964	2000

This is interpreted as meaning that compared with females (referent group), males have a 25% increased risk of dying from coronary heart disease.

Odds ratios

Relative risk requires knowledge of the disease incidence in the groups being compared; however, this is not available in case-control studies where we actively seek out cases and compare them with a set number of controls. The number of cases in the study, therefore, is not indicative of the disease incidence in the population. In this situation, researchers need to use another measure of association known as an odds ratio (OR). The odds ratio asks: 'What are the odds that a case was exposed relative to the odds that a control was exposed?' Two-by-two tables are also helpful when calculating odds ratios (see Table 5.4).

To calculate an odds ratio:

$$OR = \frac{\text{Odds that a case was exposed}}{\text{Odds that a control was exposed}} = \frac{a/c}{b/d} = \frac{ad}{bc}$$

As with relative risk, odds ratios indicate the strength of the association between the disease and exposure. Odds ratios range in value from 0 to infinity. To interpret the odds ratio:

- if OR is near or equal to 1, there is no or little association (and therefore the exposure is not related to the disease)
- if OR >1, there is a positive association (and therefore the exposure is associated with an increased risk of the disease)
- if OR <1, there is a negative or inverse association.

The way ORs are interpreted is similar to relative risks, only now you should talk in terms of the odds of exposure rather than the risk of disease. When the disease incidence is rare (present in less than 10% of the population), the OR approximates the relative risk, and then the OR can be reported in terms of disease risk.

Sources of error in epidemiological studies

A primary aim of good research design is to minimise problems, such as error and bias, which may otherwise alter the outcomes of a study. There are two main types of error: *random error* (or chance error) and *systematic error* (or bias). Random error can occur when there is random sampling variation and/or random measurement error.

Random error

If we sample a population, most of the time the characteristics of the people included in our study will be similar to the population as a whole. However, it is always possible

		Disease	
		Yes (cases)	No (controls)
Past exposure	Yes (exposed)	a	b
	No (not exposed)	c	d
Total		a + c	b + d

TABLE 5.4 Two-by-two table for a case-control study

that, by chance, the sample selected is not actually representative. This *random sampling variation* is more likely when small samples are used (less than 30), and can affect the generalisability of a study. There is no guaranteed way of preventing random sampling error, but the likelihood of it occurring is reduced when the sample size increases. Whenever possible, you should check for random sampling error if you have information on your target population (e.g. census data) with which to compare your sample.

Random measurement error refers to the random variation in measurement of key exposure or outcome variables. When you take measurements, there is a chance that there may be some sloppiness in the measurements and the data collected may vary by chance. For example, if you ask someone to recall whether they owned a pet 10 years ago, they may find it hard to accurately recall whether they had a pet at that time, unless they always have had a pet, or never had one. Another example is, if you are doing research into heart disease, you may measure blood pressure; each time blood pressure is taken, the value may be the actual blood pressure, or it could be altered slightly due to fluctuations in the instrument, the procedure used, or the timing of measurement. Random variability in measurement can be minimised by the careful training of data collectors, the use of standard protocols, and routinely tested equipment. Accuracy of a particular instrument can be assessed by repeating the measurement using a 'gold standard' instrument (i.e. one that has already been shown to be the most accurate option available). Random error cannot ever be completely removed, but the impact of random error on your results can be allowed for through the proper use of statistical methods.

Confidence intervals: We will not take you through the full range of statistical techniques that are used, but we will introduce you to the confidence interval, as each of the frequency estimates and measures of association described in this chapter should always be reported and interpreted with its associated confidence interval (CI). The CI takes into account the random error that may be present based on the sample size and the variability in the measurements taken. The CI indicates the precision of your estimate of the true population parameter (e.g. RR) you are interested in. The larger the sample and the smaller the variability in the measurements taken, the less chance there is that random error will influence the results, and therefore the narrower the CIs.

The interval itself represents the range of statistically plausible values for the measure that is being estimated. A 95% confidence interval is usually employed, meaning that 95% of the intervals computed with the appropriate formula will include the true value for the parameter you are estimating (RR, incidence, etc.). It is difficult to interpret wide confidence intervals as there is less you can 'rule out'. Always look at the full range of plausible values when interpreting a confidence interval, not just the point estimate on its own.

ACTIVITY 5.6 Issues around self-reporting

- An investigator wants to measure daily fat intake among adolescents, and asks each participant to keep a food diary that will be used to assess fat intake. Write a paragraph to describe how using a food diary might introduce error into the information the investigator is collecting.

REFLECTION 5.6

Did you consider that, even if all the adolescents are motivated and honest, and keep an accurate record of what they have eaten over the past week, it is very difficult to convert this diary into an accurate estimate of fat intake? For example, if a participant records the evening meal as spaghetti bolognaise, we do not know how large the portion was, or if the cook used lean mince, or whether they used any extra oil in the cooking. We have to make estimates about the fat content of an 'average' spaghetti bolognaise when converting the food diary into estimated fat intake. In doing so, we could easily underestimate or overestimate the fat intake of the adolescent, so the potential for random measurement error in this instrument (the food diary) is high.

Systematic error

Systematic error is a much more serious problem than random error in epidemiology. Because this error can be directional, we refer to it as *bias*. There are two types of bias to consider: *selection bias* and *information bias*. Systematic error results from any trend in the recruitment of people into different arms of a trial, or the collection, analysis, interpretation, publication or review of data that leads to conclusions that are systematically different from the truth. These types of bias can lead to incorrect results, and consequently incorrect conclusions, about the association between exposure and outcome in the study. Another type of error we need to consider is *confounding*, where factors other than those we are studying are acting to distort the study findings and can lead to incorrect conclusions.

SELECTION BIAS

Selection bias arises when there are systematic differences between people involved in a study and those not involved in a study. This could be reflected in the way the sample was selected (sampling bias) or by an individual's choice to participate after being selected by the investigators (commonly known as 'participation bias'). It also includes the influence of continued participation in a longitudinal or cohort study (known as 'loss to follow-up' or 'attrition bias'). *Sampling bias* cannot be reduced by increasing the size of a sample, nor can it be measured using statistical tests. This form of bias arises when the identification of individuals for the sample is not truly random, and can affect the generalisability of the results.

Participation bias, also known as 'volunteer bias', occurs when there are systematic differences between the people who agree to participate in a study and those who do not. In health research, population-based studies often only achieve 60% or so participation, and the people who volunteer for research studies may well have different risk factors from those who refuse. Those who decline to participate may have poorer or better health than participants, depending on the type of research or the condition under study. This can threaten the legitimacy of conclusions.

Attrition bias occurs when people who drop out of studies are systematically different from those who stay in the study. Attrition, or loss to follow-up, is primarily a problem in long-term prospective studies. There are many reasons why people do not complete research studies; they become disinterested, move address, get sicker, or die from causes directly relevant to the research or unrelated causes. Whatever the reason, it is likely that attrition will occur in most longitudinal studies; however, attrition bias only becomes an issue if one study group has a higher attrition rate than the other(s), or if the reasons for dropping out are related to the outcome under study.

INFORMATION BIAS

Information bias (also known as *measurement bias*) occurs when either outcomes or exposures are measured incorrectly in systematic ways. This can also be referred to as *misclassification* when the error in measuring exposures or outcomes results in assigning study participants to the wrong group or category. The researcher may have incorrectly classified a person as being exposed to a risk factor when in fact they were not exposed; the data may incorrectly measure the amount of exposure; a person may be classified as having a disease when they do not, or not having a disease when they do. Getting the grouping wrong in a cohort (based on exposure) or case-control study (based on case status) can result in the obscuring of important associations. If the errors are directional (e.g. the exposures are consistently under- or over-measured), then this might lead to completely spurious results that are hard to predict and impossible to detect.

Recall bias occurs when individuals with a disease are more likely to overestimate or underestimate their exposure than those without the disease. Recall bias is particularly an issue in retrospective studies, which ask participants for information about things that occurred sometime prior to the interview or survey. It is particularly an issue if the person is aware that they have the outcome of interest at the time they are recalling the exposure information (as in a cross-sectional study or a case-control study). Participants have also been known to intentionally (or non-intentionally) distort self-reported information, especially when responding to questions about personal behaviour. For example, someone who drinks alcohol excessively may under-report the level of consumption to provide a more 'socially acceptable' response.

Interviewer bias, or observer bias, occurs when the interviewer asks questions or records information in a different way for different groups being compared. Systematic error in observation, measurement, analysis and interpretation can be controlled to some extent by using only one interviewer for the whole study, making the investigator/interviewer unaware of the study participant's exposure status ('blinding'), by training the interviewer, or by using structured questionnaires or interviews and electronically recording interviews.

CONFOUNDING

Confounding can be an important source of error in epidemiological studies if it is not identified and addressed. Confounding occurs when a non-causal

---

ACTIVITY 5.7 Evaluating study results

- Is it possible that regular blood donation reduces the risk of heart disease? In 1998, a cohort study conducted in Finland reported that regular blood donors had an 88% reduction in risk of heart attack (Salonen et al. 1998). Is this proof that blood donation prevents heart disease? What else would you want to know about this study and the study participants, before you drew any conclusions?

REFLECTION 5.7

Did you consider whether there might be other factors that could explain the apparent association? For example, were the donors more healthy and health-conscious, and therefore less likely to have heart disease than non-donors?

CASE STUDY
5.8

Confounding factors

Let us consider our cat and asthma problem. Figure 5.2 shows this diagrammatically. Let us call the cat X (the exposure) and asthma Y (the outcome), and A is the confounder (some other factor that is associated with both the exposure and the outcome of interest that may be clouding the picture). Pollen is another known trigger for asthma. Many cats spend time outdoors as well as indoors; therefore, it might not be the cat itself that is associated with asthma, but the pollen it brings into the house on its fur. In order to rule out the confounding effect of pollen exposure when looking at the association between cats and asthma, you would have to measure pollen exposure and adjust for that statistically, so that you could then look at cat exposure independent of the confounding effects of pollen.

For a factor to be a confounder it must meet the following criteria: it must be a definite risk factor for the disease (Y); it must be associated with the exposure of interest (X) under study; and it must not be an intermediate step between exposure (X) and the disease (Y). For example, obesity → hypertension → heart disease. Hypertension could be part of the causal chain, rather than a confounder.

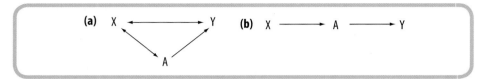

FIG. 5.2   Diagram illustrating the relationship between: (a) exposure X, disease Y, and confounder A; (b) exposure X, disease Y, and non-confounding factor on causal path A.

association between a given exposure and outcome is observed as a result of a third factor.

ACTIVITY 5.8 Alternative explanations

- Have you ever considered alternative explanations when you have heard media reports of new scientific discoveries?

REFLECTION 5.8

Next time you watch the news, or read a newspaper report about some new discovery, stop to consider whether the researchers have considered potential confounders.

Why are confounding and error important to an epidemiologist?

Confounding bias can undermine the efforts of research by leading to an over- or underestimation of association between exposure and disease. In fact, it can completely mask an association within a study or even reverse the direction of a true association. It is therefore essential to anticipate potential sources of confounding when considering your study design.

Finally, every study will be affected by some degree of error and, while strategies can be implemented to reduce chance fluctuation and bias, in practice it is impossible to eliminate all sources of error. Therefore, it is important to always consider the effects that error may have on the results of any epidemiological study.

Summing it up

Epidemiology examines health from a population level rather than an individual level. A paramedic or clinician might describe myocardial infarction in individual terms of chest pain, pulse and blood pressure, while an epidemiologist would describe myocardial infarction in terms of susceptible age groups, populations and risk factors. Both types of information are important. Current developments in epidemiology focus on the contribution of intra-individual factors (e.g. inherited genetic susceptibility) and higher-level factors (e.g. social policy and climate change). Clinical medicine is excellent for examining health issues within the confines of known aspects of the human body, but it is not equipped to infer cause in the absence of well-controlled experiments. Olsen et al. (2001) wrote:

> In its historical evolution epidemiology's successes have largely derived from its working as the investigative component of public health, studying the distribution and determinants of health and diseases in populations. This essence should continue to be preserved in the foreseeable future by incorporating into epidemiological research the new opportunities currently arising in particular fields of genetics, environmental sciences, medicine, and health care. (Olsen et al. 2001 p 15)

In order to prevent disease effectively, epidemiologists have a responsibility not only to use appropriate methods, but also to translate their findings into something of benefit to both the local and the global communities.

The end of the cat and asthma story is still being unravelled, partly because of the difficulties in designing the prefect study that we have alluded to throughout this chapter. Cat fur and dander are proven triggers for asthma attacks in those with asthma. There is some evidence that those with asthma do get rid of cats, but this is not thought to be as large an issue as previously, and may not fully account for the inverse associations we see between cat exposure and asthma (see below). The latest studies indicate that being exposed to a cat before developing asthma may indeed help some children develop tolerance, and have a protective effect. One of the pivotal papers in this field of research is by Cecile Svanes and colleagues (Svanes et al. 2006), and you can look up more of this author's work if you are interested in following this story.

A final word

This chapter has provided an introduction to some basic epidemiological concepts. As practising epidemiologists, we need to build on these concepts and also consider more complex methods of assessing evidence, taking into account various measures of association and causal inference.

REVIEW QUESTIONS

1　Define 'epidemiology' in your own words.

2　Describe how epidemiology differs from clinical medicine.

3　Describe two measures of disease frequency.

4　Discuss the differences between prevalence and incidence.

5　Explain the difference between observational and experimental study designs, giving examples of each.

6　What do relative risk and odds ratio measure?

7　What is the technical term used by epidemiologists when a third factor influences the relationship between an exposure of interest and a disease? Give an example.

8　Describe two types of systematic bias that should always be considered by epidemiologists.

9　How might you use epidemiology in your future profession?

Acknowledgements

The author would like to acknowledge those who assisted with the development of components of this chapter: Michelle Cook, Mary-Anne Kedda, Bonnie Macfarlane and Beth Newman, formerly of the School of Public Health, QUT; Diana Battistutta, Michael Dunne and Kate Halton, of the School of Public Health and Social Work, QUT; and Christopher Stevenson, School of Health and Social Development, Deakin University.

Useful websites

- Centers for Disease Control and Prevention: http://www.cdc.gov/ophss/csels/dsepd/SS1978/Glossary.html

- Epidemiology Supercourse: http://www.pitt.edu/~super1
- John Snow—a historical giant in epidemiology: http://www.ph.ucla.edu/epi/snow.html
- The James Lind Library: http://www.jameslindlibrary.org

References

Brown, W.J., Mummery, K., Eakin, E., et al., 2006. 10,000 Steps Rockhampton: evaluation of a whole community approach to improving population levels of physical activity. Journal of Physical Activity and Health 3 (1), 1–14.

Burgess, J., Matheson, M.C., Gurrin, L.C., et al., 2011. Factors influencing asthma remission: a longitudinal study from childhood to middle age. Thorax doi:10.1136/thx.2010.146845.

Burgess, J.A., Walters, E.H., Byrnes, G.B., et al., 2007. Childhood adiposity predicts adult-onset current asthma in females: a 25-yr prospective study. The European Respiratory Journal: Official Journal of the European Society for Clinical Respiratory Physiology 29, 668–675.

Clark, M.J., Purdie, J., FitzGerald, G.J., et al., 1999. Predictors of demand for emergency prehospital care: an Australian study. Prehospital and Disaster Medicine 14 (3), 167–173.

Gordis, L., 2004. Epidemiology, third ed. Elsevier Saunders, Philadelphia.

Gregory, A.T., Armstrong, R.M., Grassi, T.D., et al., 2008. On our selection: Australian longitudinal research studies. Medical Journal of Australia 189 (11/12), 650–657.

Gunes, U.Y., Eser, I., 2007. Effectiveness of a honey dressing for healing pressure ulcers. Journal of Wound, Ostomy, and Continence Nursing 34 (2), 184–190.

Jenkins, M.A., Hopper, J.L., Bowes, G., et al., 1994. Factors in childhood as predictors of asthma in adult life. British Medical Journal 309, 90–93.

Last, J.M., 1995. A Dictionary of Epidemiology, third ed. Oxford University Press, Oxford.

Olsen, J.R., Saracci, R., Trichopoulos, D., 2001. Teaching Epidemiology: A Guide for Teachers in Epidemiology, Public Health and Clinical Medicine. Oxford University Press, Oxford.

Salonen, J.T., Tuomainen, T.P., Salonen, R., et al., 1998. Donation of blood is associated with reduced risk of myocardial infarction: the Kuopio Ischaemic Heart Disease Risk Factor Study. American Journal of Epidemiology 148 (5), 445–451.

Svanes, C., Zock J.P., Antó, J., et al., 2006. Does asthma and allergy influence subsequent pet keeping? An analysis of childhood and adulthood. Journal of Allergy and Clinical Immunology 118 (3), 691–698. Highlights September.

Tenkate, T.D., Stafford, R.J., 2001. Risk factors for *Campylobacter* infection in infants and young children: a matched case-control study. Epidemiology and Infection 127, 399–404.

Webb, P., Bain, C., Pirozzo, S., 2011. Essential Epidemiology: An Introduction for Students and Health Professionals, second ed. Cambridge University Press, Cambridge.

World Health Organization, 1948. Preamble to the Constitution of the World Health Organization as adopted by the International Health Conference, New York, 19–22 June, 1946; signed on 22 Jul 1946 by the representatives of 61 States and entered into force on 7 Apr 1948. Online. Available: <http://www.who.int/about/definition/en/print.html> (3 Apr 2014).

Biological and environmental determinants CHAPTER 6

Mary Louise Fleming & Thomas Tenkate

Learning objectives

After reading this chapter, you should be able to:

- describe the complex web of determinants as part of broad causal pathways that affect health

- identify and discuss the range of physical, biological and environmental determinants that impact on health

- suggest why it is important to the practice of public health that you understand how determinants contribute to health

- understand the complexity of health and illness, and the multifaceted role of health determinants

- relate determinants of health to public health activity, and realise the need for multisectoral action and implementation of multiple approaches when working to improve health.

Introduction

This chapter describes biological and environmental determinants of the health of Australians, providing a background to the development of successful public health activity. You will recall from the introduction to Section 2 that health determinants are the biomedical, genetic, behavioural, socioeconomic and environmental factors that impact on health and wellbeing. These determinants can be influenced by interventions and by resources and systems (Australian Institute of Health and Welfare (AIHW) 2012a). Many factors combine to affect the health of individuals and communities. People's circumstances and the environment determine whether a population is healthy or not. Factors such as where people live, the state of their environment, genetics, their education level and income, and their relationships with friends and family are all likely to impact on their health. The determinants of population health reflect the context of people's lives; however, people have limited control over many of these determinants (World Health Organization (WHO) 2007).

This chapter and Chapter 7 illustrate how various determinants can relate to and influence other determinants, as well as health and wellbeing. We believe that it is particularly important to provide an understanding of determinants and their relationship to health and illness in order to provide a structure in which a broader conceptualisation of health can be placed. Determinants of health do not exist in isolation from one another. More frequently, they work together in a complex system. What is clear to anyone who works in public health is that many factors impact on the health and wellbeing of people. For example, in the next chapter we discuss factors such as living and working conditions, social support, ethnicity and class, income, housing, work stress and the impact of education on the length and quality of people's lives.

Tackling health determinants has great potential to reduce the burden of disease and promote the health of the general population. In summary, we understand very clearly now that health is determined by the complex interactions between individual characteristics, social and economic factors, and physical environments; the entire range of factors that impact on health must be addressed if we are to make significant gains in population health. Focusing interventions on the health of the population or significant subpopulations can achieve important health gains.

In Chapter 3 you were introduced to National Health Priority Areas (NHPAs): cancer control, injury prevention and control, cardiovascular health, diabetes mellitus, mental health, asthma, arthritis, musculoskeletal conditions, and, added in 2012, dementia (AIHW 2012b). As you will recall from that chapter, the NHPAs set the agenda for the Commonwealth, states and territories, local governments and not-for-profit organisations to direct attention to those areas considered to be the major foci for action. Many of these health issues are discussed in this chapter and the following chapter.

A complex web of determinants

Determinants are in complex interplay, and range from the 'upstream' background influences (e.g. culture and wealth), with many health and non-health effects that can be difficult to quantify, to immediate or direct influences with highly specific effects on particular aspects of health. They are often described as part of broad causal 'pathways' or 'chains' that affect health (Keleher & Murphy 2004).

The Public Health Agency of Canada (2013) defines 12 determinants of health (see Table 6.1). Examining these issues briefly in tabular form gives you an idea of the range of factors that impact on health. Figure 6.1 collapses these many determinants into a manageable and simple framework for your consideration. Some of these determinants are discussed further in this chapter, and the remaining determinants are considered in the following chapter.

Figure 6.1 presents a range of determinants and their pathways. The pathways are not linear, and can also occur in reverse. For example, an individual's health can influence their physical activity levels, employment status and wealth. General background

Determinants of health	Description
TABLE 6.1 Determinants of health	
Income and social status	Much research suggests poor people are less healthy than rich people; income distribution is a key element
Social support networks	Support from family, friends and community is linked to health
Education and literacy	Low literacy levels are linked to poor health
Employment/working conditions	Unemployment and poor health are related; more control over working conditions improves health
Social environments	'The importance of social support also extends to the broader community. Civic vitality refers to the strength of social networks within a community, region, province or country. It is reflected in the institutions, organizations and informal giving practices that people create to share resources and build attachments with others.'
Physical environments	Clean air and water, healthy workplaces, safe houses, communities and roads all contribute to health
Personal health practices and coping skills	Physical activity, good nutrition, smoking and drinking, and coping skills impact on health
Healthy child development	Good health in childhood has a positive influence on later life
Biology and genetic endowment	'Biology and organic make-up of the human body are a fundamental determinant of health.' Inherited characteristics play a role in determining how long we live, how healthy we will be, and the likelihood of contracting certain illnesses
Health services	Access to services that prevent diseases benefits health
Gender	Different kinds of diseases and conditions affect women and men differently
Culture	Customs and beliefs affect health

(Source: Public Health Agency of Canada, 2011. What determines health? © All Rights Reserved. Reproduced with permission from the Minister of Health, 2015.)

factors and environmental factors can determine the nature of socioeconomic characteristics, and both can influence people's health behaviour, their psychological state, and factors relating to their safety. These, in turn, can influence biomedical factors, such as blood pressure and body weight, which may have health effects through various further pathways. At all stages along the pathway these various factors interact with an individual's genetic composition. This framework then shows us a simple way of organising and examining the various pathways that may occur in a range of different contexts. In

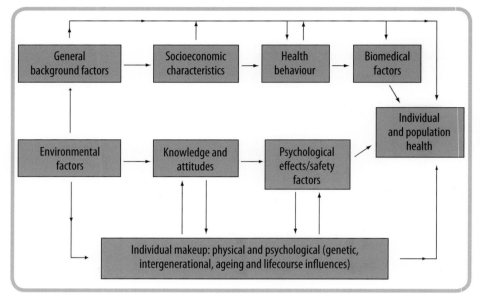

FIG. 6.1   Determinants of health.
(Adapted from AIHW 2004, Figure 3.1)

ACTIVITY 6.1 One Health

Look at the Centers for Disease Control and Prevention website and the Public Health Agency of Canada website, listed under 'Useful websites' at the at the back of this chapter, for more information about the concept of One Health. Discuss the notion of One Health with your colleagues. In particular, how is it defined? What are its major objectives? What strategies might it use? What examples are there of diseases that are common between humans and animals?

addition, the notion of 'One Health' has become more prominent, as it considers the relationship between the health of humans, the health of animals and the environment (see Activity 6.1). Some examples of this interrelationship include animals passing on some diseases to humans, known as zoonotic diseases. Zoonotic diseases include *Salmonella* poisoning. Animals are also susceptible to some diseases and environmental hazards. They can in fact serve as early warning systems for potential human illness (One Health, Centers for Disease Control and Prevention 2014).

An important use of determinants is to enable us to focus on where best to intervene. There are three broad levels of factors affecting health upon which interventions might be structured:

- *downstream factors*—include treatment systems, disease management and investment in clinical research
- *midstream factors*—include lifestyle, behavioural and individual prevention programs
- *upstream factors*—involve government policies and investment in population health research as examples (Turnock 2012, Turrell et al. 2006).

This type of approach ensures that we direct our resources upstream to focus on issues that impact on health equity. This issue will be considered in more detail in the next chapter.

Genetics and screening

Genetic determinants are important factors impacting on individual health, and they will continue to be important, as nearly every disease has constitutive and/or acquired genetic components. Identifying disease susceptibility genes, as well as identifying acquired somatic mutations underlying a specific disease such as cancer, can provide vital information for a more thorough understanding of many common illnesses. This information can then be used to determine how diseases are diagnosed and how new treatments or particular drug therapies can be identified (Europa 2014).

'Genes are the units of heredity which control the structure and function of the body by determining the structure of peptide chains that form the building blocks of enzymes and other proteins' (Harper et al. 1994 p 119). A gene's role is to ensure that the amino acids are always in the same order. Genes are located at specific points in the deoxyribonucleic acid (DNA) in the cell nucleus, and the DNA is arranged into 23 pairs of chromosomes. Of these, 22 are called autosomes, while the other pair is the sex chromosomes. One of each pair of chromosomes is derived from each parent. There are several categories of genetic disease, depending upon the location and the extent of the genetic abnormality. The categories include single-gene disorders, chromosomal disorders, disorders involving several genes and environmental influences, disorders of cytoplasmic DNA, and mutations of somatic cells.

In the case of single-gene disorders, they may be: autosomal-dominant (e.g. Huntington's disease and otosclerosis); autosomal-recessive (e.g. cystic fibrosis); or X-linked dominant or recessive, resulting in disorders such as muscular dystrophy and haemophilia.

Chromosomal abnormalities often cause fetal death and congenital disease. For example, about half of spontaneous abortions are linked to chromosomal abnormalities. Down syndrome is an example of a chromosomal abnormality.

The complex interplay of genetic and environmental factors is associated with the relationship between several genes at different loci on the chromosome, each with an additive effect and a variable environmental component. Characteristics determined in this multifactorial manner may be continuous or discontinuous. For a continuous multifactorial trait, such as blood pressure, there is a high continuous gradient from high blood pressure to normal blood pressure. An example of a discontinuous multifactorial variable is cleft lip and palate.

There is strong evidence of a genetic component to many conditions causing chronic disease and premature death. We must also keep in mind that the majority of diseases are multifactorial in aetiology and result from the interaction of multiple genetic and environmental factors. These diseases are partly the result of how genes interact with environmental and behavioural risk factors, such as diet and physical activity.

Examples of the integration of genetics into public health functions in the twenty-first century include such activities as investigating clusters of cancer in communities, developing policies for using genetic testing to prevent iron overload in the United States, population analysis of the impact of asthma interventions based on individual susceptibility, evaluating the prevention effectiveness of a national campaign for early detection of colon cancer, and a national assurance program to monitor the utilisation, effectiveness and impact of genetic testing. The implications for public health include, as examples, treatment for affected high-risk individuals, prevention for at-risk individuals, health promotion activities among the general population, and, with regard to the environment, crop modification, pharmaceuticals, and the cloning of animals. However, genetic screening raises ethical, social and legal concerns relating to the

ACTIVITY 6.2 Issues with genetic information

Consider the issue of genetic testing for breast cancer. Look at the website of the Breast Cancer Network Australia (in the reference list), and listen to Judith Maher tell the story of her daughter, Maryanne, who was diagnosed with breast cancer aged 30. Judith was subsequently diagnosed with breast cancer, as was her sister. Think about this and discuss the following issues:

- ethical, social and legal concerns relating to the privacy and confidentiality of genetic information
- fairness in the use of genetic information
- the potential psychological impact, stigmatisation and discrimination associated with the use of such information
- reproductive and clinical issues.

ACTIVITY 6.3 Diabetes

Try answering the following questions:
- What is a 'chronic disease'?
- Is diabetes a chronic disease?
- What causes diabetes?
- Is there a genetic contribution?
- Are there different types of diabetes?
- How is the condition managed?
- Can it be prevented?
- How does public health contribute to the promotion, prevention, intervention and maintenance of quality of life if a person has diabetes?

REFLECTION 6.3

Diabetes mellitus is a condition where the body cannot maintain normal blood glucose levels. There are three types of diabetes: type 1 diabetes, type 2 diabetes, and gestational diabetes. A further category of diabetes is not common and accounts for less than 1% of people with diabetes. It includes diabetes caused by a variety of distinct genetic and pathological mechanisms that are generally clearly defined.

privacy and confidentiality of genetic information, fairness in the use of genetic information, the psychological impact, stigmatisation and discrimination associated with the use of such information, reproductive and clinical issues, and uncertainties associated with gene tests for susceptibilities and complex conditions (see Activity 6.2). It will be interesting to follow modern genetics as it develops, because it will undoubtedly have implications for the choices people and populations make about their health.

The Human Genome Project (HGP) commenced in 1990 as a 15-year, large-scale, international project that involved the United States, the United Kingdom, France, Canada, Germany, Japan and China. The primary goal was to sequence the entire human genome, with other goals including identifying genes, improvements in technology and data analysis, comparative genomics, and the ethical, legal and social implications of such a project. Completed in April 2003, the HGP enables scientists to read Nature's complete genetic blueprint for building a human being.

While genomics is the study of how genes act in the body, and how they interact with environmental influences to cause disease, the fundamental question for public health is the extent to which applying this emerging knowledge will divert resources from the mission of public health, which is to prevent disease in the population.

Diabetes is a good example of the complex interplay of genetic and environmental factors. Consider the activity on diabetes as an introduction to the nature and impact of a chronic disease on health and wellbeing, and the potential role of public health. If you are not familiar with diabetes, consider looking at the Diabetes Australia website, located under 'Useful websites' at the end of this chapter, to become more familiar with the different characteristics of diabetes (e.g. type 1 and type 2 diabetes), their development, and treatment and prevention options. Then attempt the activity (Activity 6.3 and Reflection 6.3).

Diabetes is caused by resistance to, or deficient production of, the hormone insulin, which helps glucose move from the blood into the cells. When the body does not produce or use enough insulin, the cells cannot use glucose and the blood glucose level rises. This means that the body will instead start to break down its own fat and muscle for energy. Diabetes may lead to severe problems, including damage to the heart, blood vessels, eyes, nerves and kidneys (Diabetes Australia website 2014). Diabetes is defined as a chronic disease in Australia. The last section of the activity asks you how public health might contribute to the promotion, prevention and intervention and maintenance of people with diabetes. Think back to what you have learned about the nature of public health, the determinants that contribute to diabetes, and what public health strategies might be put in place as prevention and rehabilitation strategies for diabetes.

Biological and behavioural determinants

Biological determinants

Biology refers to the individual's genetic makeup, family history, and the physical and mental health problems acquired during life. Ageing, diet, physical activity, smoking, stress, alcohol or illicit drug use, injury or violence, or an infectious or toxic agent may result in illness or disability and can produce a 'new biology' for the individual (AIHW 2012a, Office of Disease Prevention 2007).

Behavioural determinants

Lifestyle or behavioural determinants are multidimensional, and are linked to a number of major health problems. Some health issues share the same determinants, such as tobacco, alcohol and nutrition.

Individual health practices are responses or reactions to internal stimuli and external conditions (see Activity 6.4). Behaviour and biology can have a reciprocal relationship, with each reacting to the other when a person is exposed to a particular health condition. Examples of the reciprocity of the relationship can be seen in the case of a family history of heart disease (biology), which may motivate an individual to add healthy eating behaviours, maintain an active lifestyle and avoid tobacco smoking (behaviours), thus preventing the development of heart disease (biology). Personal choices and the social and physical environments surrounding individuals can shape behaviours. The social and physical environments also include factors that affect the life of individuals, positively or negatively, many of which may not be under their immediate or direct control (AIHW 2012a).

TOBACCO

Tobacco is responsible for, in part, a worldwide epidemic of coronary heart disease and lung cancer. The work of researchers such as Doll and Hill (1964) clearly linked the smoking patterns of individuals with age and cause of death. The WHO *Global Burden of Disease Study* (Murray & Lopez 1996) reported that, by 2020, tobacco may account for 12.3% of deaths worldwide. Smoking rates have been declining for several decades in Australia. Between 1985 and 2007, the prevalence of smoking

> **ACTIVITY 6.4 Health issues and lifestyle behaviours**
>
> Select a health issue that is influenced by lifestyle or the behaviours of an individual.
>
> - What lifestyle or behavioural factors make a contribution to the issue?
> - Which of these does the individual have some control over?
> - Why is it difficult for an individual to have control over their health?
> - List the range of determinants that might impact on the individual as a consequence of the health condition.
> - List the social, economic and environmental factors that influence an individual's response to the health issue.

> **REFLECTION 6.4**
>
> Did you consider any of the significant factors discussed in this chapter—smoking, alcohol, injuries, etc? What factors may change if an individual could control the determinants of their health? Would it make it easier for them? Would it be more difficult? Does the environment play a role in the health issue you have selected?

ACTIVITY 6.5 Tobacco control

The Department of Health outlines five areas in its strategic plan for tobacco control. Go to the Australian Government Department of Health Tobacco Control website (the link is in the reference list) and identify and discuss each of the five aspects of the strategic plan.

declined for both males and females. Despite these trends, tobacco smoking continues to cause more ill health and death than other well-known health determinants, such as high blood pressure, over-weight/obesity and physical inactivity (AIHW 2012a). (Refer to Activity 6.5.) The impact of passive smoking, particularly on children, has become very important in recent years, increasing the likelihood of a number of illnesses, including chest and ear infections, asthma and sudden infant death syndrome (AIHW 2012a).

ALCOHOL

Alcohol plays an important role in the Australian economy, and it also has an important social role. It is a familiar part of traditions and customs in this country, and is often used for relaxation, socialisation and celebration. It is a drug that is legal, it can promote relaxation and feelings of euphoria, and it can lead to intoxication and dependence and a wide range of associated harms (Ministerial Council on Drug Strategy 2011).

Although the per capita consumption of alcohol in Australia has declined since the 1980s, it remains high by world standards. Many of the dangers of alcohol for those who drink, and those around them, are misunderstood, tolerated or ignored. The harms associated with unsafe alcohol use, including drinking to intoxication, are now well documented in the research literature.

ACTIVITY 6.6 Alcohol consumption

Get together in a group and consider the range of issues addressed in the vignette on drinking. Suggest strategies for dealing with each of the issues identified. How do the issues discussed relate to the current debate in the media about closing times for pubs and clubs in some Australian states?

Some research suggests that benefits from alcohol consumption only occur at very low levels of drinking or that there is no protective effect from drinking (National Health and Medical Research Council (NHMRC) 2009). The Australian National Preventive Health Agency report (2013 p 39) has a vignette of a state police commissioner discussing the impact of drinking to intoxication (see the ANPHA website in the reference list; and see Activity 6.6).

INJURIES

Injury affects Australians of all ages, and is the greatest cause of death in the first half of life. It leaves many with serious disability or long-term conditions. Injury was esti-mated to account for 6.5% of the burden of disease in 2010 (AIHW 2010). For these reasons, injury prevention and control was declared an NHPA (AIHW 2012b), and is the subject of three national prevention plans: the National Injury Prevention and Safety Promotion Plan: 2004–2014 (National Public Health Partnership (NPHP) 2004a); the National Falls Prevention for Older People Plan: 2004 Onwards (NPHP 2004b); and the National Aboriginal and Torres Strait Islander Safety Promotion Strategy (AIHW 2010, NPHP 2005). Injuries were responsible for almost half of the mortality for people under 45 years of age, and account for a range of physical, cognitive and psychological disabilities that seriously affect the quality of life of injured people and their families. Health costs associated with injury in Australia have been estimated to be $2.6 billion annually (AIHW 2010).

Injury usually means physical harm to a person's body, and the most common types of physical injury are broken bones, cuts, poisoning and burns. Physical injury results from harmful contact between people and objects, substances or other things in their surroundings—for example, being struck by a car, cut by a knife, bitten by a dog, or poisoned by inhaled petrol. Some physical injuries are the intended result of acts by people: harm of one person by another (e.g. assault, homicide) or self-harm (NPHP 2004a). Over recent years, Australia has achieved some significant gains in preventing a number of different types of injury where concerted efforts have been made. There have been improvements in road safety over the past 25 years. The reduction in road deaths has occurred despite significant growth in the population, vehicle numbers and kilometres travelled (see Activity 6.7). Initiatives, such as random breath-testing, compulsory wearing of seat belts, speed blitzes, car design

> **ACTIVITY 6.7 Driving campaign**
>
> Look at http://www.youtube.com/user/JoinTheDrive, and watch to some of the short video clips in the Queensland Government's 'Join the drive campaign'. Who would be the target audience for this type of campaign? What are the messages for drivers? Do you think a campaign like this can gain momentum and be a positive influence on drivers? Look also at Chapter 14 for examples of a range of promotion and prevention strategies.

and safety features (e.g. air bags), better roads, ongoing community education regarding road safety, and improved life-saving medical procedures and trauma care, have all contributed to the decline in the number of vehicle-related fatalities (NPHP 2004a).

MENTAL HEALTH

There is a wide spectrum of mental health disorders with varying levels of severity. Some examples include anxiety, depression, bipolar disorders and schizophrenia. Individuals and families suffer from the effect of mental illness, and its influence is far-reaching for society as a whole. To add to the health issues are a range of social problems commonly associated with mental illness, including poverty, unemployment or reduced productivity, violence and crime (AIHW 2012a).

In 2012 the Council of Australian Governments (COAG) established a Working Group on Mental Health Reform supported by an Expert Reference Group. The COAG's website has the latest National Mental Health Plan/Strategy and shows how the roadmap is being implemented. The national vision will be achieved through the commitment of the Commonwealth, states and territories to fundamental reform based on six action priorities, which are:

- Priority 1: Promote personal-centred approaches.
- Priority 2: Improve the mental health and social and emotional wellbeing of all Australians.
- Priority 3: Prevent mental illness.
- Priority 4: Focus on early detection and intervention.
- Priority 5: Improve access to high-quality services and supports.
- Priority 6: Improve the social and economic participation of people with mental illness (COAG 2012) (see Activity 6.8).

> **ACTIVITY 6.8 National Mental Health Plan roadmap**
>
> Consider the National Mental Health Plan roadmap document (see the COAG website in the reference list; pp. 13–29) by selecting one of the six priority areas. Summarise the major activities to be pursued under this priority. What strategies are listed? In your group, discuss the case study example provided.

DIET AND PHYSICAL ACTIVITY

A healthy diet and regular, adequate physical activity are major factors in promoting and maintaining good health. Unhealthy diets, physical inactivity and sedentary behaviour (Owen et al. 2010) are the main risk factors for raised blood pressure, raised blood glucose, abnormal blood lipids, overweight/obesity and the major chronic diseases such as cardiovascular diseases, cancer and diabetes.

ACTIVITY 6.9 National Health Priority Areas and genetic and behavioural factors

- List the National Health Priority Areas which have genetic or behavioural contributions.
- Discuss each of the priority health areas you have identified in terms of the contribution of each of the determinants outlined in this chapter.
- What priorities have the federal government set to promote and manage the health issue?

REFLECTION 6.9

When we examined the genetic determinants that contributed to a number of health issues earlier in this chapter, it became clear that many conditions can have both a genetic and a behavioural contribution. In fact, many health issues have multiple causes. Keep this in mind as you consider the environmental determinants of health.

According to *Global health risks* (WHO 2009), eight risk factors alone account for over 75% of cases of coronary heart disease, the leading cause of death worldwide. These are alcohol consumption, high blood glucose, tobacco use, high blood pressure, high body mass index, high cholesterol, low fruit and vegetable intake, and physical inactivity. Most of these deaths occur in developing countries. Worldwide, overweight and obesity causes more deaths than underweight.

A unique opportunity exists to formulate and implement an effective strategy for substantially reducing deaths and disease worldwide by improving diet and promoting physical activity. Evidence for the links between these health behaviours and later disease and ill health is strong. Effective interventions to enable people to live longer and healthier lives, reduce inequalities, and enhance development can be designed and implemented (AIHW 2012a, WHO 2004, 2009). Globally, physical inactivity is estimated to cause about 10–16% of breast, colon and rectal cancers and diabetes mellitus, and about 22% of ischaemic heart disease. Overall, 1.9 million deaths are attributable to physical inactivity.

The following activity asks you to think about the list of National Health Priority Areas discussed at the beginning of this chapter (see Activity 6.9). Can you identify those NHPAs which have genetic, behavioural or lifestyle determinants associated with them? Use some of the websites listed at the end of this chapter to help you with this exercise.

Environmental determinants

An *environmental determinant of health* can be considered to be any external agent (e.g. biological, chemical, physical, social or cultural) that can influence health status. Unfortunately, this definition is very broad, because nearly all changes in health status that are not genetically determined could be considered to result from environmental factors (Soskolne & Sieswerda 2007). Therefore, we generally restrict the scope of what is an environmental determinant to any external physical, chemical or microbiological exposure or process that can impact individuals or the community at large, and that is beyond their immediate control (i.e. it is involuntary) (McMichael et al. 2006). For example, exposure to environmental tobacco smoke (passive smoking) is considered to be an environmental determinant, whereas cigarette smoking is considered to be a behavioural determinant of health.

Like other determinants, environmental influences on health can be direct or indirect, immediate or delayed, quite obvious or very subtle. Some relationships between the environment and human health are straightforward, whereas others are much more complex (AIHW 2010). Figure 6.2 illustrates the relationship between some of these environmental determinants. When describing how the environment can impact on human health, there are two important underlying considerations (McMichael et al. 2006):

- *Natural variation versus human intervention*—Some environmental exposures occur because of natural variation (e.g. exposure to solar radiation and

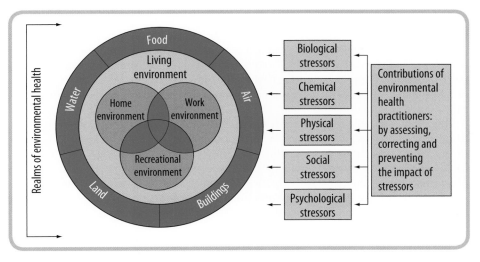

FIG. 6.2   Human interaction with the environment.
(Source: Health Development Agency 2012. Reproduced with permission)

extremes of heat and cold, due to natural variation in season, time of day, latitude and altitude), whereas other environmental hazards result directly from human activity (e.g. industrial pollution of waterways). For developed/industrialised countries, much of our effort has been on preventing chemical contamination of the air, water and food supply, and on urbanisation issues such as noise, traffic injuries, increasing residential density—the so-called 'modern environmental health hazards'. In comparison, developing countries tend to focus on 'traditional environmental health hazards', such as the microbiological quality of drinking water and food, the physical safety of housing and workplaces, indoor air pollution, and road hazards. Such hazards in developed countries are generally controlled through substantial investment in community infrastructure (e.g. drinking water supply systems, sewage systems, and solid waste collection).

• *Local versus global environmental impacts*—Until recently, prevention of environmental impacts on health have focused on localised exposures (e.g. at a household, community or city level), whereas it is clear that we are now facing more disruptions of the Earth's ecosystems on a global scale, but unfortunately our understanding of the broader implications of these complex disruptions remains limited.

The highly publicised global environmental changes will, therefore, have a lasting impact on the underlying 'environmental determinants' of human health. The global, but local, nature and complexity of these changes present unique and unparalleled health risks that are arguably the greatest challenge we face as a society. This challenge is nicely summarised in the following quote:

> The public health community needs to go beyond reacting to a changing climate. A true preventive strategy needs to ensure the maintenance and development of healthy environments from local to global levels. In the long term, sustainable development and protection of ecosystem services are fundamentally necessary for human health. (Campbell-Lendrum et al. 2007 p 236)

Human interaction with the environment

In order to make an effective contribution to dealing with global environmental issues, it is important for public health practitioners to have an understanding of the complex interactions that occur within natural and man-made environments, and how these interactions impact on human health. The following sections provide an introduction to some of the fundamental ecological process and ecosystem issues, and how these can impact on human health.

Until now we have used the term 'environment' frequently, but a more basic scientific concept is that of an ecosystem. When defining 'ecosystem', it is important to go back to the core scientific discipline, which is ecology. The term 'ecology' can be traced back to its Greek roots, and literally means 'house-study'. *Ecology*, therefore, is the study of an organism's home, and is the branch of biology that deals with the interrelationships between organisms and their environment. The concept of an *ecosystem* therefore builds on our understanding of ecology, with the following being a basic definition:

> An ecosystem is a dynamic complex of plant, animal and microorganism communities and the nonliving environment interacting as a functional unit. Humans are an integral part of ecosystems. Ecosystems vary enormously in size; a temporary pond in a tree hollow and an ocean basin can both be ecosystems. (Alcamo et al. 2003 p 3)

Biodiversity is an important concept to consider when discussing ecosystems. Biodiversity is a term that comes from the phrase 'biological diversity' and is used to describe the variety of life contained in various ecosystems. The most widely recognised definition for *biodiversity* is:

> The variability among living organisms from all sources including terrestrial, marine and other aquatic ecosystems and the ecological complexes of which they are part; this includes diversity within species, between species and of ecosystems (Secretariat of the Convention on Biological Diversity 2010).

This definition provides some insight into the many dimensions of biodiversity. For example, it recognises that every biota (i.e. all of the living organisms in a specific location or region, including animals, plants and microorganisms) can be characterised by its taxonomic, ecological and genetic diversity, and that the way in which these dimensions vary over space and time is a key feature of biodiversity. In addition to this, biodiversity should not be considered only as relating to unmanaged ecosystems (e.g. wilderness, national parks), but is also equally appropriate for managed/man-made systems. Agricultural and pastoral lands and even urban ecosystems have their own biodiversity. When it is considered that over 24% of the Earth's terrestrial surface consists of cultivated land, these ecosystems have enormous impact on biodiversity.

Ecosystem services

When functioning naturally, the Earth's ecosystems (e.g. forests, grasslands, wetlands, oceans, farmlands) provide a range of materials, conditions and processes that sustain life. The benefits that all living things obtain from ecosystems are called *ecosystem services*. Some of these services are quite familiar, such as the provision of food and timber, which are essential for life and important for the global economy. Less well known, but of equal importance, are the services provided by ecosystems that are not easy to assign a monetary value to, but are essential for living. These include the purification of air and water, the decomposition of wastes, the recycling of nutrients on land and in the oceans, the pollination of crops, and the regulation of climate (Melillo & Sala 2008).

These ecosystem services are generated by an array of natural cycles, ranging from the short lifecycles of microbes that break down toxic chemicals, to the long-term and global cycles of water and of elements such as carbon and nitrogen that are essential for life. Therefore, disruption of these cycles can have devastating effects on the life of all creatures. Ecosystem services can be categorised into (Melillo & Sala 2008):

- *Provisioning services*—These include the products that are obtained from ecosystems, such as food, fuel wood, fibre and medicines.
- *Regulating services*—These are the benefits obtained from environmental regulation of ecosystem processes, such as cleaning air, purifying water, mitigating floods, controlling erosion, detoxifying soils and modifying climate.
- *Cultural services*—These are non-material benefits that people obtain from ecosystems, such as recreation, aesthetics, intellectual stimulation and a sense of place.
- *Supporting services*—These are services that are necessary for the production of all other ecosystem services. They include the production of new organic matter by plants through photosynthesis, and the cycling of essential nutrients such as carbon, nitrogen and phosphorus.

Ecosystem services and human wellbeing

As described above, ecosystem services are the benefits that people obtain from ecosystems. The human health impacts of ecosystems are often described within the broader category of 'human wellbeing', with human health being a baseline component of wellbeing, since changes in economic, social, political, residential, psychological and behavioural circumstances all have health consequences as well (Millennium Ecosystem Assessment 2005). Ecosystem services affect human wellbeing in the following ways (Alcamo et al. 2003).

Security is affected both by changes in *provisioning services*, which affect supplies of food and other goods and the potential for conflict over declining resources, and by changes in *regulating services*, which could influence the frequency and magnitude of floods, droughts, landslides or other catastrophes. It can also be affected by changes in *cultural services* as, for example, when the loss of important ceremonial or spiritual attributes of ecosystems contributes to the weakening of social relations in a community.

Access to basic material for a good life is strongly linked to both *provisioning services*, such as food and fibre production, and *regulating services*, including water purification.

Health is strongly linked to *provisioning services*, such as food production, and *regulating services*, including those that influence the distribution of disease-transmitting insects and of pathogens in water and air. Health can also be linked to *cultural services* through recreational and spiritual benefits.

Social relations are affected by changes to *cultural services*, which affect the quality of human experience.

Freedoms and choice are largely based on the existence of the other components of wellbeing, and are therefore influenced by changes in *provisioning, regulating* or *cultural services* from ecosystems.

The interactions between ecosystem services and the constituents of wellbeing (as described above) are diagrammatically represented in Figure 6.3. This highlights, in particular, that provisioning and regulating services strongly influence wellbeing in the areas of security, basic materials for a good life, and health, with each of these also highly mediated by socioeconomic factors. Even though in some situations selected

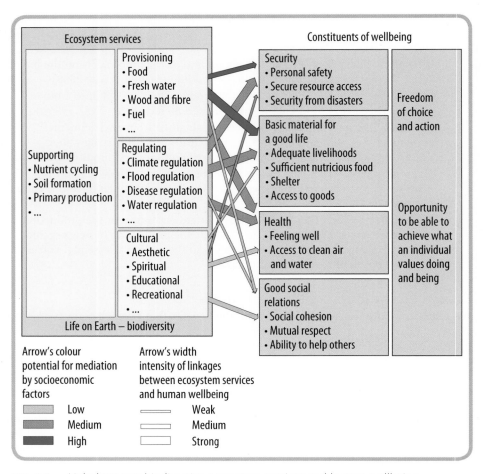

FIG. 6.3   Links between biodiversity, ecosystem services and human wellbeing.
(Source: Reproduced from Millennium Ecosystem Assessment 2005, World Resources Institute)

ACTIVITY 6.10 Ecosystems

The US Environmental Protection Agency has created the *Eco-Health Relationship Browser* as an online interactive tool that allows users to visualise the complex linkages between ecosystem services and human health (Jackson et al. 2013). For this activity, log onto http://www.epa.gov/research/healthscience/browser/index.html and then compare the different linkages for the following scenarios:

- urban ecosystems versus wetlands
- health outcomes of cancer, gastrointestinal illness, high blood pressure, and obesity
- ecosystem services of clear air versus clean water.

ecosystem services can be replaced by man-made infrastructure (e.g. water treatment facilities), in many situations natural ecosystems provide these services much more effectively or efficiently than those engineered by humans, and often they are irreplaceable. Therefore, ecosystem services contribute to making human life both possible and worth living (Levy et al. 2012). Finally, how a disruption in ecosystem services can impact human health is illustrated in Case Study 6.1 (see the case study, and then complete Activity 6.10).

Environmental burden of disease

Until now, we have focused on fundamental principles related to ecosystems, human impacts on the

CASE STUDY
6.1

Ecosystem changes and human health impacts

An example of the many potential impacts of deforestation on human disease comes from the tropical forests of South East Asia and the Amazon. In these areas, widespread logging has impacted the aquatic habitat of a range of mosquitoes, particularly the *Anopheles* mosquito, which is the vector of malaria. Some indirect impacts of deforestation include removal of the overhead trees that acidified standing water through organic acid deposition, which has led to a more neutral pH; removal of under-storey plants and litter that serve to drain standing water; and increased light and temperatures for the forest floor that have accelerated photosynthesis by algae. In addition, deforestation directly disturbs the forest floor by providing depressions that catch and hold water, and by creating new breeding sites for mosquitoes. Taken together, these changes have improved the habitat quality for the *Anopheles* larvae, and have resulted in a large increase in mosquito numbers. As malaria is the most deadly vector-borne disease, killing over 600,000 people (mainly children) worldwide each year, such ecosystem changes can only result in increased human health impacts.

(Source: Chivian 2002, WHO 2013)

environment, and the relationships between ecosystem services and human health. These sections provide a basis for discussing the impact of environmental conditions on public health status.

It is currently estimated that more than 13 million deaths each year are due to preventable environmental causes, with as much as 24% of global disease being caused by environmental exposures which can be prevented. Nearly one-third of death and disease in the least-developed regions are due to environmental causes. Well-targeted interventions are identified as being able to prevent much of this environmental risk, with over 40% of deaths from malaria and an estimated 94% of deaths from diarrhoeal diseases—two of the world's biggest childhood killers—preventable through better environmental management (Prüss-Üstün & Corvalán 2006).

> ### REFLECTION 6.10
>
> It is clear that the world's natural ecosystems are complex and provide health benefits to humans through a range of ecosystem services, while also presenting humans with the potential for adverse health effects when the systems are unbalanced or disrupted in some way. Referring back to the two important underlying considerations on how the environment can impact on human health (see 'Environmental determinants'), are you able to think of ways in which specific *regulating services* may impact on human health through local variation versus human intervention, and how disruptions to local ecosystems may have global impacts?

The four main diseases influenced by poor environments are diarrhoea, lower respiratory infections, various forms of unintentional injury, and malaria. Measures that could be taken now to reduce this environmental disease burden include: promoting safe household water storage and better hygiene measures; the use of cleaner and safer fuels; providing a safer built environment, including the better management of toxic substances in the home and workplace; and better water resource management.

Diseases with the largest total annual health burden from environmental factors, in terms of death, illness and disability—or 'disability-adjusted life years' (DALYs)—are identified as (Prüss-Üstün & Corvalán 2006):

- diarrhoea (58 million DALYs per year), largely from unsafe water, sanitation and hygiene

ACTIVITY 6.11 Environmental determinants

Go to the WHO website that contains the country profiles for environmental burden of disease (http://www.who.int/quantifying_ehimpacts/national/countryprofile/en/). Download the profiles for Australia and for Angola, a developing nation in Africa. Prepare a table that compares each country profile side-by-side, and then answer the following questions:

- How does the per capita income compare between the two countries, and what impact do you think this has on environmentally-related disease outcomes?

- What are the differences in child mortality and life expectancy between the two countries, and are there specific environmental risk factors which may account for these differences?

- Are there specific risk factors or disease outcomes that are substantially different between the two countries, and what do you think the reasons for these differences are?

REFLECTION 6.11

Depending on the quality of the natural and built environment in a local area, the health status and quality of life for residents can be substantially impacted. In developed countries such as Australia, the types of environmental determinant that impact human health are substantially different to those in developing countries; however, no matter the country, a substantial proportion of the burden of disease is associated with environmental factors. It is important to reflect on the quality of life that you have and how this is related to your local environment, while also considering the impacts on others who may be subjected to quite different environmental conditions.

- lower respiratory infections (37 million DALYs per year), largely from indoor and outdoor air pollution

- unintentional injuries other than road traffic injuries (21 million DALYs per year), with this classification including a wide range of industrial and workplace accidents

- malaria (19 million DALYs per year), largely as a result of poor water resource, housing and land use management, which fails to curb vector populations effectively

- road traffic injuries (15 million DALYs per year), largely as a result of poor urban design or poor environmental design of transport systems

- chronic obstructive pulmonary disease (COPD) (12 million DALYs per year), largely as a result of exposures to workplace dusts and fumes, and other forms of indoor and outdoor air pollution

- perinatal conditions (11 million DALYs per year).

Country-by-country analysis is now available, describing the impact that environmental factors have on the health of residents of individual countries. As expected, Australia, along with most of the industrialised countries, fares well in comparison with developing countries. However, it is still estimated that there are 22,000 deaths each year in Australia due to environmental factors, equating to 14% of the total disease burden (WHO 2007). See Activity 6.11.

To complete the discussion on environmental determinants of health and disease in Australia, the following key environmental determinants have been identified by the AIHW (2010), and each of these will be further discussed in Chapter 12.

FOOD QUALITY AND SAFETY

Despite Australia having one of the safest food supplies in the world, it is estimated that the country has between 4 million and 7 million cases of food-borne gastroenteritis each year (Hall et al. 2005). This places a considerable burden on Australian society, costing an estimated $1.2 billion annually (Abelson et al. 2006) (see Case Study 6.2).

WATER QUALITY

Ensuring a safe drinking water supply is fundamental to maintaining good public health, with the quality of the water supply dependent on controlling chemical and microbiological contamination. Water quality in Australia is generally of a very high

CASE STUDY
6.2

Hepatitis A and oysters

In early 1997, a large food-borne illness outbreak occurred across a number of states in Australia, which was traced back to the consumption of oysters harvested from Wallis Lake in New South Wales. There were over 630 cases across the country, 60 hospitalisations and 1 death due to the outbreak. The pathogen responsible for the outbreak was hepatitis A, which is associated with faecal contamination of water or food, particularly foods that are not cooked after processing. In this case, in addition to the oysters being consumed raw, oysters are 'filter-feeders', which means that they filter nutrients out of the water in which they are growing. Therefore, if the water is contaminated, the oysters will also become contaminated. Even though oyster processors have sophisticated systems that try to flush out any contamination from the oysters, hepatitis A is particularly difficult to remove. The exact source of this outbreak could not be identified. However, there was evidence of inappropriate sewage disposal from residents and houseboats, and the outbreak could have also been triggered by excessive rainfall. In response to the outbreak, a comprehensive range of initiatives were implemented, such as upgrading sewerage systems, installing improved lake-side toilets, and improving waste-disposal practices by houseboats. This outbreak highlights the environmental health links between water contamination, food processing and changed food consumption preferences.

(Sources: Conaty et al. 2000, enHealth Council 2003)

CASE STUDY
6.3

Water fluoridation

Fluoridation of public water supplies is viewed as the most effective public health measure for preventing dental decay, with the majority of Australians now living in areas that are supplied with fluoridated mains water. However, there remains quite strident debate on the safety of this chemical and whether residents should have an option to have it added to their drinking water. The distribution of fluoridated water supplies is unequal, with most of the fluoridated supplies in large cities or capital cities as compared with rural areas.

standard, with 82% of water utilities reporting full compliance with microbiological and chemical contamination standards (National Water Commission 2009) (see Case Study 6.3).

AIR POLLUTION

Outdoor air quality in Australia is relatively good by international standards, but requires continual monitoring and regulation. Even though most of the air pollutants regularly monitored have decreased considerably since air quality standards were introduced, particulates and ozone remain of most concern, and are produced by motor vehicles, power generators and other industrial activities, on which we are increasingly dependent (see Case Study 6.4).

CASE STUDY 6.4

Health impacts of bushfires

A large number of epidemiological studies have demonstrated a link between exposure to particulate air pollution and respiratory health effects. The burden of disease can be substantial, as the populations exposed are large and the detrimental effects have been shown to occur at low levels of exposure. Even though motor vehicles are a primary source for particulate air pollution, bushfires, when they occur, can provide a substantial source of air pollution. Studies conducted in Australia and overseas indicate that there may be an association between exposure to bushfire smoke and an increase in respiratory conditions. This includes an increase in asthma symptoms and medication use, increased hospital attendance and admission for respiratory conditions, and an exacerbation of symptoms for those with chronic obstructive pulmonary disease. These results highlight the public health need for effectively managing bushfires and controlled burning activities.

(Sources: Chen et al. 2006, Johnston et al. 2006)

BUILT ENVIRONMENT

Australia is one of the most urbanised countries in the world, with two-thirds of Australians living in urban areas of greater than 100,000 people, and most people (60% of the total population) living in cities of more than 1 million people (Australian Bureau of Statistics 2008). The built environment, therefore, plays a significant role in the health status of communities. For example, high-density living may create conditions that are favourable to the spread of infectious diseases, while urban sprawl that encourages motor vehicle usage contributes to traffic noise, air pollution and traffic accidents while deterring physical activity (see Case Study 6.5).

GLOBAL CLIMATE CHANGE

As discussed in previous sections of this chapter, substantial changes in the world's ecosystems have been identified, and Australia is not immune to these changes. It is now widely recognised that much of this change is due to human activities, and the implications for Australia of these changes will be discussed in detail in Chapter 12.

A final word

The determinants of health have a profound effect on the health of individuals and communities. An evaluation of such determinants is an important part of developing any strategy to improve health. In this chapter we have covered definitions of determinants of health and the range of factors that might be considered as determinants, and discussed their importance in public health planning and implementation.

We have also examined the genetic, physical and environmental determinants of health in some detail. The environmental burden of disease for Australia is at the lower end of the scale, compared with other countries; however, at 14%, environmental factors contribute substantially to our overall disease burden.

This chapter provides a discussion of the 'multicausal' role of determinants of health, and the interrelationship of genetic and environmental determinants with physical determinants. In the next chapter, we deal with the social and emotional determinants of health.

CASE STUDY 6.5

Sick building syndrome

The term 'sick building syndrome' (SBS) is used to describe situations in which building occupants experience acute health and comfort effects, but no specific illness or cause can be identified. The complaints may be localised in a particular room or may be widespread throughout the building. In contrast, the term 'building-related illness' (BRI) is used when symptoms of diagnosable illness are identified and can be attributed directly to airborne building contaminants. It has been suggested that up to 30% of new and remodelled buildings worldwide may be the subject of excessive complaints related to indoor air quality. Often, this condition is temporary, but some buildings have long-term problems. Frequently, problems result when a building is operated or maintained in a manner that is inconsistent with its original design or prescribed operating procedures. Sometimes, indoor air problems are a result of poor building design or occupant activities. The main causes of SBS have been identified as inadequate ventilation, chemical contaminants from either indoor or outdoor sources, and biological contaminants such as moulds or bacteria, which can cause outbreaks like that of Legionnaires' disease. Even though SBS is a difficult 'condition' to diagnose and determine causes for, the quality of our indoor environments is known to impact on occupant comfort and performance.

(Source: US Environmental Protection Agency website 1991)

REVIEW QUESTIONS

1 Define a 'determinant', and describe the range of determinants that impact on health.

2 Describe what is meant by the 'multicausal role' of determinants, and how they impact on health.

3 Write a paragraph about the various types of diabetes, and how genetic factors impact on environmental determinants to influence the development of the disease.

4 How are 'environmental determinants' defined?

5 What is the relationship between ecosystems and health?

6 How does the environmental burden of disease for Australia compare with that for our neighbouring countries in South East Asia?

Useful websites

- Center for Health and the Global Environment (Harvard Medical School): http://chge.med.harvard.edu/
- Centers for Disease Control and Prevention—Office of Genomics and Disease Prevention: www.cdc.gov/genomics

- Centers for Disease Control and Prevention—One Health: http://www.cdc.gov/onehealth/about.html
- CDC Chronic Disease: www.cdc.gov/nccdphp
- Department of Health (Australia)—National Chronic Disease Strategy: https://www.health.gov.au/internet/main/publishing.nsf/Content/pq-ncds-strat
- Department of Health (Australia)—Nutrition and Physical Activity: https://www.health.gov.au/internet/main/publishing.nsf/Content/Nutrition+and+Physical+Activity-1
- Diabetes Australia Diabetes Information: http://www.diabetesaustralia.com.au/Understanding-Diabetes/
- Human Genome Project: http://www.genome.gov/10001772
- Millennium Ecosystem Assessment: www.millenniumassessment.org
- National Center for Biotechnology Information (NCBI): http://www.ncbi.nlm.nih.gov/
- National Human Genome Research Institute (NHGRI): http://www.genome.gov/
- Public Health Agency of Canada: www.publichealth.gc.ca
- US Department of Energy Genomics websites: http://genomics.energy.gov/
- World Health Organization: Health and development: http://www.who.int/hdp/en/
- World Health Organization—Noncommunicable diseases: http://www.who.int/topics/noncommunicable_diseases/en/
- World Health Organization—Quantifying environmental health impacts: www.who.int/quantifying_ehimpacts/en
- World Resources Institute: www.wri.org
- Worldwatch Institute: www.worldwatch.org

References

Abelson, P., Potter Forbes, M., Hall, G., 2006. The Annual Cost of Foodborne Illness in Australia. Australian Government Department of Health, Canberra.

Alcamo, J., Hassan, R.M., Bennett, E., 2003. Ecosystems and Human Wellbeing: A Framework for Assessment/Millennium Ecosystem Assessment. World Resources Institute, Washington DC.

Australian Bureau of Statistics (ABS), 2008. Census of population and housing (CDATA Online). Online. Available: <http://www.abs.gov.au/CDataOnline> (28 Feb 2014).

Australian Government Department of Health, 2014. Tobacco control. Online. Available: <http://www.health.gov.au/internet/main/publishing.nsf/Content/tobacco> (25 Aug 2014).

Australian Institute of Health and Welfare, 2004. Australia's Health 2004. AIHW Cat. No. AUS 44. AIHW, Canberra.

Australian Institute of Health and Welfare, 2010. Australia's Health 2010. AIHW Cat. No. AUS 122. AIHW, Canberra.

Australian Institute of Health and Welfare, 2012a. Australia's Health 2012. AIHW Cat. No. AUS 156. AIHW, Canberra.

Australian Institute of Health and Welfare, 2012b. National Health Priority Areas. Online. Available: <http://www.aihw.gov.au/national-health-priority-areas/> (29 Apr 2014).

Australian National Preventive Health Agency, 2013. State of Preventive Health 2013: Report to the Australian Government Minister for Health. ANPHA, Canberra. Online. Available: <http://www.anpha.gov.au/internet/anpha/publishing.nsf/Content/state-of-prev-health-2013> (25 Aug 2014).

Breast Cancer Network Australia website, 2010. Breast cancer in the family. Online. Available: <https://www.bcna.org.au/understanding-breast-cancer/breast-cancer-in-the-family/> (22 Aug 2014).

Campbell-Lendrum, D., Corvalan, C., Neira, M., 2007. Global climate change: implications for international public health policy. Bulletin of the World Health Organization 85 (3), 235–237.

Centers for Disease Control and Prevention, 2014. One Health. Online. Available: <http://www.cdc.gov/onehealth/about.html> (29 Apr 2014).

Chen, L., Verrall, K., Tong, S., 2006. Air particulate pollution due to bushfires and respiratory hospital admissions in Brisbane, Australia. International Journal of Environmental Health Research 16 (3), 181–191.

Chivian, E. (Ed.), 2002. Biodiversity: Its Importance to Human Health. Center for Health and the Global Environment, Harvard Medical School, Cambridge, MA.

Conaty, S., Bird, P., Bell, G., et al., 2000. Hepatitis A in New South Wales, Australia, from consumption of oysters: the first reported outbreak. Epidemiology and Infection 124, 121–130.

Council of Australian Governments (COAG), 2012. The roadmap for national mental health reform 2012–2022. Online. Available: <http://www.coag.gov.au/sites/default/files/The%20Roadmap%20for%20National%20Mental%20Health%20Reform%202012-2022.pdf.pdf> (29 Apr 2014).

Diabetes Australia, 2014. Understanding diabetes. Online. Available: <http://www.diabetesaustralia.com.au/Understanding-Diabetes/> (29 Apr 2014).

Doll, R., Hill, A.B., 1964. Mortality in relation to smoking: ten years' observations of British doctors. British Medical Journal 1, 1399–1467.

enHealth Council, 2003. Guidelines for Economic Evaluation of Environmental Health Planning and Assessment. Department of Health and Ageing, and enHealth Council, Canberra.

Europa Gateway to the European Union, 2014. Online. Available: <http://ec.europa.eu/health/index_en.htm> (23 Apr 2014).

Hall, G., Kirk, M.D., Becker, N., et al., 2005. Estimating foodborne gastroenteritis, Australia. Emerging Infectious Diseases 11 (8), 1257–1264, Online. Available: <http://www.cdc.gov/ncidod/EID/vol11no08/pdfs/04-1367.pdf> (7 Mar 2014).

Harper, A.C., Holman, C.D.J., Dawes, V.P., 1994. The Health of Populations: an Introduction. Churchill Livingston, Melbourne.

Health Development Agency, 2012. Environmental Health 2012: A Key Partner in Delivering the Public Health Agenda. NICE, London. Available: <www.nice.org.uk>.

Jackson, L.E., Daniel, J., McCorkle, B., et al., 2013. Linking ecosystem services and human health: the Eco-Health Relationship Browser. International Journal of Public Health 58, 747–755.

Johnston, F.H., Webby, R.J., Pilotto, L.S., et al., 2006. Vegetation fires, particulate air pollution and asthma: a panel study in the Australian monsoon tropics. International Journal of Environmental Health Research 16 (6), 391–404.

Keleher, H., Murphy, B. (Eds.), 2004. Understanding Health: A Determinants Approach. Oxford University Press, Melbourne.

Levy, K., Daily, G., Myers, S.S., 2012. Human health as an ecosystem service: a conceptual framework. In: Ingram, J.C., DeClercke, F., Rumbaitis del Rio, C. (Eds.), Integrating Ecology and Poverty Reduction: Ecological Dimensions. Springer, New York, pp. 231–251.

McMichael, A.J., Kjellstrom, T., Smith, K.R., 2006. Environmental health. In: Merson, M.H., Black, R.E., Mills, A.J. (Eds.), International Public Health: Diseases, Programs, Systems, and Policies, second ed. Jones and Bartlett Learning, Sudbury, MA, pp. 393–443.

Melillo, J., Sala, O., 2008. Ecosystem services. In: Chivian, E., Bernstein, A. (Eds.), Sustaining Life: How Human Health Depends on Biodiversity. Oxford University Press, New York, pp. 75–116.

Millennium Ecosystem Assessment, 2005. Ecosystems and Human Wellbeing: Biodiversity Synthesis. World Resources Institute, Washington DC.

Ministerial Council on Drug Strategy, 2011. National Drug Strategy 2010–2015. Commonwealth of Australia, Canberra.

Murray, C.J.M., Lopez, A., 1996. The Global Burden of Disease: A Comprehensive Assessment of Mortality and Disability from Disease, Injuries and Risk Factors in 1990 and Projected to 2020. Harvard University Press, Cambridge, MA.

National Health and Medical Research Council, 2009. Australian Guidelines to Reduce Health Risks from Drinking Alcohol. NHMRC, Canberra.

National Public Health Partnership, 2004a. The National Injury Prevention and Safety Promotion Plan: 2004–2014. NPHP, Canberra. Online. Available: <http://www.health.gov.au/internet/main/publishing.nsf/content/health-pubhlth-strateg-injury-index.htm> (28 Feb 2014).

National Public Health Partnership, 2004b. The National Falls Prevention for Older People Plan: 2004 onwards.

National Public Health Partnership, 2005. National Aboriginal and Torres Strait Islander Safety Promotion Strategy. Online. Available: <http://www.health.gov.au/internet/main/publishing.nsf/content/health-pubhlth-strateg-injury-index.htm> (28 Feb 2014).

National Water Commission, 2009. National Performance Report 2007–2008: Urban Water Utilities. NWC, Canberra.

Office of Disease Prevention, 2007. Healthy People 2010. US Department of Health and Human Services, Washington. DC.

Owen, N., Healy, G.N., Matthews, C.E., et al., 2010. Too much sitting: the population health science of sedentary behavior. Exercise and Sport Sciences Reviews 38 (3), 105–113.

Prüss-Üstün, A., Corvalán, C., 2006. Preventing Disease Through Healthy Environments: Towards an Estimate of the Environmental Burden of Disease. World Health Organization, Geneva.

Public Health Agency of Canada, 2011. What determines health? Online. Available: <http://www.phac-aspc.gc.ca/ph-sp/determinants/index-eng.php>.

Secretariat of the Convention on Biological Diversity, 2010. Global Biodiversity Outlook 3—Executive Summary. Secretariat of the Convention on Biological Diversity, Montréal.

Soskolne, C., Sieswerda, L.E., 2007. Environmental determinants of health. Encyclopedia of Public Health. Online. Available: <http://www.answers.com/topic/environmental-determinants-of-health> (30 Apr 2014).

Turnock, B.J., 2012. Essentials of Public Health. 2nd ed. Jones and Bartlett Learning, Sudbury, MA.

Turrell, G., Stanley, L., de Looper, M., et al., 2006. Health Inequalities in Australia: Morbidity, Health Behaviours, Risk Factors and Health Service Use. Queensland University of Technology and AIHW, Canberra.

US Environmental Protection Agency, 1991. Indoor Air Facts No. 4 (revised): Sick Building Syndrome. Online. Available: <http://www.epa.gov/iaq/pdfs/sick_building_factsheet.pdf> (29 Apr 2014).

World Health Organization, 2004. Global strategy on diet, physical activity and health. Online. Available: <http://www.who.int/dietphysicalactivity/strategy/eb11344/strategy_english_web.pdf> (29 Apr 2014).

World Health Organization, 2007. Country profiles of environmental burden of disease. Online. Available: <http://www.who.int/quantifying_ehimpacts/countryprofiles> (29 Apr 2014).

World Health Organization, 2009. Global Health Risks: Mortality and Burden of Disease Attributable to Selected Major Risks. WHO, Geneva.

World Health Organization, 2013. World Malaria Report 2013. WHO Global Malaria Programme, WHO, Geneva.

CHAPTER 7

Social and emotional determinants of health

Elizabeth Parker

Learning objectives

After reading this chapter, you should be able to:

- describe what is meant by socioeconomic differences in health, and the social and emotional determinants of health

- understand how health inequalities are affected by the social and economic circumstances that people experience throughout their lives

- discuss how factors such as living and working conditions, income, place and education can impact on health

- identify actions for public health policymakers that have the potential to make a difference in improving health outcomes within populations

- appreciate the concepts of social cohesion and social capital, and their role as potential protective factors in health

- understand conceptual models that can assist in analysing these issues.

Introduction

In Chapter 6, you were introduced to the concept of the determinants of health, and, specifically, the biological and environmental determinants of the health of Australians. In this chapter, we extend this to include the social, economic and emotional determinants of health. After reading both of these chapters, you should understand the interactions that people's biological, environmental, social and emotional life circumstances have on their health. This information is important for all health professional students.

In exploring the central theme of why some people are healthy and others are not, Evans et al. (1994 p 3) claimed that 'top people live longer'. That is, there is a gap between the health of those at the top of the socioeconomic scale and those at the bottom (Evans et al. 1994). In Australia, there are differences between the health of urban and rural Australians, between Aboriginal and Torres Strait Islander peoples and non-Indigenous Australians, and between different ethnic groups. The observation by Evans et al. (1994) regarding the gap in health status between those at the top of the socioeconomic scale and those at the bottom still holds in Australia (Turrell et al. 1999) and in most other countries; furthermore, the gap in health status is widening in many countries (Marmot & Bell 2006).

The Australian Institute of Health and Welfare (Australian Institute of Health and Welfare (AIHW) 2010) also claims that people's general backgrounds influence their levels of security, hygiene, nourishment, technology, information and freedom, and the morale of societies, and thus their health status. It is difficult to quantify these factors, let alone assess their impact precisely. 'Many things affect how healthy we are, ranging from the macro to the molecular: from society-wide influences, right down to highly individual factors such genetic make up …' (AIHW 2012 p 11). 'Some of these actions can be direct (such as being burnt by the sun), whereas others are less direct (such as education improving our understanding of health information …)' (AIHW 2012 p 11). Over the past 20 years, the evidence regarding health inequalities both within and between countries, and how these inequalities are linked to socio-economic position in society, is irrefutable (Australian Bureau of Statistics (ABS) 2010a; Marmot 2006; Wilkinson & Marmot 2003). The ongoing challenge for public health is to translate this research into effective policies and programs to close this health status gap, and to explain more clearly the factors implicated in mortality (death) and morbidity (illness). Indeed, Baum et al. (2013 p 503) acknowledged the newly elected Coalition Government's commitment to medical research, but exhorted the National Health and Medical Research Council to 'give greater emphasis in its grant allocation priorities to research on public health and social determinants research'.

Socioeconomic determinants and the health inequalities jigsaw

Health status both influences and is influenced by a variety of socioeconomic factors, such as income and education. For example, if you are disabled, you may have limited work opportunities, and this will have an impact on your income. The AIHW suggests that the socioeconomic characteristics that influence health include not only income and education, but also 'occupation, marital and family status, labour force participation, housing, ethnic origin and characteristics of the area of residence' (AIHW 2006 p 153). We will discuss these factors to help you to understand how they could impact on the health of your patients and communities.

This association of socioeconomic characteristics with health inequities began to receive the attention it deserved with the release of the *Black Report* (Black et al. 1980). The report had three components: a description of differences between occupational classes in mortality, morbidity, and use of health services; an analysis of likely explanations and recommendations for further research; and a strategy to reduce health inequalities or their consequences (Macintyre 1997). The findings revealed 'marked differences in mortality rates between occupational classes for both sexes and at all ages, and a class[1] gradient can be observed for most causes of death, a lack of improvement and in some cases deterioration of the health experience of unskilled and semi-skilled manual classes and inequalities exist in the utilisation of health services, especially preventive services' (Townsend & Davidson 1992 p 198).

These findings were echoed in the United Kingdom's *Whitehall Study of Civil Servants* that began in 1967 (Langenberg et al. 2005). It examined the 25-year mortality of men (aged 40–69 in 1967), showing the social gradient[2] by type of occupation within the civil service (Langenberg et al. 2005). Marmot (2006) claims that men second from the top of the occupational hierarchy within the civil service had a higher rate of death than men at the top, while those who were third from the top had a higher rate of death than those second from the top. In *Whitehall II*, launched 20 years after the first Whitehall study, women were included, and the gradient in mortality applied to most of the major causes of death, especially heart disease.

In the Whitehall study, all of the respondents were employed, yet those in the bottom tier of the workforce had the worst health. It makes sense that unemployment would lead to poorer health, because of the lack of funds to enable the purchase of some of the requirements for good health, such as good-quality foods and healthcare. The reverse may also hold—that is, those who are ill become unemployed or are forced to leave the labour force.

The evidence of social and economic determinants and health inequalities is compelling, whether within developed countries such as Canada and Australia, newly developed countries such as Brazil and India, or developing countries such as in Africa (Marmot & Bell 2006). While health is multifactorial and influenced by one's genetic makeup and biology (as discussed in Chapter 6), there is a strong correlation between social conditions and a person's position within society, and their health. As Turrell and Kavanagh (2004) put it:

> While health inequalities often differ in magnitude among these countries (reflecting in part differing social, political, economic and cultural systems) the overall picture is very similar. Illness and death are patterned in ways that indicate that those with the least access to social and economic resources are the most disadvantaged in terms of their health. (Turrell & Kavanagh 2004 p 393)

ACTIVITY 7.1 Social gradient of health

- Write down your answers to the following questions: What is meant by a 'social gradient in health'? Research further the findings of the *Black Report* and the Whitehall studies—are they still relevant? Do you believe less healthy behaviour is more prevalent in circumstances of social and economic disadvantage? If so, why should that occur, particularly if knowledge about risk behaviours (e.g. tobacco smoking) is widely disseminated through the media and health centres?

Marmot (2006) gives an example of these differences in a study on health disparities. There was a large difference in male life expectancy between two areas in London even though they were within close proximity of each other—Somers Town (70 years) and Hampstead (81 years) (Marmot 2006).

Increasingly, there is evidence that people's health is shaped by the social and economic circumstances that they experience differentially throughout their life. 'Those at the lower end of the socioeconomic hierarchy have poorer health partly as a consequence of material disadvantage such as living on a low income or working in a hazardous job, partly as a result of less healthy behaviours, and partly as a result of psycho-social factors such as anxiety, stress, social isolation and feelings of lack of control' (Turrell &

Kavanagh 2004 p 392). This is called the *social gradient in health*, one that runs across society, with the most profound differences in health seen between the most and the least disadvantaged members of society. For example, those in the upper middle levels of 'least disadvantage' will have better health than those in the lower middle levels of 'least disadvantage' (World Health Organization (WHO) 2003).

In the next section, we discuss various characteristics of socioeconomic position and how these influence people's health. Although discussed separately, each of these characteristics and their health effects are interrelated.

> **REFLECTION 7.1**
>
> Did you suggest that a social gradient in health is about the fact that inequalities in population health status are related to inequalities in social status? What should the role of public health be in addressing these challenges? Search online for the nineteenth-century doctor William Farr. Can you see the relevance of his work to current public health issues? Is less healthy behaviour more prevalent in circumstances of social and economic disadvantage?

Socioeconomic characteristics that influence health

Education

Education is an important determinant of health, as it enhances skills, job opportunities and workforce mobility. One measure of the level of education within society is retention rates in Year 12. In Australia, the retention rate of students in high school has increased over the past 30 years. In 1980, 32% of males and 37% of females completed Year 12 (AIHW 2005). In 2008, the national retention rate was 75% (ABS 2009), an increase from 72% in 1998. Rates were higher for females (81%) than for males (69%) (AIHW 2010 p 79). And education levels in Australia are increasing. The proportion of people with non-school qualifications increased from 51% in 2001 to 59% in 2010–11 (ABS 2012). Of those employed, almost two-thirds (65%) held a qualification, compared with 45% of those who were unemployed, and 38% of those not in the labour force held no qualification (ABS 2012). While Aboriginal and Torres Strait Islander Australians' education levels increased, they were less likely to complete their final years of schooling than non-Indigenous students (49% compared with 81%) in 2011 (ABS 2010b). There was a steady improvement in the retention rates of Aboriginal and Torres Straits Islander Australians in Years 7 and 8 to Year 12, from 35% in 1999 to 45% in 2009 (Purdie & Buckley 2010).

Why do you think education is important to health? Analysis of data from the Swedish Census showed 'a remarkable social gradient in mortality' (Erikson 2001 p 2084). Erikson (2001) discovered that in men, the higher the educational level, the lower the mortality risk. What is it about having an education that has a protective effect against behavioural risk factors such as tobacco smoking and being overweight, and risk conditions (sometimes called 'material circumstances') such as poor and unstable housing, lower income and fewer work choices? Other authors also report a correlation between higher levels of education and lower mortality, with reduced levels of smoking and alcohol consumption, and increased likelihoods of using preventive care such as immunisation and cancer screening (Cutler & Lleras-Muney 2008, Cutler & Frisvold 2009). A US study found that those who do not have a high-school degree have poorer health compared with those who have completed college (Hummer & Hernandez 2013).

Clearly, there is a link between education and improved health outcomes and opportunities. The Organisation for Economic Co-operation and Development (OECD) claims that upward mobility is a significant feature of Australia's education system, for as many as 41% of 25–34-year-old non-students have attained tertiary education despite being from socioeconomically disadvantaged backgrounds and having parents with low levels of education (OECD 2013). 'Forty-nine per cent of young Australians in this group have attained a higher level of education than their parents, and families with low levels of education enjoy better than average educational opportunities' (OECD 2013 p 4). This is the fifth highest level of upward mobility out of 29 OECD countries with available data.

In summary, education provides opportunities for income and job security, and gives people a sense of control over their life choices, and, as the research indicates, this has consequences for better health opportunities and outcomes.

We now introduce income as one of the interrelated socioeconomic characteristics under discussion.

Income

The AIHW (2006) claims that income is related strongly to health, particularly in lower-income countries, and that it provides psychological benefits, such as feeling in control. This makes intuitive sense, and is borne out in Australian data—for example, socioeconomic disadvantage is associated with 19% per cent of the mortality burden for males and 12% for females (AIHW 2006). The challenge for public health researchers, policymakers and planners is to build evidence about the interrelationships between income and the other socioeconomic characteristics in order to understand how they influence health.

Work and employment status

There has been an increase in unemployment in Australia from 5.2% in 2006 (AIHW 2006) to 5.8% in December 2013 (ABS 2014). At the latter time, there were 722,000 unemployed persons in Australia (ABS 2014). The increase in unemployment was most marked in Victoria (6.2%) and in Western Australia (4.3%) (ABS 2014). There is continuing evidence that unemployment is linked to health status (AIHW 2006). Draper et al. (2004, in AIHW 2006 p 155) claimed that there is evidence of an association between occupation and mortality: 'persons employed in manual occupations have higher mortality rates for most causes of death than those employed in clerical or managerial professional occupations'. This could be related to more hazardous work, such as in factories, farming and mining, where there is a higher risk of injury. Research is ongoing into the impact of occupational status above and beyond those workplace hazards. There is a change in the workforce profile in Australia with the increased 'casualisation' of the workforce. About 2.2 million, or one in five of all workers in Australia, are employed as 'casuals' (Sheen 2012). A casual job is one without paid leave entitlements, or redundancy packages, and employees are paid on an hour-to-hour, week-to-week, year-to-year basis. Does casual work and perceived job insecurity have an impact on health? Research with a small cohort ($n = 1071$), surveyed at age 32 and 40, revealed that perceived job insecurity can lead to adverse health effects in both permanent and temporary employees (Virtanen et al. 2011).

We now examine the influence of place or location on health inequalities.

Place or geographical location

Did you know that your health and health-related behaviours can be affected by the neighbourhood in which you live? (Botticello 2009, Chum 2011, Godley et al. 2010, Marmot 2006, Turrell et al. 2010, Turrell et al. 2012). Godley et al. (2010) discovered a link between self-reported poorer health status and socioeconomically disadvantaged neighbourhoods in Calgary, Canada. In addition, in a multilevel longitudinal study of physical activity (PA) in middle-aged men and women (40–65 years) in 200 neighbourhoods in Brisbane, Turrell et al. (2010 p 2) concluded that 'levels of PA varied significantly across Brisbane's neighborhoods, and neighborhood disadvantage accounted for some of this variation', and 'neighborhoods may exert a contextual effect on residents' likelihood of participating in PA'.

A number of authors have proposed hypotheses about the relationship between geographical location and health. For example, a cross-sectional analysis of 4286 women aged 60 to 79 years old from 457 British electoral areas found that the odds of coronary heart disease was 27% greater for those women living in electoral 'wards' (electorates) that were 'deprived' (Lawlor et al. 2005). The more deprived an area, the higher the odds of coronary heart disease. In a study of residence and socioeconomic status and its impact on children's health in South Australia, Spurrier et al. (2012) discovered that four-year-old Aboriginal children were more overweight and obese compared with their non-Aboriginal peers. The authors declare that 'a significant investment is required to optimise the health of Aboriginal women before pregnancy and throughout pregnancy, and dietary management in early childhood' (Spurrier et al. 2012). Giskes et al. (2006) followed a group of 404 smokers in 83 areas in the Netherlands for six years. They concluded that the socioeconomic factors of the areas where people live impact on their ability to stop smoking (Giskes et al. 2006).

Contextual effects are the collective aspects of local areas where people live that impact on their health and wellbeing. *Compositional effects* describe the socioeconomic position we hold in terms of income, education and employment status; and these are generally predictors of positive health behaviours and subsequent health outcomes. However, contextual area effects can exert more influence than compositional effects on health, although there is varying opinion on explanations for the causes of such differences. Is it because there are better and more accessible 'collective resources in better-off neighbourhoods or is worse/better health because of the discrepancy between an individual's situation and those around them?' (Stafford & Marmot 2003 p 357).

A range of authors corroborate the evidence that 'place' does matter in influencing health behaviours and outcomes (Carroll et al. 2007, 2008, Kamphuis et al. 2008, Kavanagh et al. 2007, King et al. 2006). Area of residence and neighbourhood are significant for encouraging health behaviours, such as cycling in Melbourne (Kamphuis et al. 2008); and overweight/obesity in Australia is influenced by social disadvantage and place of residence (King et al. 2006). The health of rural Australians is an example of area effects and health. Thirty-two per cent of Australians live in rural and/or remote communities (NRHA 2013). One would assume that access to health services such as doctors and hospitals would be an influential factor, but, even accounting for that factor, health profile differences between rural and urban Australians are significant (AIHW 2006). On average, 'people who live in regional and remote areas have shorter lives and higher levels of some illnesses than people who live in major cities' (AIHW 2008 p 81). 'And are more likely to engage in behaviours that are associated with poorer health, such as tobacco smoking and physical inactivity' (AIHW 2012 p 49). While there would be individual socioeconomic differences between individuals in these communities, the collective health profile of rural Australians is poorer than that of urban areas. Studies examining the contextual and compositional effects of living in rural Australia are warranted.

Gender

Gender is another interrelated socioeconomic characteristic. Gender has been used to refer to 'attributes, characteristics, stereotypes, social environments as well as genetic status' (Davidson et al. 2006 p 733). While women's life expectancy is higher than men's in Australia, women tend to report more physical illness, more psychological distress, and more psychiatric symptoms than do men (AIHW 2006). Women living in socioeconomically disadvantaged areas and Indigenous women have higher fertility rates than those in areas of least socioeconomic disadvantage

---

ACTIVITY 7.5 Contextual and compositional factors

- With a group of students, write a short summary of the difference between *contextual* and *compositional* factors, and their influence on health. Can you speculate as to why living in a disadvantaged area is linked to poor health? Apart from poor access to health services, including hospitals, health behaviours are poor for many rural and remote Australians. Discuss whether contextual and/or compositional factors could influence health in rural and remote communities.

REFLECTION 7.5

Remember that public health is about populations. There will be differences in the health status of specific individuals within the populations and subpopulations, but it is the *overall* population health profile between and among groups that public health is interested in, and why these differences occur.

(AIHW 2012). Women in lower socioeconomic areas 'also reported consulting doctors more often, but dentists less often. Women who live in these areas were also less likely to report having had a recent pap smear' (AIHW 2006 p 233).

Interestingly, educational qualifications are particularly good predictors of women's self-assessed health. An education enhances both women's sense of self and their self-reported health status. However, men's unemployment has adverse consequences for the health of their wives, due to the family living in disadvantaged material circumstances. Women's participation in employment and their family role have undergone substantial changes over the past 40 years, so approaches to measuring inequalities in women's health need to reflect changes in women's employment participation, and changes in marital status and living arrangements (Arber 2002). To expand your knowledge about gender and health, see Bird (2008).

The next section tries to unravel the intricacies of the social and emotional determinants of health by examining a number of propositions, and presents frameworks to assist public health in addressing these issues.

> **ACTIVITY 7.6 Health profiles**
>
> - Consolidate your understanding of the above issues by writing a paragraph on the following statement: research shows undeniably that being socially and economically disadvantaged is hazardous to your health. Find examples from the literature to argue your point.
> - With a group of students, research the difference in health profiles of unemployed young adult men (18–25 years) and young adult women (18–25 years).

> **REFLECTION 7.6**
>
> If you were the Minister of Health for the state you live in and were shown some of this evidence, what other government departments would you recommend your staff work with to plan public health actions? In thinking this through, what would be the strengths and limitations of such an approach?

A public health framework to address the social determinants of health

Reducing health inequalities

Reducing health inequalities is not an easy task for public health. Turrell and Kavanagh claim that 'meeting this challenge requires will and commitment on the part of politicians, all government departments (not only health), non-government organisations, private sector companies and other groups and organisations' (2004 p 392). Specific actions to reduce social gradients should include:

- changes to macro-level social and economic policies
- improving living and working conditions
- strengthening communities for health
- improving behavioural risk factors
- empowering individuals and strengthening their social networks
- improving responses from the healthcare system and associated treatment services (Oldenburg et al. 2000a, 2000b).

Frameworks help us investigate complex issues. The frameworks in this chapter assist us to analyse the characteristics of the social determinants of health to provide options for actions to tackle these inequalities and to design policies and programs to create improved health opportunities for all segments of the community.

Turrell et al. (1999) developed a framework that illustrates how all the pieces of the health inequalities jigsaw fit together, and how public health might address the unequal patterning of health in the community (see Figure 7.1). The framework has

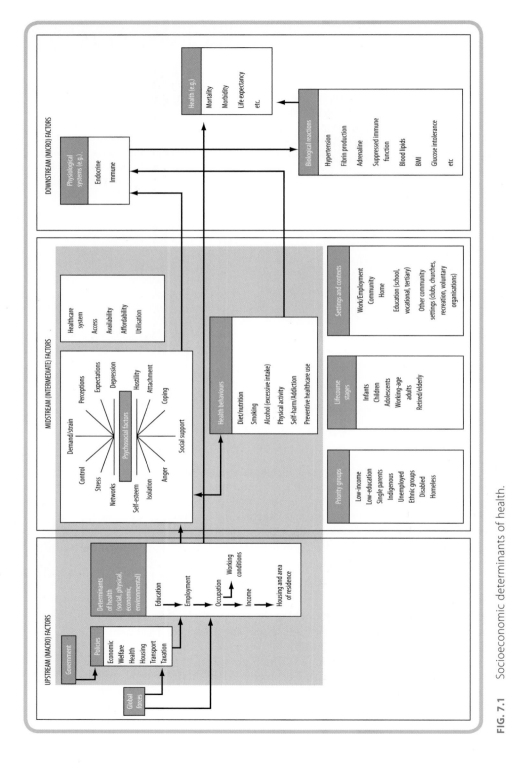

FIG. 7.1   Socioeconomic determinants of health.

(Source: Reproduced from Turrell et al. 1999, © Queensland University of Technology, School of Public Health, Centre for Health Research)

three dominant features: upstream, midstream and downstream factors. These factors, while discrete, are interconnected. These terms are also discussed in Chapter 14.

UPSTREAM FACTORS

Upstream factors (or macro-level) factors include international influences, government policies and the fundamental social, physical, economic and environmental determinants of health. The government policies that can be influential in creating health opportunities are access to housing, transport, economics and welfare (e.g. unemployment benefits and family allowances).

MIDSTREAM FACTORS

You can see the range of 'midstream or intermediate-level factors' on the framework, such as diet/nutrition, smoking, lack of physical activity and the intake of excess alcohol. Other midstream factors could include mental health and depression. These midstream-level factors are often called 'behavioural risk factors'.

DOWNSTREAM FACTORS

These are the micro-level factors that are influenced by the upstream and midstream factors. The downstream factors include biological and physiological reactions to all of these influences, which in turn shape health outcomes, such as mortality, morbidity, quality of life and life expectancy.

Mackenbach and Stronks (2002) argue that a combination of strategies at the three levels is needed to reduce health inequalities. Upstream measures include improving physical and psychosocial work environments, reducing smoking in lower socioeconomic groups, improving nutrition (preferably through universal measures such as healthier school meals), and reducing childhood poverty. Turrell et al. (1999) would view these as midstream, under health behaviours. Downstream policies include healthcare policies that 'improve accessibility for lower socioeconomic groups' (Turrell et al. 1999 p 104). The point of Mackenbach and Stronks's (2002) argument is that it is a *combination* of strategies that is needed at these three levels to make a difference.

The purpose of Case Study 7.1 is for you to think about how the Turrell et al. (1999) model could be used in practice to examine policy and program options to improve health.

ACTIVITY 7.7 Influence of upstream, midstream and downstream policies

- Complete the following activities with a group of students. List two upstream policies that are not identified in the Turrell et al. (1999) framework that could potentially have an impact on people's opportunities for health. One of the 'risky' health behaviours is low physical activity (PA). To increase PA, should municipal swimming pools be free-of-charge to those who are unemployed or on a pension? Or should they be free for everyone? Should there be more publicly-funded gyms open free-of-charge to the public? If you think so, why aren't they free now?

REFLECTION 7.7

What options did you propose in order to provide accessible PA opportunities? Would these make a difference? Walking paths are 'free', yet not everyone uses them! Working on midstream factors to reduce risky behaviour requires more than a single strategy, such as having free entry to pools. In Chapter 14, a range of health promotion success stories are presented. Essentially, public health policies and actions have to work across upstream, midstream and downstream factors to make a difference.

ACTIVITY 7.8 Social and psychosocial determinants of health

- What characteristics of disadvantage can you identify in Case Study 7.1? Can you make any connections between the social and psychosocial determinants of health? Using the Turrell et al. (1999) *framework— socioeconomic determinants of health*, plot the links between each of your identified characteristics so that you get a full picture of the issues. What range of public health policies and programs would you implement to assist Leila and other refugee families?

CASE STUDY 7.1

Leila, a refugee

You are a 34-year-old woman called Leila, and have arrived in Australia as a refugee with your four children. You are part of a group of refugee women who have arrived in Australia together. Your husbands were killed in a civil war in your country. You had your last child in the refugee camp, where you waited for food trucks each week to deliver food and medical supplies. You have been waiting for three years to be settled somewhere outside your country. You speak three languages, but not English. You have finally been granted refugee status in Australia, and now are settled in a suburb with one other family from your country of origin—people you do not know very well. The local bus goes infrequently during the day to the shopping centre, where the food is totally different from what you know, and it is difficult to understand the cooking instructions on the labels. You pick up your children from the local school in the afternoon, a 15-minute walk from your house. On days when you shop, you have to take the bus to the shopping centre, pick up some groceries, and time your trips to ensure you are home to pick up your children.

You have decided to make contact with the other family in the suburb—neither of you has a car, but you have made telephone contact. Both you and the other woman feel stressed and depressed, are homesick and are grieving for your husbands. You are both really keen to begin English classes at the local TAFE (Technical and Further Education) college, and wonder how you will manage it all. Your family allowance covers some basic essentials, yet you realise that without English it will be difficult to get work. Your children want Australian sporting equipment, like a cricket bat and a soccer ball, and you know that having these is important for them to fit in.

REFLECTION 7.8

Were there connections between the social and psychosocial determinants of health? When you mapped your identified characteristics, could you see how the upstream or macro-level policies—such as transport and access to English language classes—had the potential to improve refugees' quality of life? What happens when people who do not speak English seek healthcare in a local clinic?

Social and economic disadvantage and emotional health

We now turn to a brief examination of the impact of social and economic disadvantage on *emotional health*. Social and economic disadvantage can affect the emotional health of many vulnerable populations—for example, refugees who have experienced trauma in war and dispossession. We discuss specifically the impact of this disadvantage on children, as universally they are the most vulnerable. It makes intuitive sense that patterns of health established in childhood will have some bearing on an individual's adult health, for example through the establishment of good nutrition, exercise, structured and orderly lives, play and emotional security. Moreover, there is a substantial body of research that suggests that parental socioeconomic disadvantage is associated with mental health problems in children (Najman et al. 2004). In a large study following mothers and their children at 3–5 days, 6 months, 5 and 14 years, the children from low-income families were 'found to have higher rates of problems with language and reasoning ability, and these were observed at 5 and 14 years of age' (Najman et al. 2004 p 1155). The authors conclude that 'at ages 5 and 14, children born to mothers in the lowest socio-economic status group have a much greater likelihood of manifesting cognitive development problems, and their mental and emotional health is more likely to be impaired' (Najman et al. 2004 p 1156). Teenage maternity was associated with an increased risk of child mental health impairment at five years of age, but not necessarily at an older age. Thus, socioeconomic disadvantage in childhood has the potential to have a deleterious effect on adult health (Najman et al. 2004). In an analysis of two sets of data from the Longitudinal Study of Australian Children (LSAC) up to age seven, Nicholson et al. (2012 p 81) claim that 'disadvantage was associated with poorer outcomes across most measures of physical and developmental health and showed no evidence of either strengthening or attenuating at older compared to younger ages. Findings confirm the importance of early childhood as a key focus for health promotion and prevention efforts.'

This research corroborates a review of eight studies that examined the relationship between socioeconomic status and mental and psychosocial morbidity among children (Turrell et al. 1999). Children from lower-socioeconomic-status backgrounds were more likely to experience behavioural disturbances and social problems, or be diagnosed as autistic, and infants were more likely to experience a shorter duration of breastfeeding or none at all (Turrell et al. 1999).

> **ACTIVITY 7.9 Social and economic disadvantage**
>
> - Can you identify from your readings what aspects of social and economic disadvantage potentially compromise children's health? Research the types of program that are available in your local area to assist families who have children and are under financial and/or housing stress—for example, food banks and children's toy libraries.

> **REFLECTION 7.9**
>
> Did you know that many programs for families and children are provided by agencies, such as education, churches, libraries, social and service clubs, parks and recreation? Thus, the health of the community is everybody's business. This reinforces the concept you were introduced to early in the book about public health functioning across all sectors in the community.

The lifecourse approach

A lifecourse approach traces health outcomes across the lifecycle, and socioeconomic variability in adult disease 'is due to adverse exposure experienced in both early and later life' (Turrell & Kavanagh 2004 p 402). Adolescence is a vulnerable time of transition between the family-determined social status and adulthood, and health patterns adopted in childhood may continue or be altered in a more positive or negative direction.

Can socioeconomic status have an impact on adolescent depression and obesity, both of which increase the risk of cardiovascular disease? Goodman et al. (2003) analysed a large sample in the United States. The attributable risk of depression and obesity in the lowest-income households was profound. The impact of socioeconomic status and the social and environmental backgrounds of adolescents as 'risk factors' are often ignored when examining adolescent behavioural choices (Goodman et al. 2003). In other words, public health efforts need to focus on socioeconomic status in designing programs for adolescents, as it is a strong determinant of lifestyle choices.

Keleher and Murphy (2004) pose a number of questions that need to be answered when examining mental health—for example, what is the extent to which literacy and education affect people's mental illness experience? What social support is available?

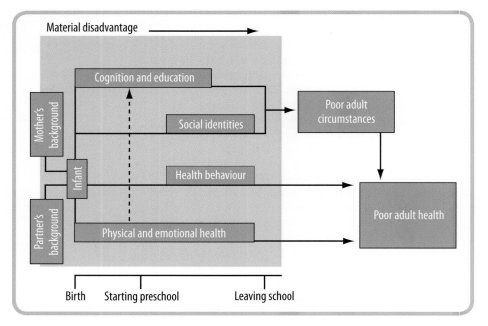

FIG. 7.2   Lifecourse framework.
(Source: Health Development Agency 2004. Reproduced with permission.)

They argue for a comprehensive approach: the need for accessible mental health services, early diagnosis of mental illness, and upstream factors that provide strong public health policy directions and investment in mental health awareness, such as the national depression initiative. Mental health is a National Health Priority Area (see Chapter 3).

Figure 7.2 demonstrates the connections between material disadvantage—poor income, limited education, limited work opportunities or unemployment—and physical and emotional health, from the early developmental years of childhood through to leaving school. The model provides a glimpse of the pathways to health and the interrelationships between contextual factors, such as material disadvantage and physical and emotional health, and how these patterns are connected across the lifecourse. While Turrell et al. (1999) provide an overarching framework in which to examine upstream, midstream and downstream factors at the macro- or 'big picture' level, Graham and Power (2004) focus specifically on the early years of life, and how material disadvantage has the potential to affect early childhood development. You can trace the links between cognition (intellectual development) and education, social identity, health behaviour and

> **ACTIVITY 7.10 Lifecourse approach to health**
>
> - With other students, identify why you think family income is linked to children's mental health. What is a lifecourse approach, and why is it used? Would a lifecourse approach be useful to analyse the health of the middle and later years of life? If you were a public health manager making recommendations in government, what advice would you give about the impact of disadvantage and emotional health, and where public investments should occur in order to make a difference?

physical and emotional health, and those patterns are potentially linked to poor adult circumstances and poor adult health. Nicholson et al. (2004) claim that family contexts exert a strong influence on health.

In studying this chapter, note that although poor health and the factors that influence this are more likely to be experienced by socioeconomically disadvantaged groups, health professionals should not inadvertently use these patterns as a basis for stereotyping and labelling individuals from disadvantaged backgrounds (Turrell & Kavanagh 2004). We now discuss the concepts of social cohesion and social capital as potential mediating factors in health inequalities.

> **REFLECTION 7.10**
>
> A lifecourse approach can be helpful in mapping policies and programs across the lifespan. In thinking about middle and older adulthood, did you consider that there are many potential public health issues that arise with the ageing of the population, such as having adequate recreation, and programs to reduce social isolation and loneliness?

Role of social cohesion and social capital

Can the social disadvantages that contribute to health inequalities be improved? There are a number of protective factors, such as psychosocial midstream factors. Note the psychosocial factors of support, self-esteem and social networks in the Turrell et al. (1999) framework. We are going to expand on these support factors by examining social cohesion and social capital—protective factors can have an impact on health and quality of life.

Social cohesion

Social cohesion is the connections and relations between societal units, such as individuals, groups and associations, or the glue that holds communities together (AIHW 2005). The majority of Australians are confident that they can rely on their support network in times of crisis, and make contact with family and friends on a weekly basis. Three-quarters of Australians donate to money to charities and non-profit organisations. Markedly smaller percentages are civically engaged, in terms of being regularly involved in the activities of political advocacy or a community organisation. However, less than half of Australians are socially trusting (of less well-known acquaintances and strangers) (AIHW 2005).

Interestingly, Marmot (2006) makes a point about the powerful influence of social cohesion on the stability of societies by pointing to countries such as Sri Lanka, Costa Rica and the state of Kerala in India. For example, the United States is the richest country in the world (apart from Luxembourg), but the life expectancy for males is similar to that of Costa Rica or Cuba. While the income levels across Costa Rica and Cuba are not high, and the material conditions for good health may not appear evident, as people may be relatively poor, the disparity between the highest-earning and the lowest-earning is relatively narrow, and social cohesion within these societies seems to play some part (Marmot 2006). Social cohesion includes social networks, and social networks keep people engaged with others. Being involved in social networks is good for health, as networks can provide social support, trust, friendship and mutual obligations, and there is evidence that social networks are linked to individual health outcomes (Berkman 2000). Social networks and social support include being in supportive families, relationships and organisations, and participating in informal networks through volunteering, playing group sport or participating in group cultural events. Social isolation, often part of being alone in old age, reduces contact with others, and therefore the experience of connectedness that is normally gained through a variety of social networks (Berkman 2000). There are challenges in research on social determinants and health, as most of the research is cross-sectional. There is also a need for further cohort studies to enrich our knowledge (see Chapter 5).

Social capital

One of the features of a socially integrated or cohesive society is that it has social capital (Berkman 2000). *Social capital* combines the concept of 'capital', an economic concept, with social concepts, such as fairness and trust (Pearce & Davey Smith 2003). Social capital is about people's trust and sense of belonging to networks and communities, which can strengthen social cohesion within communities. It represents trust and reciprocity within social networks and relationships (Winter 2000, Ziersch 2005). Putnam (1993) argues that people's networks, norms and human connections in the form of trust that can be transferred from one social setting to another, as well as community resources and civic engagement, are important for strengthening social ties and opportunities, and hence health.

In a study of 39 states in the United States, Kawachi et al. (1997) found that membership in voluntary groups and levels of social trust impact positively on mortality data. Mutual trust, a sense of belonging and reciprocity—that is mutual give-and-take and sharing—are all concepts of social capital.

Think about the natural disasters that Australia has faced in the past few years—the Victorian bushfires in 2009, the Queensland and Victorian floods in 2011, Cyclone Yasi in 2011, and the Blue Mountains bushfires in 2013. Thousands of volunteers assisted those in need, with donations of food, clothing and shelter, fund-raising, and cleaning up streets and houses. This surely is evidence of people's trust and sense of belonging, both of which are some of the hallmarks of social capital.

We need to be knowledgeable about of the impacts of social disadvantage on health, and, importantly, the protective role that social support, trust, reciprocity and social cohesion play in building social capital in our communities.

Can social capital have a negative effect? Healthy, positive uses of social capital include trust, cooperation, understanding, empathy, openness to new ideas, and alliances across differences. Unhealthy uses of social capital are racism, fear of the unknown, dislike of change and new ideas, and an 'us and them' mentality (Baum 1999). Additionally, entrenched norms of behaviour do not necessarily build 'trust and reciprocity', and may militate against advancing health. For example, in some groups violence against women is acceptable (Baum 1999). However, the evidence is increasingly compelling that, in general, social cohesion and social capital are protective factors for health.

These social forces can be examined as possible avenues and starting points for interventions, programs and policies to redress socioeconomic disadvantage, and improve physical and emotional health. Chapter 14 contains a community development model that can help you with your initiatives.

ACTIVITY 7.11 Social cohesion, social capital and health

- Find two articles on social cohesion and social capital, and health inequalities. With other students, discuss how the concepts have been applied to recent natural disasters in Australia. Are the concepts valid, in your view? Are there other public health problems and aspects that could benefit from integrating these concepts to improve health outcomes for the population?

REFLECTION 7.11

In your own life, do you have strong social networks of friends, family and neighbours? What were your thoughts on the US study that showed volunteering as a mechanism for building strong community social cohesion?

A final word

This chapter has introduced you to the social and emotional determinants of health by examining the influence of socioeconomic disadvantage on inequalities in health in populations. This is an overview of this complex field, and it is advisable that you read widely to gain a better understanding of the literature that is emerging in this area. We began by describing some of the characteristics of socioeconomic disadvantage, and the impact that these *interrelated* factors have on health. The framework by Turrell et al. (1999) identified the multilevel and diverse determinants of socioeconomic health inequalities. The links between compromised health in childhood, social and economic disadvantage, poor health behaviours, and the potential for poor health across the lifespan were introduced using visual representations of a lifecourse approach. Finally, concepts of social cohesion and social capital as potential protective factors for maintaining and promoting health were explained. Public health has always faced challenges that reach across all sectors of society, all levels of government, and the private and non-government sectors, and the problem of population health inequalities is a significant one. Ongoing international and national research is attempting to unravel the dynamics of inequalities in health and, significantly, the public health actions for all levels of society that can make a difference to improving health.

REVIEW QUESTIONS

1   What do you understand by the term 'socioeconomic disadvantage'?

2   What are the main messages from the *Black Report* and the Whitehall study?

3   Why are education, employment, income, area of residence, and gender important characteristics in health inequalities?

4   Low income and its link to potentially poor emotional health in children were introduced. Can you identify some of the risk factors that can affect positive growth over the lifecourse?

5   What do the terms 'downstream', 'midstream' and 'upstream' mean, and what are some of their key components?

6   How can 'social cohesion' and 'social capital' be helpful in understanding health inequalities, and what are the healthy and unhealthy uses of these concepts?

7   What implications does understanding socioeconomic disadvantage and health have for you as a health professional in counselling patients; or in designing a public health nutrition program for a community?

8   Imagine you are a health planner. You have learned that neighbourhood and area of residence can influence health. How would you assess the compositional and contextual factors to improve health in a poorer neighbourhood in the city/town/rural community where you live?

9   Changes are planned to Australia's car-manufacturing industry, with the closures of the General Motors and Toyota plants and their subsidiaries over the next few years. Knowing there is a link between work and health, what implications could these closures have for the health of the affected workers? What services could be needed?

10   Would you move to a rural area to become a farmer over the next five years? Explore further the health of rural Australians.

Endnotes

1   'Class' refers to social strata in societies, where members share certain social, economic or cultural attributes.

2   '*The socioeconomic gradient in health* refers to the worse health of those who are at a lower level of socioeconomic position—whether measured by income, occupational grade or educational attainment—even those who are already in relatively high socioeconomic groups' (Kawachi et al. 2002 p 649).

Useful websites

- Australian Institute of Health and Welfare: http://www.aihw.gov.au
- Australian Women's Health Network: http://www.awhn.org.au/
- World Health Organization: http://www.who.int/en

References

Arber, S., 2002. Comparing inequalities in women's and men's health: Britain in the 1990s. Social Science and Medicine 44 (6), 773–787.

Australian Bureau of Statistics, 2009. Australian Social Trends, Data Cube—Education and Training. ABS Cat. No. 4102.0. ABS, Canberra.

Australian Bureau of Statistics, 2010a. Health and Socioeconomic Disadvantage. Australian Social Trends 4102.0, Mar 2010. ABS, Canberra. Online. Available: <http://www.abs.gov.au/AUSSTATS/abs@.nsf/Lookup/4102.0Main+Features30Mar+2010> (30 Mar 2014).

Australian Bureau of Statistics, 2010b. The Health and Welfare of Australia's Aboriginal and Torres Strait Islander Peoples, October 2010. ABS, Canberra. Online. Available: <http://www.abs.gov.au/ausstats/abs@.nsf/mf/4704.0/> (15 Feb 2014).

Australian Bureau of Statistics, 2012. Qualifications and the Labour Market. 4235.0—Learning and Work, Australia, 2010–11. ABS, Canberra. Online. Available: <http://www.abs.gov.au/AUSSTATS/abs@.nsf/Lookup/4235.0Main+Features32010-11> (15 Feb 2014).

Australian Bureau of Statistics, 2014. 6202.0—Labour Force, Australia, Jan 2014. ABS, Canberra. Online. Available: <http://www.abs.gov.au/ausstats/abs@.nsf/mf/6202.0> (15 Feb 2014).

Australian Institute of Health and Welfare, 2005. Australia's Welfare 2005. AIHW Cat. No. AUS 65. AIHW, Canberra.

Australian Institute of Health and Welfare, 2006. Australia's Health 2006. AIHW Cat. No. AUS 73. AIHW, Canberra.

Australian Institute of Health and Welfare, 2008. Australia's Health 2008. AIHW Cat. No. AUS 99. AIHW, Canberra.

Australian Institute of Health and Welfare, 2010. Australia's Health 2010. AIHW Cat. No. AUS 122. AIHW, Canberra.

Australian Institute of Health and Welfare, 2012. Australia's Health 2012. AIHW Cat. No. AUS 156. AIHW, Canberra.

Baum, F., 1999. The role of social capital in health promotion: Australian perspectives. Health Promotion Journal of Australia 9 (3), 171–178.

Baum, F., Fisher, M., Trewin, D., et al., 2013. Funding the 'H' in NHMRC. Australian and New Zealand Journal of Public Health 37 (6), 503–505.

Berkman, L., 2000. Social support, social networks, social cohesion and health. Social Work in Health Care 31 (2), 3–14.

Bird, C., 2008. Gender and Health: The Effects of Constrained Choices and Social Policies. Cambridge University Press, Cambridge.

Black, D., Morris, J., Smith, C., et al., 1980. Inequalities in Health: Report of a Research Working Group. Department of Health and Social Security, London. ('The Black Report'.).

Botticello, A., 2009. School contextual influences on the risk of adolescent alcohol misuse. American Journal of Community Psychology 43 (1/2), 85–97.

Carroll, J.A., Adkins, B.A., Parker, E., 2007. 'Blogging about jogging': digital stories about physical activity from residents in a new urban environment with implications for future content and media choices in population health communication. In Proceedings 57th Annual Conference of the International Communication Association, San Francisco.

Carroll, J., Adkins, B., Parker, E., et al., 2008. My place through my eyes: a social constructionist approach to researching the relationships between socioeconomic living contexts and physical activity. International Journal of Qualitative Studies in Health and Well-Being 3, 204–218.

Chum, A., 2011. Policy implications of neighbourhood effects on health research: towards an alternative to poverty deconcentration. Health and Place 17, 1098–1104.

Cutler, D., Lleras-Muney, A., 2008. Education and health: evaluating theories and evidence. In: House, J., Schoeni, R., Kaplan, G., et al. (Eds.), Making Americans Healthier: Social and Economic Policy as Health Policy. Russell Sage Foundation, New York.

Cutler, J., Frisvold, D., 2009. Higher education and health investments: does more schooling affect preventive health care use? Journal of Human Capital 3 (2), 144–176.

Davidson, K., Trudeau, K., van Roosmalen, E., et al., 2006. Perspective: gender as a health determinant and implications for health education. Health Education and Behavior 33, 731–743.

Draper, G., Turrell, G., Oldenburg, B., 2004. Health Inequalities in Australia: Mortality. Health Inequalities Monitoring Series No. 1. Cat. No. 55. Queensland University of Technology and the Australian Institute of Health and Welfare, Canberra.

Erikson, R., 2001. Why do graduates live longer? In: Jonsson, J.O., Mills, C. (Eds.), Cradle to Grave: Life-course Change in Modern Sweden. Sociology Press, Durham, pp. 211–227.

Evans, R.G., Barer, M.L., Marmor, T.R. (Eds.), 1994. Why Are Some People Healthy and Others Not? The Determinants of Health of Populations. De Gruyter, New York.

Giskes, K., van Lenthe, F.J., Turrell, G., et al., 2006. Smokers living in deprived areas are less likely to quit: a longitudinal follow-up. Tobacco Control 15, 485–488.

Godley, J., Haines, V., Hawe, P., et al., 2010. Small area contextual effects on self-reported health: evidence from Riverside, Calgary. BMC Public Health 10, 264.

Goodman, E., Slap, G., Huang, B., 2003. The public health impact of socioeconomic status on adolescent depression and obesity. American Journal of Public Health 93 (11), 1844–1850.

Health Development Agency, 2004. Childhood disadvantage and adult health: a lifecourse framework. NICE, London. Available: <www.nice.org.uk>.

Hummer, R.A., Hernandez, E.M., 2013. The effect of educational attainment on adult mortality in the United States. Population Bulletin 68 (1), 1–15. Online. Available: <http://www.prb.org/pdf13/us-education-mortality.pdf> (7 Feb 2014).

Kamphuis, C.B.M., Giskes, K., Kavanagh, A.M., et al., 2008. Area variation in recreational cycling in Melbourne: a compositional or contextual effect? Journal of Epidemiology and Community Health 62 (10), 890–898.

Kavanagh, A., Thornton, L., Tattam, A., et al., 2007. Place Does Matter for Your Health: A Report of the Victorian Lifestyle and Neighbourhood Environment Study. University of Melbourne, Melbourne.

Kawachi, I., Kennedy, B.P., Lochner, K., et al., 1997. Social capital, income inequality and mortality. American Journal of Public Health 87, 1491–1498.

Kawachi, I., Subramanian, S., Almeida-Filho, N., 2002. A glossary for health inequalities. Journal of Epidemiology and Community Health 56 (9), 647–652.

Keleher, H., Murphy, B. (Eds.), 2004. Understanding Health: A Determinants Approach. Oxford University Press, South Melbourne.

King, T., Kavanagh, A.M., Jolley, D., et al., 2006. Weight and place: a multilevel cross-sectional survey of area-level social disadvantage and overweight/obesity in Australia. International Journal of Obesity 30, 281–287.

Langenberg, C., Martin, J., Shipley, G., et al., 2005. Adult socioeconomic position and the association between height and coronary heart disease mortality: findings from 33 years of follow-up in the Whitehall Study. American Journal of Public Health 95 (4), 628–632.

Lawlor, D., Davey Smith, G., Patel, R., et al., 2005. Life-course socioeconomic position, area deprivation, and coronary heart disease: findings from the British Women's Heart and Health Study. American Journal of Public Health 95 (1/January), 91–97.

Macintyre, S., 1997. The Black Report and beyond: what are the issues? Social Science and Medicine 64 (6), 723–745.

Mackenbach, J., Stronks, K., 2002. A strategy for tackling health inequalities in The Netherlands. British Medical Journal 325, 1029–1032.

Marmot, M., 2006. Health in an unequal world. Lancet 368, 2081–2096.

Marmot, M., Bell, R., 2006. The socioeconomically disadvantaged. In: Levy, B.S., Sidel, V.W. (Eds.), Social Injustice and Public Health. Oxford University Press, New York, pp. 25–45.

Najman, J., Aird, R., Bor, W., et al., 2004. The generational transmission of socioeconomic inequalities in child cognitive development and emotional health. Social Science and Medicine 58, 1147–1158.

National Rural Health Alliance, 2013. NRHA Priority Recommendations from the 12th National Rural Health Conference 2013 National Rural Health Alliance. Online. Available: <http://ruralhealth.org.au/sites/default/files/documents/nrha-policy-document/positions/nrha-priority-recommendations-17-june-2013.pdf> (12 Feb 2014).

Nicholson, J., Carroll, J.-A., Brodie, A., et al., 2004. Child and youth health inequalities in Australia: the status of Australian research 2003. Paper prepared for the Health Inequalities Research Collaboration, Children, Youth and Families Network.

Nicholson, J.M., Lucas, N., Berthelsen, D., et al., 2012. Socioeconomic inequality profiles in physical and developmental health from 0–7 years: Australian National Study. Journal of Epidemiology and Community Health 66, 81–87. doi: 10.1136/jech.2009.103291.

Oldenburg, B., McGuffog, I.D., Turrell, G., 2000a. Socioeconomic determinants of health in Australia: policy responses and intervention options. Medical Journal of Australia 172, 489–492.

Oldenburg, B., McGuffog, I.D., Turrell, G., 2000b. Making a difference to the socioeconomic determinants of health; policy responses and intervention options. Asia-Pacific Journal of Public Health 12 (Suppl.), s51–s54.

Organisation for Economic Co-operation and Development (OECD), 2013. Education at a glance 2013: OECD indicators. OECD Publishing. Online. Available: <http://www.oecd.org/edu/eag2013%20%28eng%29–FINAL%2020%20June%202013.pdf> (15 Feb 2014).

Pearce, N., Davey Smith, G., 2003. Is social capital the key to inequalities in health? American Journal of Public Health 93 (1), 122–128.

Putnam, R., 1993. Making Democracy Work: Civic Traditions in Modern Italy. Princeton University Press, Princeton.

Purdie, N., Buckley, S., 2010. School attendance and retention of Indigenous Australian students. Issues Paper No. 1 produced for the Closing the Gap Clearinghouse, September 2010. Online. Available: <http://www.aihw.gov.au/uploadedFiles/ClosingTheGap/Content/Publications/2010/ctg-ip01.pdf> (Feb 7 2014).

Sheen, V., 2012. Labour in vain: casualisation presents a precarious future for workers. The Conversation. 25 Jul 2012.

Spurrier, N.J., Volkmer, R.E., Abdallah, C.A., et al., 2012. South Australian four-year-old Aboriginal children: residence and socioeconomic status influence weight. Australian and New Zealand Journal of Public Health 36 (3), 285–290.

Stafford, M., Marmot, M., 2003. Neighbourhood deprivation and health: does it affect us all equally? International Journal of Epidemiology 32, 357–366.

Townsend, P., Davidson, N. (Eds.), 1992. Inequalities in Health: The Black Report. Penguin, London.

Turrell, G., Oldenburg, B., McGuffog, I., et al., 1999. A Framework of Socioeconomic Determinants of Health: Towards a National Research Program and a Policy and Intervention Agenda. Queensland University of Technology, School of Public Health and Ausinfo, Canberra.

Turrell, G., Kavanagh, A., 2004. Socioeconomic determinants of health: from evidence to policy. In: Moodie, R., Hulme, A. (Eds.), Hands-on Health Promotion. IP Communications, Melbourne.

Turrell, G., Kavanagh, A., Draper, G., et al., 2007. Do places affect the probability of death in Australia? A multi-level study of area-level disadvantage. Journal of Epidemiology and Community Health 61, 13–19.

Turrell, G., Haynes, M., Burton, N.W., et al., 2010. Neighborhood disadvantage and physical activity: baseline results from the HABITAT multilevel longitudinal study. Annals of Epidemiology 20 (3), 171–181.

Turrell, G., Hewitt, B.A., Miller, S.A., 2012. The influence of neighbourhood disadvantage on smoking cessation and its contribution to inequalities in smoking status. Drug and Alcohol Review 31 (5), 645–652.

Virtanen, P., Janlert, U., Hammarstrom, A., 2011. Exposure to temporary employment and job insecurity. a longitudinal study of the health effects. Occupational and Environmental Medicine 68 (8), 570–574.

Wilkinson, R., Marmot, M., 2003. The Solid Facts: Social Determinants of Health. Centre for Urban Health, World Health Organization, Copenhagen.

Winter, I., 2000. Major themes and debates in the social capital literature: the Australian connection. In: Winter, I. (Ed.), Social Capital and Public Policy in Australia. Australian Institute of Family Studies, Melbourne, pp. 17–42.

World Health Organization (WHO) Europe, 2003. The Solid Facts: Social Determinants of Health, second ed. WHO, Geneva.

Ziersch, A.M., 2005. The health implications of access to social capital: findings from an Australian study. Social Science and Medicine 61, 2119–2131.

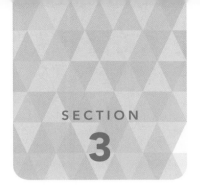

ETHICS, EVIDENCE AND PRACTICE

Introduction

- **An ethical approach** to practice is essential for health workers who see the importance of maintaining a high standard of professional practice in their day-to-day work. Chapter 8 discusses the development of public health ethics, and the factors that underpin an ethical approach. The field of public health ethics has now been firmly established, and we regularly see academic and policy-based contributions that expand and challenge the philosophical, political and ethical underpinning of public health. Prior attempts to investigate and analyse the ethical problems inherent in public health practice, theory and research using traditional bioethical approaches put a predominant emphasis on autonomy and individual rights, and were found to be inadequate and limiting. Chapter 8 covers the key ethical systems, theories and concepts that predicate ethical decision-making, and then discusses and applies those to public health practice. Too often, health practitioners do not have a clear understanding of ethical practice, nor an opportunity to explore the range of circumstances that may impact on how they do their job. This chapter explores all of these issues, leading from the theoretical to the practical, and exploring the range of ways in which ethics applies to public health.

- **Chapter 9 follows on** from the previous chapter, in that ethical practice should be based on evidence, not on habit nor the practices of those who have come before us. Evidence-based practice began as evidence-based medicine, and has evolved and developed into a process that centres on evidence-gathering and exploring the limitations of such evidence. It focuses on the *barriers* and *facilitators* to identifying and implementing *best practice*. The chapter discusses the key components of evidence-based public health, including making decisions on the basis of the best available scientific evidence, systematic use of data and information systems, applying program planning frameworks, engaging the community in decision-making, conducting sound evaluation, and disseminating what is learned (Brownson 2011). The chapter also discusses the limitations of evidence-based practice, and the potential use of other sources of information to guide practice.

- **In the final chapter** in this section, using an ethical approach to practice and the evidence that should be used to guide practice come together in a discussion of the importance of planning and evaluation to public health practice. Chapter 10 links planning with evaluation, and stresses the importance of evaluating the planning and implementation processes to ensure that practitioners can decide on what works and what needs to be modified. Evaluation is an essential element in the planning and implementation process because, at the very least, it gives the practitioner an idea of where changes or modifications might need to be made. Chapter 10 also addresses the stages of undertaking a needs assessment to assist in the planning process. Public health plans are based on identifying and assessing needs. This chapter identifies the variety of ways in which needs can be defined, and then discusses the program planning and implementation process. Some planning models are presented and discussed, and the advantages and disadvantages of each are considered. This chapter includes a conversation with the reader about the implications for practice, and an understanding of the difficulties associated with the processes of implementing and evaluating a program or intervention.

Reference

Brownson, R.C., 2011. Evidence-Based Public Health. Oxford University Press, New York.

Ethics and public health

CHAPTER 8

Trish Gould

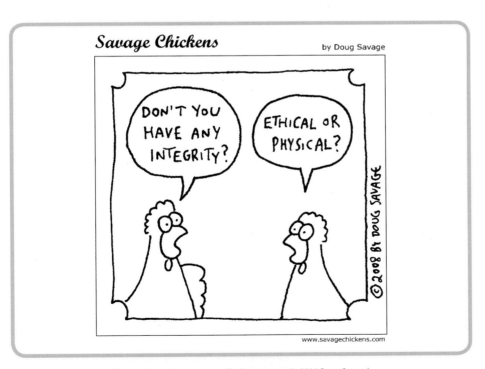

'Integrity'. (Source: Savage Chickens cartoon © 2008 Doug Savage)

Learning objectives

After reading this chapter, you should be able to:

- recognise that the word 'ethics' is often defined and applied in different ways

- explain why ethics is actually at the very core of public health

- describe the foundations and development of public health ethics

- summarise some systems or philosophies of ethics, and their relevance to public health practice

- critique some examples of formal, published codes of ethics in health

- recognise, evaluate and communicate ethical issues in public health work and policy

- apply ethical principles in your public health practice.

Introduction

While there has been more dialogue on public health ethics recently, the field is still underdeveloped compared with ethics in other professional disciplines. Ethics are important for health professionals and their clients, but also for politicians, law-makers and policymakers, who depend on health professionals for guidance about health-related issues. For example, as human populations increasingly become part of a global monoculture, with the consequent increase in pandemic and epidemic risks, decision-makers need help from health professionals to grapple with difficult and controversial decisions arising from those risks. As public health continues to develop, health practitioners need to be aware that their professional ethical obligations with regard to the population's health will also change.

This chapter introduces you to the basic ethical principles that underpin public health practice. One of the pivotal challenges in public health ethics is balancing the rights of the individual with the wellbeing of the population as a whole. For example, a person with an infectious disease might have their right to liberty suspended to protect the rest of the population. Thus we are confronted by the question of how we should go about deciding when it is fair or acceptable to restrict the rights of one category of people to ensure the wellbeing of others.

Questions such as this demonstrate the importance of such factors as power, fairness and values in public health ethics. The themes examined in this chapter include the characteristics of 'ethics', the advantages of exploring ethics, the foundations of public health ethics, and how we can apply ethics to our practice. These themes are illustrated by some typical ethical challenges in professional health practice. It is argued that ethics is more than an abstract philosophical concern. Rather, it is a practical field intimately tied up with effective health service delivery to consumers, and is of great concern to health professionals, politicians and, not least, the public.

Should we be more ethical? There is already an implicit expectation from the public and health professions that health and wellbeing services be ethical, because clearly there is likely to be an outcry if such health services, service delivery or policy is perceived to be unfair, corrupt or self-serving. Given that public health is already expected to be ethical, the question is how do we become more conscious and *effective* in both our understanding and our practice of ethics? And what do we need to *do* to be more aware of public health areas where ethical matters should be specifically considered?

The bulk of public health ethics work has tended to concentrate on two main areas: research ethics and responses to infectious diseases (Kenny et al. 2006). However, public health ethics must also consider such things as: population health, safety and wellbeing; impartiality in service delivery; and the rights of both individuals and groups (Gostin 2003).

It is vital that the core concerns of ethics—including the 'common good' and the corresponding key functions of public health practice—are identified and explored (Kenny et al. 2006), and that a variety of ethical analyses are applied in order to encapsulate the diversity and depth of public health (Bayer et al. 2007). Failure to do so means that critical public health decisions are made thoughtlessly or unconsciously, and without due regard to the ethical matters likely to be of concern within the client population.

What relevance do ethics have to your own practice? As the considerable expenditure and work hours that go into public health initiatives and policies are, at root, ethically motivated (an intention to 'do good'), health professionals are constantly making explicit or implicit ethical decisions. Health professionals are regularly confronted by ethical dilemmas, and selecting the correct course of action is often challenging. For example, as well as yielding improvements in health, an intervention may cause harm, such as where 'justice' is violated by imposing more of a burden on one subpopulation than on others (see Activity 8.7).

What is your understanding of 'ethics'? Does it have positive, negative or neutral connotations? Is your ethical perspective influenced by other factors, such as your religious or cultural background? Activity 8.1 will help you to explore this concept.

Debates on various cultural, environmental, economic and political issues (all of which have the potential to impact on health) raise themes related to ethical and fair conduct, even though these issues may not be openly identified. For example, with worldwide concerns over dwindling energy resources, it seems that we must choose between different types of pollution, such as the toxic chemicals associated with 'fracking' versus radioactive waste from nuclear energy production, both of which carry risks to the environment and to people's health. One of the ethical questions raised is who should shoulder the burden—for example, is it fair that people living near these industries may have higher health risks than the rest of the population?

Activity 8.1 Ethical practice

- Discuss with your classmates how you would define 'ethical practice'. Imagine and discuss some instances of unethical conduct within your professions.

REFLECTION 8.1

Some of your classmates' ideas may have been very different to your own. Nonetheless, you may find that if you look at the underlying basis for their arguments, many people had similar ideas—for example, 'do no harm' or 'treat others as you would like to be treated'. If there were major differences, do you think you can work effectively with those people?

This chapter alerts you to the likelihood of ethical issues arising in your practice, and the varied perspectives, theories and approaches to these, rather than trying to provide solutions for every potential ethical dilemma.

The next section introduces you to some of the relevant ethical concepts.

Ethical frameworks, theories and concepts

Many of the key ideas, concepts and theories that are employed in public health ethics are derived from the field of ethics within the discipline of philosophy. Therefore, a brief overview of ethics philosophy is essential for those who are likely to be involved in potentially controversial public health-related decisions.

The discipline of ethics typically enquires into a wide range of concerns: *normative* ethics tries to ascertain what are good or right actions and motives; *applied* ethics involves exploring and resolving particular dilemmas; *descriptive* ethics explores the ethics people actually believe in and/or put into practice; and *meta-ethics* analyses the essential nature of ethical principles and whether they can be objectively validated.

Normative ethics in public health

Given the objective of finding out how to determine what are good and right actions and motives in practice, normative ethics has direct relevance to public health practice. However, as we might expect with such controversial questions, there are differing positions on how to decide what is good or right. The following are five common normative ethical positions:

1   *Consequences—Consequentialism* claims that an action's rightness depends on its consequences (Cribb & Duncan 2002). An example is *utilitarianism*, where the best action is said to be the one that brings about the greatest amount of pleasure and the least amount of pain for the maximum number of people. While this might sound good in theory, dreadful suffering might be inflicted on a minority in the name of the common good.

2   *Duties and Rights—Deontology* maintains that every individual has absolute or fundamental duties and rights—and it is these that should form the basis of ethical decisions. In other words, the consequences of actions do not determine their merit; rather, it is other elements such as your intent (Beauchamp & Childress 2001). For example, in Kant's *Categorical Imperative*, it states that you should only carry out any action if you would accept that same action as a universal law.

3   *Character—Virtue ethics* emphasises an individual's intrinsic qualities (whatever people agree are desirable characteristics; e.g. compassion and honesty) in preference to rules or consequences.

4   *Liberty and Human Rights—Liberalism's*: focus is usually rights, equality, freedom and

---

ACTIVITY 8.2 Issues around quarantining

- Discuss the following with your classmates. The age-old methods of preventing the spread of infection are quarantine and isolation. Imagine a situation where there is an emerging infectious disease with a high mortality rate—for example, avian influenza A (H7N9, first identified in China in 2013) (World Health Organization 2013). Furthermore, there is the possibility that H7N9 will become transmissible between people, and the Australian Government's response in this case is to mandate isolation and quarantine.

- What do you think would be an appropriate response to the threat of a virulent new virus? Should you isolate sick people and quarantine people who only *might be* infected?

- Do you think one ethical perspective is better than the others? Or is it more useful to use all five as complementary viewpoints that have relevance, and require skilful balancing?

democracy. Such concepts, particularly 'rights', are the basic premise of many influential public health documents (Parker et al. 2007). For example, the *Declaration of Alma-Ata* states that health 'is a fundamental human right' (World Health Organization (WHO) 1978).

5 *Community—Communitarianism* recognises humans as social beings, thus emphasising relationships and shared values (Sindall 2002). This perspective requires enforcing limits on individual autonomy for the benefit of the community (Callahan & Jennings 2002).

Activity 8.2 applies each of these five viewpoints to demonstrate how different beliefs and theories in normative ethics have real-world practical impacts.

The usefulness of these various normative positions can only be realised if their relationships to each other are understood, just as ethics can only be grasped in terms of the relationships between people, groups and their total environment. While we cannot employ a one-size-fits-all approach, we need to agree upon the meanings of the ethical theories and approaches to help us communicate in our efforts to apply ethics in public health endeavours. Arguably, Activity 8.2 illustrates that these normative theories offer a range of perspectives on the ethics of any particular public health action, and thus all should be considered when assessing the ethics of any given public health research or intervention.

The next section explores the development of public health ethics.

> **REFLECTION 8.2**
>
> - A *consequentialist* might argue that it is right to isolate someone with a highly lethal, infectious disease because of the *consequences* of not doing so—a probable epidemic, and subsequent deaths.
> - In contrast, a *deontologist* might claim that, regardless of the possible outcomes, there is a *duty* to protect people, and everyone has a *right* to be protected from disease.
> - A *virtue ethicist* might defend isolation based on the good intentions of those enforcing isolation and quarantine.
> - *Liberalists* might argue against enforced isolation and quarantine, and make a case for education in order to persuade infectious people to isolate themselves from others.
> - *Communitarians* may argue that it is justifiable to limit individual freedoms—that is, isolating an infected person—if it benefits the whole community.
>
> Clearly, there are many differences between these examples of normative ethics—for example, the divergence between the 'rights' of the individual (liberalism) and the 'good' of the community (communitarianism). Nevertheless, they also have things in common—for example, utilitarianism and communitarianism both tend to favour the community over the individual.

Themes and debates in the development of ethics in public health

Many authors have differentiated between medical ethics and bioethics (Bayer et al. 2007, Thompson et al. 2003). Medical ethics generally refers to a health professional's ethical responsibility towards their (individual) patient. Bioethics developed in the middle of the twentieth century as a discipline separate from medical ethics, and from medical ethics' emphasis on individual autonomy and the right not to be harmed (Bayer et al. 2007, Thompson et al. 2003). While also individualist in its focus, bioethics has tended to concentrate more on the ethics of such issues as research, genomics, stem cell therapies and cloning, rather than medical treatment (Azétsop & Rennie 2010, Thompson et al. 2003). This is not surprising, in view of the development of the discipline of bioethics as a reaction to some questionable research practices, such as the Tuskegee Syphilis Study (see Activity 8.6); and the Nazi 'medical' experiments, brought to the public's awareness through the Nuremberg Trials[1] (Beauchamp & Steinbock 1999, Coleman et al. 2008, Fairchild & Johns 2012, Thompson et al. 2003).

Chapter 1 discussed the influence of the biomedical perspective on health. Similarly, although frameworks for public health ethics have partially derived from the bioethical tradition, public health ethics is now a distinct, albeit overlapping, discipline, thus limiting the use of bioethical models to public health practice (Callahan & Jennings 2002, Fairchild & Johns 2012, Thomas et al. 2002, Thompson et al. 2003). That is, the core values of the public health tradition often insist on giving priority to the needs and rights of the population (many individuals) over those of specific individuals (Bayer & Fairchild 2004, Fairchild & Johns 2012). In addition, public health, unlike medicine, focuses more on preventing disease than on treating it (Callahan & Jennings 2002, Thomas et al. 2002). Paradoxically, at the same time, public health ethics has to keep in mind that those populations are made up of specific individuals, and thus individual rights remain relevant, too.

Public health law and human rights

There is an intricate relationship between public health, law, political philosophy and human rights. Although distinct social institutions, ethics and law are crucial tools for regulating behaviour; they work in partnership to provide guidance for public health. Practitioners must use their judgement to make decisions within the boundaries of the law. Ethics is a reflective procedure best performed with other people, and entails evaluating any proposed strategy, together with giving good reasons for any action—particularly when the law has nothing specific to say about the issue until after action has already been taken. There are often no 'correct' solutions, especially when the scientific data are limited. Thus, being able to collaborate with others to reflect on all the potential actions and their ethical implications will enable acceptable decisions to be identified (Bernheim 2005). In addition, if a legal or political controversy arises over a particular public health decision or policy, the fact that an explicit ethical assessment was done as part of that decision process or policy analysis may provide reassurance to both the public and the court.

One of the challenges with a rights-based framework for public health is that expressions such as 'the right to equal opportunity' and 'the right to health' are imprecise; they cannot be clarified without making it clear who has a duty to ensure access to each theoretical right (Leeder 2004, O'Neill 2002). Moreover, 'rights' has a different meaning in a legal context, in contrast to its meaning in a political or rhetorical context. Additionally, rights often intersect or clash—for example, the right to privacy may be in opposition to the right of the public to be protected from infectious disease.

When talking about the 'right to equal opportunity', we also need to distinguish between 'equity' and 'equality'. Essentially, equity is about fairness (WHO 1996), and about having equal opportunities to health-enhancing factors, not equal health status.

The basis for human rights is the International Bill of Human Rights (IBHR) (Office of the High Commissioner for Human Rights). The Universal Declaration of Human Rights was adopted in 1948 by the General Assembly of the United Nations (United Nations 1948) as part of the IBHR. This edict provides a rights-based model for a public health code of ethics (see Chapter 3 for Article 25).

Mann (1997) claims that a human rights-based paradigm provides a more practical framework and language for contemporary public health ethics than do frameworks modified from medical, biomedical or earlier public health ethics. Thus, the language of human rights may be more appropriate for dealing with the determinants of health that are also external to the health sphere, such as housing, education and transport (Mann 1997). In addition, a human rights-based approach focuses on action and advocacy, thus making it relevant for 'global public health' (Annas 2010 p 189), as the aim of both human rights and public health is to create environments that facilitate human wellbeing.

Applied ethics

The health practitioner needs not only an awareness of their own values, but also the values that are fundamental to public health practice, as these values, whether explicit or not, will impact on public health policy and practice. The next section outlines some codes of ethics, and provides examples of the application of ethical analyses to a range of issues.

Codes of ethics

A 'code of ethics' is a published collection of standards for practitioners and organisations that dictates certain benchmarks as to their practice and their character while demonstrating their values to the public, as well as the standards of care that the public can expect (Gostin 2003).

> **ACTIVITY 8.3 Principles of ethical practice**
>
> • Examine the *Principles of the Ethical Practice of Public Health* (Public Health Leadership Society, 2002). These guidelines were developed for US political, economic and cultural conditions. Would you change anything to better suit them to conditions in Australia?

> **REFLECTION 8.3**
>
> These principles are a good starting point for discussion about a public health ethics code in Australia, which at the time of writing has no code of ethics specifically for public health practice.

A number of ethical codes for public health have been proposed or adopted. In 2002, the American Public Health Association (APHA) agreed to adopt a code of ethics for public health practice (Thomas et al. 2002). Activity 8.3 examines this code of ethics.

Many health practitioners will be 'covered' by their organisations' codes of ethics. For example, all employees of the Queensland Government are covered by the Code of Conduct for the Queensland Public Service (2011). In addition, Australia does have guidelines for ethical conduct in research with humans. These include the National Health and Medical Research Council's (NHMRC) National Statement on Ethical Conduct in Human Research (NHMRC 2014), and Values and Ethics: Guidelines for Ethical Conduct in Aboriginal and Torres Strait Islander Health Research (NHMRC 2003). All health researchers in Australia are obliged to conform to these guidelines.

The NHMRC (2003) research guidelines concerning Aboriginal and Torres Strait Islander peoples emphasise six core values:

1 *spirit and integrity*—the continuity of the cultural heritage of past, present and future generations
2 *reciprocity*—the research must both benefit, and be valued by, the community
3 *respect*—there must be respect for, and acceptance of, dignity and diverse values
4 *equality*—there must be a commitment to justice and equality
5 *survival and protection*—the research and researchers must not harm Aboriginal and Torres Strait Islander cultures, identity or languages
6 *responsibility*—researchers must ensure that they do not harm Aboriginal and Torres Strait Islander peoples or the things they treasure, and must be accountable to the people (NHMRC 2003).

Similar guidelines are also in place for research with Indigenous peoples in other countries; for example, Canada and New Zealand (Canadian Institutes of Health Research et al. 2010, Health Research Council of New Zealand 2005). Activity 8.4 investigates the application and suitability of the *Values and Ethics* (NHMRC 2003) guidelines to a range of situations.

ACTIVITY 8.4 Application of research ethics to health work

- The *Values and Ethics* (NHMRC 2003) guidelines were developed to guide health researchers in their *research* activities with Aboriginal and Torres Strait Islander Australians. Do you think they can be applied more generally to any *health-related work* undertaken with Aboriginal and Torres Strait Islander Australians, such as health promotion programs?
- Can these same precepts be used with non-Indigenous populations?
- Do you understand the principles, or are they too abstract? How can you determine whether you have complied with the guidelines? Can you see any potential conflicts between the various principles?

REFLECTION 8.4

Although devised for health *research*, the NHMRC guidelines—with their emphasis on such concepts as respect, reciprocity and responsibility—might also offer a positive model for implementing *public health programs* with Aboriginal and Torres Strait Islander communities. More importantly, however, Aboriginal and Torres Strait Island peoples need to have ownership of, and control over, any research or health initiative for it to be worthwhile and appropriate (Onemda VicHealth Koori Health Unit 2008). These guidelines might also be suitable for any group with whom you work in partnership, especially different ethnic groups or nations (Parker et al. 2007). However, there may be difficulties reconciling the views of practitioners from different cultural traditions—from the perspective of many non-Indigenous practitioners, the good of the community can often conflict with that of the individual. Conversely, for many Aboriginal and Torres Strait Island people an individual would never be considered in isolation from his or her community. (See Chapter 16 for an analysis of Aboriginal and Torres Strait Islander Australians' health issues.)

Another code of ethics is that of the Pharmaceutical Society of Australia (PSA 2011). The code outlines nine principles for pharmacists. A pharmacist:

1 recognises the health and wellbeing of the consumer as their first priority
2 pays due respect for the autonomy and rights of consumers and encourages consumers to actively participate in decision-making
3 upholds the reputation and public trust of the profession
4 acknowledges the professional roles in and responsibilities to the wider community
5 demonstrates a commitment to the development and enhancement of the profession
6 maintains a contemporary knowledge of pharmacy practice and ensures health and competence to practise
7 agrees to practise only under conditions which uphold the professional independence, judgement and integrity of themselves or others
8 conducts the business of pharmacy in an ethical and professional manner
9 works collaboratively with other health professionals to optimise the health outcomes of consumers (PSA 2011). (See Activity 8.5.)

While useful for communicating expected standards of professional conduct for professionals and the public, codes of conduct cannot provide instructions for resolving specific ethical issues. Decision-making frameworks, such as Gostin's (2003) outlined below, are not able to cover every eventuality, but will clarify many concerns. That is, you will need to assess:

- the nature, probability and severity of the risk
- the likelihood that the proposed action will be effective in meeting its objectives
- the economic costs entailed, including opportunity costs
- the burdens on human rights
- the fairness, including a just allocation of benefits and burdens (Gostin 2003 pp 185–186).

There are other existing and proposed ethical codes, models or frameworks for public health ethics—for example, the Nuffield Council's *Stewardship Model* (2007). The aim of this model is to accomplish preferred 'social goals while minimising significant limitations on individual freedom' (Nuffield Council on Bioethics 2007 p 26). See the Nuffield Council website in the reference list for more on this model.

Clearly, ethics should underlie all of our actions. Some of the conflicts—for example, between the individual and the population, between treatment and prevention—will become more obvious as we examine more examples.

The application of ethics in public health practice

These examples of ethical problems—from a range of health domains—will help you to integrate and apply the theories to your profession, and demonstrate the relevance of ethics to your practice.

PUBLIC HEALTH RESEARCH

When undertaking research projects, you are required to obtain ethical approval from at least one institution (e.g. a university ethical board). In addition to your responsibility to respect confidentiality and the participants' rights to informed consent, there are many other associated issues and risks. These include paying people to participate in a study, and the implications for the notion of voluntary consent (Fry et al. 2004); and research funding and the potential conflict of interest—for example, a cigarette company funding research on whether plain packaging of tobacco products reduces smoking rates. Case Study 8.1 raises a number of ethical issues associated with research.

ACTIVITY 8.5 PSA Code of ethics

- Read the Pharmaceutical Society of Australia (PSA) *Code of Ethics for Pharmacists*. Can you apply this code, in its entirety, to Australian public health practice, or are there some sections that might need to be modified?

REFLECTION 8.5

All of the principles in the PSA code of ethics (PSA 2011) could be applied to public health practice. The major difference is that—unlike public health practitioners—pharmacists still tend to have as their focus the treatment of illness rather than prevention, and the individual consumer rather than the whole population. However, more pharmacists are beginning to participate in public health and health promotion activities, such as advising on smoking cessation (Saba et al. 2013). Looking at the normative ethics in the previous section, what changes might be made to the PSA code to make it more applicable to public health practice?

CASE STUDY 8.1

The Tuskegee Syphilis Study

Beginning in 1932, the Tuskegee Syphilis Study took place in Tuskegee, Alabama. The participants were mainly underprivileged African-Americans. When the study began, the accepted treatments for syphilis were not very effective and had toxic side-effects. The researchers wanted to establish whether outcomes were better if patients were not treated with these dangerous medications. By the mid-1940s, penicillin was the orthodox therapy for syphilis, but, instead of ending the study and giving penicillin to all of the participants, the researchers withheld penicillin and the relevant information. The study finally ended in the 1970s, when details were disclosed through the press. By this time, many of the participants had died from syphilis, and their families had become infected (Centers for Disease Control and Prevention website, University of Virginia Health Sciences Library 1996).

ACTIVITY 8.6 Issues arising from the Tuskegee Syphilis Study

- Imagine you are part of the Tuskegee study research team. From the point of view of the social and ethical environment of today, are the issues any different? Can the researchers' actions be justified, considering that laws, practices and attitudes were very different at that time?

REFLECTION 8.6

At the time that the study began, doctors frequently did not disclose information to patients about their illness, as the doctors thought they 'knew best' or did not want to 'worry' their patients. Furthermore, the medical ethics of that period did not have the rigorous requirements for informed consent that exist today. As a consequence of this and similar studies, many African-Americans have little confidence in medical and public health authorities (Centers for Disease Control and Prevention website, University of Virginia Health Sciences Library 1996), which can have negative consequences for both the individuals and the population as a whole. Despite the differences, there is also a large amount of overlap between medical ethics (the physician's duty towards his or her patient), bioethics (medical research ethics), and public health ethics, as you could utilise all of these approaches together in exploring the above example.

ANTHROPOLOGICAL RESEARCH

On 13 September 2007, the United Nations General Assembly adopted the (non-binding) *Declaration on the Rights of Indigenous Peoples* (United Nations Permanent Forum on Indigenous Issues 2010). Article 31 acknowledges the rights of Indigenous peoples to:

> … maintain, control, protect and develop … *the manifestations of their sciences, technologies and cultures, including human and genetic resources, seeds, medicines, knowledge of the properties of fauna and flora, oral traditions* … [emphasis added] (United Nations 2008)

ACTIVITY 8.7 Ethical issues arising from the Genographic Project

- A study of genetic anthropology, The Genographic Project aimed to collect 100,000 DNA samples from Indigenous peoples to investigate human migration (The Genographic Project website). The project ran into opposition from some Indigenous groups, with Harry (2009 p 10) commenting that it 'is a highly invasive continuation of the NGS's [National Geographic Society's] practice of exploiting, objectifying, and capitalizing on the lives of Indigenous peoples'.
- Why do you think people would protest about this research?
- For the Indigenous peoples of the Pacific region, what are the likely advantages and/or disadvantages to participating?
- Who owns the samples and resources, the research outcomes and the intellectual property rights? (Nicholas & Hollowell 2009, United Nations 2008).

REFLECTION 8.7

Did you consider principles of privacy, autonomy and ownership? Despite the potential benefits, there are many possible pitfalls with this project. In many societies, the human body is 'sacred', and must be kept 'whole'; to remove blood or any other body part is inappropriate. Peoples' own knowledge of their creation, ancestors, oral histories and languages, and their cultural and spiritual beliefs, may be damaged by the (Western) interpretation of any data acquired (Kanehe 2007, Nicholas & Hollowell 2009), and this can impact on health. Furthermore, if the results indicate that some Indigenous peoples did not arrive as early as their own histories indicate, the research could have negative consequences for their land and resource rights, and their sovereignty (Kanehe 2007; Tallbear 2013), which might negatively impact on their socioeconomic status and, therefore, their wellbeing. In addition, the researchers have not explained whether there are any direct benefits (health or other) for the participants. Therefore, it is likely that a social, spiritual and/or emotional burden is imposed on the people, with no guarantee of receiving any benefits. Do the *means* (collecting samples from Indigenous groups) justify the *ends* (a more comprehensive picture of human migration patterns)? Finally, the importance given to a group's genetic inheritance could result in people being stigmatised as 'being somehow inherently flawed', and disregards other factors that impact on health status (Harry 2009 p 154), such as the social, political and economic environment (see Chapters 4 and 7).

Activity 8.7 demonstrates some of the downsides for Indigenous peoples who are 'researched'.

SCREENING

In Australia, prostate cancer is the second leading cause of cancer-related mortality in Australian males (after lung cancer) (AIHW 2012). If found early, prostate cancer can be treated; however, the treatments have significant and common side-effects, including impotence and incontinence. In addition, many prostate cancers are very slow-growing and are unlikely to kill the patient (Brawley et al. 2009). There is screening available for prostate cancer, although there are limitations, including high rates of false positives and false negatives (Etzioni et al. 2002). Activity 8.8 examines some of the issues surrounding screening.

DISEASE CONTROL

Disease control (see Chapter 11) sometimes involves the enforcement of rules and/or control of individuals' behaviour for the good of the population as a whole. While diseases such as HIV/AIDS (McMichael & Butler 2007), TB (tuberculosis), H1N1 (swine flu), EVD (Ebola), and constantly emerging viruses are important public health problems, they also raise critical ethical issues. Activity 8.9 explores the ethics of enforcing treatment for someone with an infectious disease who refuses to cooperate with the health professional's advice—should they be detained and treated against their will?

In Australia, at the time of writing, there is no federal law covering compulsory detention and treatment, with each state having the autonomy to create its own laws; however, the states generally adhere to federal *guidelines*. For example, in New South Wales the chief health officer can order the detention and treatment of a patient with an infectious disease for a period of up to 28 days; this applies to non-compliant patients with category 4 diseases (e.g. SARS and TB) or category 5 diseases (e.g. HIV/AIDS) (New South Wales Consolidated Acts Public Health Act). Clearly, utilising a public health order fails to sort out any ethical tensions; it just allows for the *legal* confinement of an infectious person who refuses treatment (Senanayake & Ferson 2004).

ACTIVITY 8.8 Screening issues

Download the audio or the transcript of the ABC Radio *National Health Report* of 19 April 2010, regarding screening and commercial sponsorship (the link is in the reference list).

- Is it ethical to screen for any particular condition or disease predisposition if there is not always an effective and acceptable treatment, or if the side-effects of treatment are significant and irreversible? Which normative approach are you applying in your answer?

- Conversely, is it ethical not to screen when there is the potential to save lives, whatever the magnitude of that potential?

- What are the issues involved in a commercial organisation sponsoring screening, particularly when that organisation provides merchandise to manage the problems that can result from the treatment that may follow screening?

REFLECTION 8.8

Did you consider any of the following issues? A false negative may give the person peace of mind when it is unwarranted, while a false positive may lead to unnecessary diagnostic tests and anxiety. Should the participants be advised of the rates of false positives/negatives? Is it ethical to spend limited health funds on screening a subpopulation, where the number of positives identified may be minimal? How would you respond if a screening program had the potential to save 1 life for every 10,000 people screened? Should we ignore the life of that one individual? What about commercial sponsorship of medical screening? Some would say that there is a conflict of interests in such cases. For example, in the *Test for Prostate Cancer* report, the diaper (nappy) manufacturer who is sponsoring prostate cancer screening stands to profit financially from the possible negative outcomes of treatments that may follow the screening tests.

Heavy-handed use of such legal powers might be considered wrong or unethical by the general public. This example raises many other issues. Is it possible, or desirable, to protect people from this type of state intrusion into what are essentially private affairs—that is, a person's right to receive or refuse medical treatment? What limits to national or state authorities are reasonable? Can you find a balance between the

ACTIVITY 8.9 Population versus individual rights

- Imagine you are chief health officer in New South Wales. You have tried all other avenues to get an individual with active, infective pulmonary TB to comply with a treatment regimen, but the patient still refuses, thus posing a health risk to others. Now you are required to initiate proceedings to serve a public health order, which may mandate the person's detention and treatment (NSW Department of Health website).

- Can you envision any alternatives to the patient's (enforced) confinement and treatment?

- Is it acceptable to detain and treat someone against their will?

- What, if any, are some of the ethics and/or rights that are in conflict in the above example?

- If you were responsible for drafting laws or policies to deal with such situations, which options would you support?

REFLECTION 8.9

With regard to conflicting rights, did you consider the duty to protect the community, the collective good and/or the right to privacy and liberty (Gostin et al. 2007 p 261)? If you said 'no' to detaining someone against their will, would you still oppose such a public health order if the person also had HIV/AIDS, given that, worldwide, infection with HIV significantly increases susceptibility to TB infection, and TB is a leading cause of mortality in people with HIV (Australian Government Department of Health 2012)? All these issues demonstrate the complexity of decision-making in such cases.

communal good and that of the individual in a situation such as this, or must the needs of one outweigh the other? If you say that the needs of a population should be put ahead of those of an individual what sort of ethical theory are you applying?

Another aspect of disease control is contact tracing (see Chapter 11), which involves finding people who may have had contact with someone who has an infectious disease. However, these people have not in any way sought diagnosis and treatment, nor given their consent to be traced. Do people have rights in this instance to privacy and confidentiality? Conversely, do they have a right to be informed of their possible risk status? Which right, if any, should take precedence? What about protecting the public? Unquestionably, one of the core issues for public health ethics is the necessity to use authority to protect 'the people's' health, while also averting the abuse of such power (Thomas et al. 2002).

SOCIAL NETWORKING FOR PUBLIC HEALTH

Worldwide, there are already billions of people and groups using social networking (Mandeville et al. 2014), and with the growth in 'smart' technologies there are increasing opportunities for health promotion and education, research, and disease control (such as contact tracing) (Mandeville et al. 2014, Stein et al. 2014). Clearly, social networking, such as Facebook, is a useful setting for educating populations about protecting themselves from infectious diseases, and for researching 'infection rates, behaviours, and risk perceptions' (Stein et al. 2014 p 57). For instance, the Centers for Disease Control and Protection (CDC) use social media and networking for 'health communication campaigns, activities and emergency response efforts' (CDC 2014). However, there are ethical dilemmas associated with utilising social networking for some public health objectives (Mandeville et al. 2014, Stein et al. 2014), particularly relating to individuals (Mandeville et al. 2014).

Mandeville et al. (2014) discuss a case where a person with meningococcal septicaemia was comatose, thus unable to tell the health authorities who he had been in contact with. Without consulting the relevant authorities, a friend decided to post the information on the patient's Facebook account, where it could be seen by all the person's Facebook friends, in order to inform possible contacts of their risk (Mandeville et al. 2014). Activity 8.10 examines such issues as the right to privacy, consent, and the rights of people to be protected from disease.

Health promotion

As discussed in other chapters in this book, health professionals must consider not only individuals' responsibility for their own health, but also the range of other factors that impact on health. Importantly, in order to prevent unethical (and unproductive) victim blaming, they need to recognise that there are numerous, interrelated health determinants (Kenny et al. 2006).

Furthermore, health promotion interventions have the potential to be patronising and coercive, and the practitioner's definition of 'health' may not be congruent with the community's (see Chapter 1 for an exploration of 'health'). Activity 8.11 explores an example of some ethical and practical issues related to health promotion.

Advocacy

As we have seen in Chapters 4 and 7, deprivation and inequality have a strong relationship with ill health, and there is ample evidence that people's social and economic environments impact on their health (Gostin 2003, Wise 2001). This raises the question of whether health professionals have a duty to advocate for equity with regard to the direct determinants of health, in addition to the broader determinants such as housing and employment. The WHO (1998 p 5) claims that people in the health professions have an obligation to 'act as advocates for health at all levels in society'. What does this mean? One definition of 'advocacy' is where individuals or groups endeavour to change some of the factors that shape people's environments and health behaviours by restructuring a range of elements, such as institutions, policies and laws (Chapman 2001, Wise 2001).

Use the following example to reflect on advocacy and how you may be able to contribute to improving people's environments. The Australian movement *BUGA-UP* (Billboard Utilising Graffitists Against Unhealthy Promotions) began in 1979. It targeted billboards advertising harmful products: namely, tobacco and alcohol (BUGA-UP website, Chapman 1996). BUGA-UP activists defaced billboards, often making witty observations about the concealed intentions and effects of the advertised products. BUGA-UP contributed to tobacco control by helping to change the focus from an individual responsibility paradigm to one where individuals' behaviours were influenced by their environment—in this case, policies controlling the tobacco industry's advertising (Chapman 1996). Keep the BUGA-UP example in mind as you complete Activity 8.12.

Ethical relativism

There are some ethical rules or laws that seem to apply in all human cultures, such as those against murder and theft. These systems or laws enable people to live together

---

ACTIVITY 8.10 Privacy versus the public interest

Imagine you are diagnosed with an infectious disease—for example pertussis (whooping cough), which is the 'least well controlled of all vaccine-preventable diseases' in Australia (Australian Government Department of Health 2014) and is a particular risk for young unvaccinated infants. The public health authorities ask you if they can contact your Facebook and Twitter friends, in order to trace anyone who has been in contact with you before the pertussis diagnosis.

- How would you react? Would you feel that your right to privacy would be violated, or would you be relieved that your friends would be informed and tested?

- What if you were unconscious, and thus unable to provide consent, as in the case described by Mandeville et al (2014)?

REFLECTION 8.10

Clearly, there is a conflict between safeguarding your privacy and the needs of your friends who may have been infected (Mandeville et al. 2014). Such a case would require a careful balancing of the rights and responsibilities of the relevant authorities, the patient and the public.

Imagine you work with a community that has a high rate of type 2 diabetes. You provide information to the community about the role of diet and exercise in controlling diabetes, and you establish an exercise group. However, the results are disappointing—community members seem indifferent. Those people with diabetes and pre-diabetes (blood glucose levels higher than normal, although not sufficiently high to be labelled diabetes) are not paying more attention to their diets, nor are they exercising more than they were previously.

- What do you think went wrong?
- Do people not care, or do they think that diabetes is 'no big deal'?

Did you consider the people's own perceptions of their problems? There could be other issues that they considered more urgent. If you identified a health issue and its solution without consulting the community, not only have you ignored the precepts of effective health promotion practice (see Chapter 14), but you have also disregarded people's autonomy. Perhaps people did want to address their health problems, but had limited access to affordable, suitable food, or had inadequate exercise facilities (e.g. no safe area to exercise). As well as these more practical issues, it also raises problems of meaning—perhaps your idea of 'health' or 'diabetes' did not accord with theirs. Importantly, there is the possibility that your approach may have been interpreted as coercive and paternalistic—that is, there may have been a perception that you imposed your own views of what the community priorities should be, regardless of the perceptions of community members.

- Do you think a similar approach today to that taken towards tobacco—changing the focus from individual responsibility to individuals' behaviours being influenced by their environment—would influence policies on the advertising and availability of alcohol? Worldwide, alcohol is responsible for 4% of all deaths, more than that caused by HIV/AIDS or TB (WHO 2011). Alcohol misuse in Australia is responsible for '3.2 per cent of the total burden of disease and injury in Australia' (National Preventative Health Taskforce 2010 p 24), and cost the Australian community more than $14 billion in 2010 (this figure does not include the harmful effects on other people) (Manning et al. 2013). Furthermore, risky alcohol use is increasing in teenagers and young people throughout the world (WHO 2011), and there is mounting evidence of a direct relationship between advertising and underage drinking (Jones & Jernigan 2010).
- Do you think that alcohol companies should be subject to the same advertising limitations as tobacco companies? What other ethical obligations should be required of such powerful organisations?
- Was the behaviour of BUGA-UP ethical or unethical, given the alcohol and tobacco companies' rights (at the time) to advertise?

(Gostin et al. 2007) by minimising conflict. However, different cultures can have very different values and traditions. Does this mean that ethics should be analysed from a culturally-relative perspective? That is, should we make the assumption that certain behaviours are acceptable in some cultures but not in others, and must be considered in their specific context (Bayer et al. 2007)? Activity 8.13 examines the notion of cultural relativism.

Contemporary and future public health ethics

There is a vital need for more research and discussion on public health ethics, especially on the subject of research and practice with vulnerable or marginalised populations,

REFLECTION 8.12

If you think alcohol policies should be changed, did you think about lobbying the government, or developing media campaigns? Did you consider whether there are any risks to yourself? For example, if your employer does not support your viewpoint, any public action that you take could endanger your employment. Is there any way you can lobby or protest as a 'private individual'? If you think current Australian policies about the availability and advertising of alcohol are fine, can you justify your stance, given the problems of alcohol misuse? Do you think it is about individual freedom of choice versus the 'nanny state' or paternalism (i.e. where the state tries to control your actions for your own benefit)? What the BUGA-UP activists did may not have been legal—that is, defacing signs that did not belong to them—but should it be argued that it was ethical as they had good intentions (*deontological* ethical argument) and actually contributed to a healthier environment for all Australians (*consequentialist* ethical argument)?

ACTIVITY 8.13 Cultural impacts on health

- In some societies it is not acceptable for women and girls to be seen by non-related males, which means they may be denied healthcare if there are no female health professionals available. Similarly, they may not be permitted to attend school: a lack of education not only impacts on their health and the health of their children, but also on that of the whole population.
- Does this mean that it is ethical within that particular culture for about half the population to have little or no access to healthcare or education?

REFLECTION 8.13

If you said it is not ethical, can you say why? Conversely, if you said that it is—because we should respect other people's culture and traditions—what about when people migrate to countries where everyone takes good healthcare and education for granted? Do the new arrivals have the same rights as they would if they were still in their country of origin, or do they have the same rights as everyone else in their new country? If we accept ethical relativism, we may also have to accept some abhorrent consequences—for example, some groups have beliefs about the worth or 'humanity' of other groups. Does that mean that it is ethical for the former to kill the latter if they think they are not fully human? Agreeing to ethical relativism excludes the possibility of condemning or questioning the behaviour of other groups, or our own, and learning from this process (Bayer et al. 2007).

including Indigenous peoples, refugees, and people on low incomes. Moreover, health professionals need to consider more than just public health-related ethical concerns—they need to contend with all of the factors that promote or damage health, including the social, environmental, political and economic determinants, and the ethical challenges associated with them. Health professionals also have a duty to advocate for change, in order to address the factors that contribute to unhealthy environments.

A thorough exploration of values and analyses from a range of philosophies will illuminate beliefs and judgements, and this will produce more valuable and equitable health policies, systems and procedures.

A final word

In this chapter we have considered definitions of ethics and introduced you to a variety of ethical theories relevant to public health ethics. We have emphasised that public health professionals need to stay up-to-date on any changes to their own ethical obligations, in both a legal and a professional sense. We presented some practical examples of ethics in action to illustrate some of the dilemmas that confront organisations and professionals in their attempts to protect and promote the health of the public.

This chapter has endeavoured to unite ethics and public health to demonstrate that good public health practice is intrinsically ethical, and that ethics should be an ordinary part of our day-to-day public health activities. As health professionals, your understanding of ethical practice is a significant aspect of your professional training. This knowledge and insight will enable you to anticipate and address any potential ethical issues prior to taking action, and practise in such a way that your motives and values are clearly apparent to others. Anyone working in a public health-related environment should realise that diverse individuals and disciplines might take separate directions in managing similar ethical challenges. There may be more than one correct solution in any given situation, a range of equally unattractive compromises, or none at all. Nevertheless, if you practise systematically, and reflect on your practice, you can be confident that the approach you take will be, in your professional opinion, the best possible strategy in that particular place and time. Furthermore, you will be able to justify your actions, both to yourself and to others.

REVIEW QUESTIONS

1 What is the best theoretical approach to public health ethics—for example, consequence- or rule-based? Is there only one best approach, or must all be applied in a balanced way? Justify your response.

2 Think of an example of a conflict between the principles of autonomy and of the good of the community. Why is there a conflict, how would you approach it, and is there an outcome where both principles can be respected?

3 Do you think it is possible to ethically practise in, or research with, a culture or community different from your own? Do you see any likely ethical dilemmas?

4 Identify some key contemporary challenges for public health ethics, and outline their significance.

5 After reading each chapter in this book, try to identify an ethical dilemma that could potentially arise as a result of public health actions (or lack of action). Explain why they would be problems, and outline your solutions.

6 Why should health professionals be concerned with policies and programs external to the health sector, such as economic and welfare policies?

7 Outline two of the main differences between public health ethics and bioethics.

8 What is meant by 'cultural relativism', and is it a concept that we need to utilise in public health practice?

9 Why does the WHO (1998 p 5) claim that people in the health professions have an obligation to 'act as advocates for *health* at all levels in society'?

10 What are some of the challenges with utilising a rights-based framework for public health ethics?

Acknowledgement

Special thanks to Briin Gould for his perceptive editorial comments.

Endnote

1   The Nuremberg Trials refer to the prosecution in the 1940s of some of the leaders of the Nazi movement, following World War 2, for war crimes and crimes against humanity, in Nuremberg, Germany (Holocaust History Project 2008).

References

ABC Radio National, 2010. Test for prostate cancer. The Health Report 19 April 2010. Online. Available: <http://www.abc.net.au/rn/healthreport/stories/2010/2875054.htm> (5 Sep 2014).

Annas, G.J., 2010. Worst Case Bioethics: Death, Disaster and Public Health. Oxford University Press, New York.

Australian Government Department of Health, 2012. The strategic plan for control of tuberculosis in Australia: 2011–2015, 2012. Communicable Diseases Intelligence 36 (3), E286–E293. Online. Available: <http://www.health.gov.au/internet/main/publishing.nsf/Content/cda-cdi3603i.htm> (5 Sep 2014).

Australian Government Department of Health, 2014. Australian immunisation handbook, 10th edn, 2013. Online. Available: <http://www.health.gov.au/internet/immunise/publishing.nsf/Content/handbook10-4-12> (21 Sep 2014).

Australian Institute of Health and Welfare, 2012. Australia's Health 2012. AIHW Cat. No. AUS 156. AIHW, Canberra.

Azétsop, J., Rennie, S., 2010. Principlism, medical individualism, and health promotion in resource-poor countries: can autonomy-based bioethics promote social justice and population health? Philosophy, Ethics, and Humanities in Medicine 5, 1.

Bayer, R., Fairchild, A.L., 2004. The genesis of public health ethics. Bioethics 18 (6), 473–492.

Bayer, R., Gostin, L.O., Jennings, B. (Eds.), 2007. Public Health Ethics: Theory, Policy, and Practice. Oxford University Press, New York.

Beauchamp, T.L., Childress, J.F., 2001. Principles of Biomedical Ethics, fifth ed. Oxford University Press, New York.

Beauchamp, D., Steinbock, B. (Eds.), 1999. New Ethics for the Public's Health. Oxford University Press, New York.

Bernheim, R.G., 2005. Moderator's Comment. In: Melnick, A., Kaplowitz, L., Lopez, W.F. et al. (Eds), Public Health Ethics in Action: Flu Vaccine and Drug Allocation Strategies. Journal of Law, Medicine and Ethics 33 (4/Suppl.): 102–105.

Brawley, O.W., Ankerst, D.P., Thompson, I.M., 2009. Screening for prostate cancer. CA: A Cancer Journal for Clinicians 59, 264–273.

BUGA-UP (Billboard Utilising Graffitists Against Unhealthy Promotions) website, 2012. Online. Available: <http://www.bugaup.org/> (18 Mar 2014).

Callahan, D., Jennings, B., 2002. Ethics and public health: forging a strong relationship. American Journal of Public Health 92, 169–176.

Canadian Institutes of Health Research, Natural Sciences and Engineering Research Council of Canada, Social Sciences and Humanities Research Council of Canada, 2010. Tri-Council Policy Statement: Ethical Conduct for Research Involving Humans. Online. Available: <http://www.pre.ethics.gc.ca/pdf/eng/tcps2/TCPS_2_FINAL_Web.pdf> (18 Mar 2014).

Centers for Disease Control and Prevention website. U.S. Public Health Service syphilis study at Tuskegee. Online. Available: <http://www.cdc.gov/tuskegee/timeline.htm> (18 Mar 2014).

Centers for Disease Control and Prevention, 2014. CDC social media tools, guidelines and best practices. Online. Available: <http://www.cdc.gov/socialmedia/tools/guidelines/socialmediatoolkit.html> (4 May 2014).

Chapman, S., 1996. Civil disobedience and tobacco control: the case of BUGA UP. Tobacco Control 5 (3), 179–185.

Chapman, S., 2001. Advocacy in public health: roles and challenges. International Journal of Epidemiology 30, 1226–1232.

Coleman, C.H., Bouësseau, M.-C., Reis, A., 2008. The contribution of ethics to public health. Bulletin of the World Health Organization 86 (8), 578–579.

Cribb, A., Duncan, P., 2002. Health Promotion and Professional Ethics. Blackwell Science, Oxford.

Etzioni, R., Penson, D.F., Legler, J.M., et al., 2002. Overdiagnosis due to prostate-specific antigen screening: lessons from U.S. prostate cancer incidence trends. Journal of the National Cancer Institute 94 (13), 981–990.

Fairchild, A.L., Johns, D.M., 2012. Beyond bioethics: reckoning with the public health paradigm. American Journal of Public Health 102 (8), 1447–1450.

Fry, C.L., Peerson, A., Scully, A., 2004. Raising the profile of public health ethics in Australia: time for debate. Australian and New Zealand Journal of Public Health 28 (1), 13–15.

The Genographic Project website, 2014. Online. Available: <https://genographic.nationalgeographic.com/> (18 Sep 2014).

Gostin, L.O., 2003. Public health ethics: tradition, profession, and values. Acta Bioethica 9 (2), 177–188.

Gostin, L.O., Bayer, R., Fairchild, A.L., et al., 2007. Ethical and legal challenges posed by severe acute respiratory syndrome: implications for the control of severe infectious disease threats. In: Bayer, R., Gostin, L.O., Jennings, B. (Eds.), Public Health Ethics: Theory, Policy, and Practice. Oxford University Press, New York, pp. 261–278.

Harry, D., 2009. Indigenous peoples and gene disputes. Chicago-Kent Law Review 84 (1), 147–196. Online. Available: <http://scholarship.kentlaw.iit.edu/cklawreview/vol84/iss1/8> (5 May 2014).

Health Research Council of New Zealand/Te Kaunihera Rangahau Hauora o Aotearoa, 2005. Guidelines on ethics in health research May 2002 (revised 2005). Online. Available: <http://www.hrc.govt.nz/sites/default/files/HRC%20Guidelines%20on%20Ethics%20in%20Health%20Research.pdf> (21 Apr 2014).

Holocaust History Project, 2008. The trial at Nuremberg. Online. Available: <http://www.holocaust-history.org/> (18 Mar 2014).

Jones, S.C., Jernigan, D.H., 2010. Alcohol advertising, marketing and regulation. Editorial. Journal of Public Affairs 10 (1–2), 1–5.

Kanehe, L.M., 2007. From Kumulipo: I know where I come from—an Indigenous Pacific critique of the Genographic Project. In: Mead, A.T.P., Ratuva, S. (Eds.), Pacific Genes and Life Patents—Pacific Indigenous Experiences and Analysis of the Commodification and Ownership of Life. Call of the Earth Llamado de la Tierra and The United Nations University Institute of Advanced Studies, Wellington, pp. 114–127.

Kenny, N.P., Melnychuk, R.M., Asada, A., 2006. The promise of public health: ethical reflections. Canadian Journal of Public Health 97 (5), 402–404.

Leeder, S.R., 2004. Ethics and public health. Internal Medicine Journal 34 (7), 435–439.

McMichael, A.J., Butler, C.D., 2007. Emerging health issues: the widening challenge for population health promotion. Health Promotion International 21 (Suppl. 1), 15–24. doi: 10.1093/heapro/dal047.

Mandeville, K.T., Harris, M., Thomas, H.L., et al., 2014. Using social networking sites for communicable disease control: innovative contact tracing or breach of confidentiality? Public Health Ethics 7, 47–50.

Mann, J.M., 1997. Medicine and public health, ethics and human rights. The Hastings Center Report 27 (3), 6–13.

Manning, M., Smith, C., Mazerolle, P., 2013. The societal costs of alcohol misuse in Australia. Trends and Issues in Crime and Criminal Justice 454 (April), 1–6. Online. Available: <http://www.aic.gov.au/media_library/publications/tandi_pdf/tandi454.pdf> (18 Mar 2014).

National Health and Medical Research Council (NHMRC), 2003. Values and Ethics: Guidelines for Ethical Conduct in Aboriginal and Torres Strait Islander Health Research. NHMRC, Canberra. Online. Available: <https://www.nhmrc.gov.au/_files_nhmrc/publications/attachments/e52.pdf> (18 Sep 2014) (under review).

National Health and Medical Research Council (NHMRC), 2007 (updated March 2014). National Statement on Ethical Conduct in Human Research. NHMRC, the Australian Research Council and the Australian Vice-Chancellors' Committee. Commonwealth of Australia, Canberra. Online. Available: <http://www.nhmrc.gov.au/guidelines/publications/e72> (21 Sep 2014).

National Preventative Health Taskforce, 2010. Taking preventative action—a response to Australia: the healthiest country by 2020—the report of the National Preventative Health Taskforce 2010. Online. Available: <http://www.preventativehealth.org.au/internet/preventativehealth/publishing.nsf/Content/6B7B17659424FBE5CA25772000095458/$File/tpa.pdf> (21 Sep 2014).

New South Wales Consolidated Acts. Public Health Act 2010: sect. 62. Online. Available: <http://www.austlii.edu.au/au/legis/nsw/consol_act/pha2010126/s62.html> (31 Mar 2014).

New South Wales Department of Health website. Online. Available: <http://www.health.nsw.gov.au/Infectious/controlguideline/Pages/tuberculosis.aspx#9> (31 Mar 2014).

Nicholas, G., Hollowell, J., 2009. Decoding Implications of the Genographic Project for Archaeology and Cultural Heritage: Transcript of a Panel Discussion Held at the Chacmool Conference 'Decolonizing Archaeology. University of Calgary, Alberta, Canada. November 2006. International Journal of Cultural Property 16(2): 141–181.

Nuffield Council on Bioethics, 2007. Public health: ethical issues. Online. Available: <http://nuffieldbioethics.org/project/public-health/> (15 Sep 2014).

Office of the High Commissioner for Human Rights. Online. Available: <http://www.ohchr.org/Documents/Publications/FactSheet2Rev.1en.pdf> (31 Mar 2014).

O'Neill, O., 2002. Public health or clinical ethics: thinking beyond borders. Ethics and International Affairs 16 (2), 35–45.

Onemda VicHealth Koori Health Unit, 2008. We Can like Research … in Koori Hands: a Community Report on Onemda VicHealth Koori Health Unit's Research Workshops in 2007. Onemda VicHealth Koori Health Unit, University of Melbourne, Melbourne.

Parker, E., Gould, T., Fleming, M.L., 2007. Ethics in health promotion—reflections in practice. Health Promotion Journal of Australia 18 (1), 69–72.

Pharmaceutical Society of Australia, 2011. Code of ethics for pharmacists. Online. Available: <http://www.psa.org.au/download/codes/code-of-ethics-2011.pdf> (21 Sep 2014).

Public Health Leadership Society, 2002. Principles of the ethical practice of public health. Online. Available: <http://phls.org/CMSuploads/PHLSposter-68526.pdf> (20 Sep 2014).

Queensland Government, 2011. Code of conduct for the Queensland public service. Online. Available: <http://www.psc.qld.gov.au/includes/assets/qps-code-conduct.pdf> (20 Sep 2014).

Saba, M., Bittoun, R., Kritikos, V., et al., 2013. Smoking cessation in community pharmacy practice—a clinical information needs analysis. SpringerPlus 2, 449. doi: 10.1186/2193-1801-2-449.

Senanayake, S.N., Ferson, M.J., 2004. Detention for tuberculosis: public health and the law. Medical Journal of Australia 180 (11), 573–576.

Sindall, C., 2002. Does health promotion need a code of ethics? Health Promotion International 17 (3), 201–203.

Stein, M.L., Rump, B.O., Mirjam, E.E., et al., 2014. Social networking sites as a tool for contact tracing: urge for ethical framework for normative guidance. Public Health Ethics 7 (1), 57–60.

Tallbear, K., 2013. Native American DNA: Tribal Belonging and the False Promise of Genetic Science. University of Minnesota Press, Minneapolis.

Thomas, J.C., Sage, M., Dillenberg, J., et al., 2002. A code of ethics for public health. American Journal of Public Health 92 (7), 1057–1059.

Thompson, A., Robertson, A., Upshur, R., 2003. Public health ethics: towards a research agenda. Acta Bioethica 9 (2), 157–163.

United Nations General Assembly, 1948. Universal declaration of human rights. Adopted and proclaimed by General Assembly resolution 217 A (III) of 10 December 1948. Online. Available: <http://www.un.org/Overview/rights.html> (19 Sep 2014).

United Nations, 2008. United Nations declaration on the rights of Indigenous peoples. Online. Available: <http://www.un.org/esa/socdev/unpfii/documents/DRIPS_en.pdf> (17 Apr 2014).

United Nations Permanent Forum on Indigenous Issues, 2010. Available: <http://www.un.org/esa/socdev/unpfii/index.html> (18 Sep 2014).

University of Virginia Health Sciences Library, 1996. Final report of the Tuskegee Syphilis Study Legacy Committee (20 May 1996). Online. Available: <http://exhibits.hsl.virginia.edu/badblood/report/> (18 Sep 2014).

Wise, M., 2001. The role of advocacy in promoting health. Promotion and Education 8 (2), 69–74.

World Health Organization, 1978. Declaration of Alma-Ata. International Conference on Primary Health Care, Alma-Ata, USSR, 6–12 September 1978. Online. Available: <http://www.who.int/publications/almaata_declaration_en.pdf> (26 Sep 2014).

World Health Organization, 1996. Equity in Health and Health Care. WHO, Geneva.

World Health Organization, 1998. Health Promotion Glossary. WHO, Geneva. Online. Available: <http://whqlibdoc.who.int/hq/1998/WHO_HPR_HEP_98.1.pdf> (19 Sep 2014).

World Health Organization, 2011. Global status report on alcohol and health. Online. Available: <http://www.who.int/substance_abuse/publications/global_alcohol_report/msbgsruprofiles.pdf> (18 Sep 2014).

World Health Organization, 2013. China–WHO Joint Mission on Human Infection with Avian Influenza A (H7N9) Virus 18–24 Apr 2013 mission report. Online. Available: <http://www.who.int/influenza/human_animal_interface/influenza_h7n9/ChinaH7N9JointMissionReport2013u.pdf?ua=1> (5 Sep 2014).

CHAPTER 9

Evidence-based practice

Mary Louise Fleming & Gerry FitzGerald

Learning objectives

After reading this chapter, you should be able to:

- define the terms used to describe evidence-based practice in public health

- identify the major challenges associated with the application of evidence-based practice

- describe the need for evidence-based practice, and the links between research, practical experience, and evidence-based practice or policy

- appraise the quality of research, and evaluate its application to evidence-based practice

- identify the factors that impact on applying research to evidence-based practice or policy.

Introduction

This chapter traces the history of evidence-based practice (EBP) from its roots in evidence-based medicine to contemporary thinking about its usefulness to public health practice. It defines EBP and differentiates it from 'evidence-based medicine', 'evidence-based policy' and 'evidence-based healthcare'. As it is important to understand the subjective nature of knowledge and the research process, this chapter describes the nature and production of knowledge. This chapter considers the necessary skills for EBP, and the processes of attaining the necessary evidence. We examine the barriers and facilitators to identifying and implementing 'best practice', and when EBP is appropriate to use. There is a discussion about the limitations of EBP and the use of other information sources to guide practice, and concluding information about the application of evidence to guide policy and practice.

The evolution: evidence-based medicine

Health and medical research has always informed the development of clinical practice. However, translating research into practice has often been prolonged and disjointed. Medical and other health professionals are attached to the value of experience. Thus, standards of clinical practice were traditionally formulated through a combination of research, analysis and the collective wisdom of the profession, and individual practice was reliant on clinicians' own experiences.

In 1972, an epidemiologist, Dr Archie Cochrane, criticised the medical profession for not providing reviews of clinical interventions so that policymakers and organisations could base their practice on empirically proven evidence (Killoran & Kelly 2010, Mazurek Melnyk & Fineout-Overholt 2005, Oliver & McDaid 2002).

Similarly, researchers from McMaster University in Canada felt that the medical profession was too reliant on clinical experience and personal judgement, rather than empirically supported evidence (Hamer 2005). It was this group of researchers who first coined the term 'evidence-based medicine', defined as 'the conscientious, explicit, and judicious use of current best evidence in making decisions about the care of individual patients' (Sackett et al. 1996 p 71). This definition implies an organised process applied to a particular circumstance, and recognises the clinicians' expertise. *Conscientious use* of evidence implies a systematic and organised approach to the identification of the evidence. *Judicious use* implies the wise application of the evidence to the particular clinical circumstances, and recognises the value of the clinician's cumulative experience, education and skills in applying the evidence to the particulars of the patient (Fink 2013).

Launched in 1993, the Cochrane Collaboration aimed to provide up-to-date systematic reviews of healthcare interventions, and to ensure the accessibility of these reviews, so that consumers could make informed decisions about their healthcare (Mazurek Melnyk & Fineout-Overholt 2005) (Box 9.1).

The impact of evidence-based medicine has been, first, to develop the means of accumulating the evidence in a systematic manner, analysing the evidence, and converting that evidence into clinical guidelines, which translate the often enormous quantities

---

BOX 9.1

THE COCHRANE COLLABORATION

Dr Archie Cochrane observed that thousands of low-birth-weight premature infants were dying needlessly. He was able to exemplify his argument for the need for reviews of intervention trials by locating, analysing and synthesising results from several randomised controlled trials (RCTs) that tested the effectiveness of corticosteroid therapy to halt premature labour in high-risk women. His systematic review of these trials demonstrated that corticosteroid therapy significantly reduced the likelihood of premature infants dying.

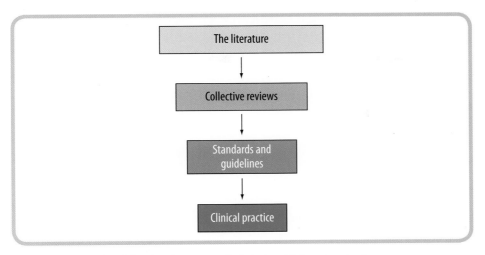

FIG. 9.1 Example of the development of clinical guideline standards.

of data available in the literature into an accessible and usable format for clinicians (Figure 9.1).

Second, an emphasis on evidence-based medicine has served to reduce the previous reliance on 'opinion' as unqualified 'evidence' in its own right.

The principles have been applied to public health, health policy, planning and management (Bali 2013, Fink 2013, Flitcroft et al. 2011, Gerrish 2006).

The nature of evidence, and key concepts of evidence-based practice

What defines 'evidence', and 'EBP'? How does EBP fit into the complex nature of public policy, public health and healthcare?

We are currently living in an 'information age' (Bali 2013, Hamer 2005, Mazurek Melnyk & Fineout-Overholt 2005). Technological advancement means increased accessibility of information (Bali 2013). For example, the internet brings information from all over the world into our homes—literally at our fingertips (see Activity 9.1).

The nature and scope of knowledge

Underpinning the quest for evidence are questions about the nature of knowledge—'epistemology' (Topping 2006). Epistemology is the branch of Western philosophy that is concerned with reality— that is, the nature and scope of knowledge and how it is produced (Topping 2006). Over time, different perspectives of reality have dominated. These

ACTIVITY 9.1 Appraising the evidence

- A family member's favourite celebrity is campaigning against mobile phone towers being placed near schools. The family member asks you about the health impact of mobile phone towers, as you are studying for a health degree. Because your studies have taught you to base your decisions on evidence, you research information on the health impact of mobile phone towers. What sources might you consult and trust? What sources do you think would interest your family member the most?

REFLECTION 9.1

There is a range of information sources—journals, textbooks, newspapers, magazines, editorials, internet newspapers, telecommunications industry/associations' reports, blogs written by companies or individuals, and government and private health agencies' websites and reports. Some information sources are more trustworthy than others. Information from the internet or in news clips may not be as reliable as that provided by rigorous scientific studies. There has been a significant increase in the number of research studies being conducted, papers being published, and journals available. Technological advancements have meant that the quality of research methodologies has improved, and research findings are more accessible (Killoran & Kelly 2010, Smith 2013).

This abundance of information justifies EBP. However, we need to know how to interpret information and critically analyse it for its value. Values and beliefs influence how evidence is applied, sometimes at the expense of the research outcomes. Is there a single truth? How is knowledge created? Is it neutral, or is it influenced by social, economic and political factors?

While we are lucky to have so much information at our disposal, it does mean that there is more information to assess to determine what constitutes evidence. Information must be sorted, analysed and then given meaning, or moulded into knowledge by describing its practical application in specific settings (Dawes 2005, Head 2010, Mozaffarian 2012).

This process can be very time-consuming, and other factors increase the complexity of identifying and implementing 'best practice', including problems with dissemination and communication of the implications of research, and the methods employed to obtain these results (Mozaffarian 2012). Political pressure might influence what research is conducted, published and used to influence practice, and organisational barriers might hinder health professionals who are implementing EBPs within their organisations (Brownson et al. 2009b).

perspectives, or 'worldviews', are referred to as *paradigms*. A change in the dominant perspective is referred to as a *paradigm shift* (Taylor & Roberts 2006).

Professional groups may have different paradigms; what constitutes evidence for one profession may not be considered so for another. Even within healthcare and health research, individuals may have different perspectives about what forms sound knowledge (Rychetnik & Wise 2004, Taylor & Roberts 2006). Knowledge and evidence are, therefore, socially constructed.

Research is influenced by assumptions underlying the current paradigm of the profession and individual researchers, and is not an isolated or objective process (Topping 2006). Using 'rigorous' research to guide practice is a requirement of the current scientific paradigm. Corcoran and Vandiver (2004) claim that this approach is now considered the industry standard. Where well-established practices would have once constituted 'evidence', contemporary EBP requires that the efficacy of the intervention is demonstrated in practice (Frommer & Rychetnik 2003, Smith 2013).

The concept of *rigour* and the methods required for rigorous research are also socially constructed, influenced by the researchers' *worldviews*. Traditionally, science has taken a positivist approach, believing in absolute and objective truths (Topping 2006). Positivists are concerned about the frequency and distribution of an event or phenomenon, and attempt to use standardised methods and maintain objectivity, primarily through distancing themselves from the subjects under study, to reach a 'truth' (Liamputtong & Ezzy 2005). But evidence is imperfect, so practitioners will have to seek the best evidence available at the time (Brownson et al. 2009b).

The use of qualitative methods means that researchers focus on an understanding of human behaviour through exploration of feelings, values, perspectives and interpretations of individuals and social groups. Qualitative research aims to provide an in-depth, information-rich account of human experience, and researchers argue that reality is not objective, rather it is socially constructed. Therefore, there is no single truth (Brownson et al. 2010, Topping 2006).

The perspectives of the individual researcher, the science, and the health professions will influence how research is carried out and what is established as 'evidence'. The shift of focus away from quantitative methods to utilising a combination of methods is an example of a paradigm shift (Brownson et al. 2009a, Taylor & Roberts 2006, Topping 2006). Many health researchers argue that using a combination of perspectives and methods can provide a more comprehensive account of the phenomenon under study, and that different methods may be more useful for answering different questions (Hall et al. 2010, Topping 2006). (See Activity 9.2.)

Key concepts of evidence-based practice

Evidence-based practice originated in growing concerns to improve healthcare and health outcomes by basing practice on the best available evidence (Gray 2009, Hall et al. 2010, Rosenthal & Sutcliffe 2002).

EBP should not be confused with 'research utilisation', which refers to using knowledge gained from a single study (Hall et al. 2010, Mazurek Melnyk & Fineout-Overholt 2005). While there may not be sufficient research on a particular topic to conduct a systematic review, there are risks in using the results of only one study to guide practice (see Case Study 9.1).

One of the most successful public health interventions of the twentieth century led to the recognition that smoking was associated with an increased risk of lung cancer. Despite it being widely accepted by the public and health professionals alike that tobacco use is responsible for many cases of lung cancer, this has not been empirically proven, and it is unlikely that it ever will be. It would be unethical to subject some individuals to tobacco smoke and not others, which would be required in order to conduct a randomised controlled trial (RCT).

In some cases there is no research available on a certain topic. In a practice setting, it is not feasible to send clients away just because there has been no prior research conducted about their problems. EBP must also consider the expertise of the health professional, as well as the values and preferences of the client (Hall et al. 2010, Mazurek Melnyk & Fineout-Overholt 2005).

ACTIVITY 9.2 Evaluating evidence

- For a public health professional, evidence is some form of data—including quantitative data, results of program or policy evaluations, and qualitative data—for use in making judgements or decisions. While evidence is usually the result of a complex web of observation, theory and experiment, the 'evidence' is in the eye of the beholder. For example, a Scottish study of five men who ate 227 g of carrots for breakfast for three weeks revealed that their average cholesterol had decreased by 11%. Due to the limitations of the study design, the researchers could not say whether it was the carrots, not eating their usual breakfast, or the Hawthorne effect that caused the reduction (Schardt 2011).

- What do you think were the problems with the study? Do you think the sample size was large enough? Do you know what else they were eating or if they changed their diet? What is the Hawthorne effect?

REFLECTION 9.2

The problems are related to the small size of the sample, no comparison or control group, no randomisation of participants in the study, no discussion of other activities or dietary changes, and no blinding to treatment.

If we had not 'renegotiated' evidence and the processes we used to construct evidence, we might still think that: cigarette smoking is harmless; disease is a punishment from God; or homosexuality is a disease. In some cultures, these beliefs and the processes used to establish the 'evidence' to 'prove' such beliefs may not yet be contested and, therefore, still prevail. Can you think of other examples of 'evidence' that have been subsequently falsified over time?

In practice, what does an 'evidence base' mean? Is it about using strategies that the research suggests are the best means for achieving the stated aims? Is it about changing practice? Is it about a systematic appraisal of the best available evidence? The answer to all of these questions is 'yes'. However, in practice there is never absolute certainty, as programs that are implemented even in similar circumstances are never quite the same. In addition, research is not always reliable and valid, even if it is available on a particular issue. Several authors refer to the approach to EBP being more like a journey

CASE STUDY
9.1

Dangers of 'research utilisation'

Kraaijenhagen et al. (2000) reported that a study they had conducted revealed that travellers were not at an increased risk from deep vein thrombosis (DVT) compared with the general population. Shortly after, other research studies reported that travellers were at increased risk. In 2001, Scurr et al. (2001 p 1485) reported that 'symptomless DVT might occur in up to 10% of long-haul airline travellers'. Public opinion was further persuaded by reports of a woman who was travelling by air to Australia and died from a pulmonary embolus.

According to Dawes (2005), several studies published over a six-month period reported conflicting data. Consumers who sought advice from their general practitioner on the health risks of travelling may have received an incomplete picture of the risk if the healthcare professional relied only on the first article published.

REFLECTION ON CASE STUDY 9.1

Should health professionals use only the results obtained from randomised controlled trials (RCTs) to guide their practice? Not all health topics could ethically be tested using an RCT. When there are differences of opinion about an issue in the scientific literature, what information should health professionals use to guide their practice? How much evidence should be collected before making a decision?

towards more effective practice, and along this journey the practitioner must become more open-minded (Brownson et al. 2010, Fink 2013, Naidoo & Wills 2005) (see Box 9.2).

What is 'evidence-based practice'?

Using evidence to make decisions about practice is very similar to undertaking primary research. There are five steps involved:

1 identifying the problem
2 identifying evidence that relates to the problem

BOX 9.2

WHAT IS AN 'EVIDENCE-BASED PRACTITIONER'?

If you are an evidence-based practitioner, you can use problem-solving skills to determine:

- what it is that you need to know
- whether the intervention is effective, acceptable, equitable, implemented consistently and safely, and is cost-effective
- whether you have the best available evidence
- whether the quality of the evidence is good
- whether the evidence is appropriate for the population and context in which you will use the evidence (adapted from Naidoo & Wills 2005).

3 finding the evidence

4 determining how useful the evidence is through critical appraisal

5 synthesising the available evidence into a practical application.

To become an evidence-based practitioner, you need to critique the evidence and be willing to change your practice if doing so is indicated by the evidence.

Identifying the problem. First, the problem must be defined sufficiently and specifically so that it will be useful for the search for evidence. Examine Activity 9.3 and consider how you might identify the problem in order to ensure that your focus is on the most appropriate evidence.

There are two major issues to be considered when thinking about the evidence that might suggest a particular way of approaching an intervention. First, what sources should you be looking for as evidence? And second, how should you use evidence to make an informed decision? To answer the first question, most EBP relies on primary research from academic or professional journals, textbooks, published and unpublished reports, conference papers and presentations. The second question is about the range of evidence that might inform practice, which might include how effective the intervention was in meeting its goals, whether there is evidence available on the transferability of the intervention to other settings and with other populations, what the positive and negative effects of the intervention were, and what the barriers to implementing the intervention were (Hall et al. 2010, Naidoo & Wills 2005, Smith 2013). (See Activity 9.3.)

The scientific model has gained prominence as a quantitatively objective method for *finding the evidence*; contextual factors, such as environment, socioeconomic factors or education, are considered as *confounding variables*, and study designs often try to eliminate their effects. RCTs are viewed as the 'gold standard', but when we are dealing with populations it becomes very difficult if not impossible to adopt an RCT methodology (Naidoo & Wills 2005, Smith 2013). Research findings are graded according to an established *hierarchy of evidence* (see Table 9.1), according to how valid and reliable the methodology for the research is considered to be.

How useful is this paradigm when population health research does not fit neatly into an RCT? Does this mean that there is no evidence base for public health? A focus on scientific experimental evaluation would ignore a large body of emerging work related to public health in community settings and interventions (Killoran & Kelly 2010). Desirable methodological characteristics of research into the effectiveness of interventions include issues such as whether:

- the level of detail of an intervention would enable it to be replicated
- the participants who are the target of the intervention are fully described
- the size and effect of non-respondents is detailed
- there are clear outcomes, and these outcomes are compared with baseline measurements taken before the intervention commences (Killoran & Kelly 2010).

TABLE 9.1 Hierarchy of evidence	
Type 1 evidence	Systematic reviews and meta-analyses including two or more RCTs
Type 2 evidence	Well-designed RCTs
Type 3 evidence	Well-designed controlled trials without randomisation
Type 4 evidence	Well-designed observational studies
Type 5 evidence	Expert opinion, expert panels, views of service users and carers

RCT = randomised controlled trial.
(Source: Naidoo & Wills 2005)

TABLE 9.2 Systematic review process	
The systematic review search should be:	
Explicit	Use key terms, record your search, ensure that it is transparent so that others can assess value, and it can be replicated
Appropriate	Look where evidence is likely to be
Sensitive	Collect all information that is relevant to your question
Specific	Collect only information that is relevant to the question
Comprehensive	Include all available information

There are a number of ways in which evidence can be sourced. Table 9.2 shows the five characteristics involved in systematic reviews.

Numerous sources of evidence can be used to guide practice, such as bibliographical databases (e.g. Medline, Cinahl, Scopus) and the Cochrane and Campbell collaborations. The Cochrane Collaboration focuses on a health and medical perspective, whereas the Campbell Collaboration examines systematic reviews of the effectiveness of social and behavioural interventions. Searches need to be systematically undertaken, using consistent key words or phrases, and they need to be transparent to ensure that others can gauge their suitability and comprehensiveness (Hall et al. 2010).

Determining the usefulness of the evidence is termed *critical appraisal.* This process determines the quality of the research process. It is the systematic evaluation of the relevance of the study, and the ability to critically appraise a range of study types. To undertake this process it is crucial to understand the epidemiological concepts discussed in Chapter 5, not only to be able to understand the results as they have been presented, but also to be able to have a systematic approach to the appraisal (Guillemin & Gillam 2006, Hall et al. 2010). Standard checklists are available to support the systematic appraisal of different types of study design, to help determine the validity of the study findings and whether they can be generalised to other populations. Critical appraisal has to be pragmatic—the focus should be on studies that reach a certain standard of rigour and relevance. Pragmatism is important, because it is usually possible to identify flaws in published research studies and the ways in which the context of the research and one's own practice differ (Brownson et al. 2009a, Brownson et al. 2010, Gray 2009).

Putting evidence into practice

Now that you have been introduced to the reasoning behind EBP, and the skills for finding, evaluating and translating research evidence, it is important that you consider how the ideal compares with reality, in both practice and policy. In this section we discuss the evidence–practice gap, and review current research regarding the reasons why research findings are frequently not translated into action. Techniques for analysing barriers to EBP are described, as is the role of evidence in decision-making.

Although you might assume that having the research evidence required will lead to rational practices and policies, this is often not the case. Examples 9.1, 9.2 and 9.3 demonstrate how the evidence is only slowly incorporated into practice.

Advising on smoking cessation in pregnancy

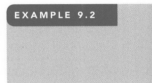
EXAMPLE 9.1

Although evidence from a number of trials strongly suggests that smoking cessation programs can effectively reduce rates of smoking among pregnant women, data showed that 90% of protocols and policies developed and used by antenatal care providers in Australia did not include written advice about smoking cessation (National Institute of Clinical Studies (NCIS) 2008. This material is licensed under Creative Commons Attribution 3.0 Australia license, <https://creativecommons.org/licenses/by/3.0/au/deed.en>).

Measuring glycated haemoglobin in diabetes management

EXAMPLE 9.2

Two major trials have shown that assessing diabetes by glycated haemoglobin (HbA$_{1c}$) measurement can improve diabetes control. However, the Australian Institute of Health and Welfare estimates that less than one-quarter of people with diabetes have these tests performed as frequently as recommended (NICS 2008. This material is licensed under Creative Commons Attribution 3.0 Australia license, <https://creativecommons.org/licenses/by/3.0/au/deed.en>).

Placing infants to sleep on their back to reduce the risk of SIDS

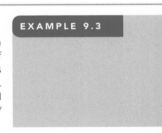
EXAMPLE 9.3

Although public awareness campaigns have successfully reduced the number of infants being placed on their stomach to sleep (the highest-risk position for sudden infant death syndrome (SIDS)), large numbers of infants, particularly Indigenous infants, are still being placed on their side. Evidence shows that, although this position is not as high risk as the stomach, lying infants on their backs provides greater protection from SIDS. Public campaigns need to emphasise the risks of both stomach and side sleeping (NICS 2008. This material is licensed under Creative Commons Attribution 3.0 Australia license, <https://creativecommons.org/licenses/by/3.0/au/deed.en>).

It has been estimated that there is an average delay in conversion of evidence into practice of up to 17 years. The consequence of this delay is that limited clinical practice is in accordance with the latest evidence.

Many of the advances in knowledge occur within research teams whose principal aim is to conduct the research and publish the results. This situation has been aggravated by problems with health workforces, which has resulted in the movement of many 'leading lights' out of traditional teaching roles into research only, or combined clinical and research roles. Thus the diffusion even to new practitioners has been limited.

Why is there a gap between research and practice?

There are many views about the reasons for the gap between research and practice. The research may be unrelated to the clinical concerns or situations, and may not apply to the process of clinical decision-making. Research is standardised, whereas real practice

CASE STUDY 9.2

Handwashing in hospitals

Proper washing of hands by personnel in hospitals has been shown to be highly effective in preventing the transmission of infection from patient to patient. A number of initiatives have been introduced to increase handwashing rates, such as increasing the number of sinks and raising awareness of the need for handwashing. However, studies reveal that hand hygiene is still poor in some departments, particularly between staff consultations (Michie et al. 2005).

REFLECTION FOR CASE STUDY 9.2

A number of reasons could be proposed to explain why staff did not wash their hands appropriately, such as forgetting to or not really thinking it is important. The Michie et al. (2005) model is useful, as it provides a framework to understand the reasons why EBP is not performed, which might suggest avenues to pursue to change this behaviour. Michie et al. (2005) suggest handwashing is not performed because of:

- resources, facilities and time—these are *organisational reasons* (reasons at the higher-order, social and systems levels)
- group norms that prioritise patient throughput over hygiene, or view repeated handwashing as obsessive, or beliefs that rates of infection are not linked to handwashing— these are *motivational factors* (in that they explain why individuals have not yet established an intention to change)
- staff being aware of the need for handwashing, but forgetting to always perform the behaviour—this is *action initiation* (explains the behaviour of those who are motivated to change).

Viewing behaviour in this way suggests avenues to change behaviour, such as local quest to action (e.g. reminders) (Michie et al. 2005). Alternatively, more in-depth educational campaigns may be needed to re-educate hospital staff, if motivational factors are involved.

occurs in diverse settings and circumstances. The research may be inaccessible, confusing or contradictory, and, finally, there are practical limitations to keeping up-to-date in a busy practice.

The causes of the evidence–practice gap are multiple, and vary from setting to setting; one of the simplest models was developed by Michie et al. (2005), who propose three overarching groups (see the reflection for Case Study 9.2).

A number of surveys of health practitioners have been conducted to assess attitudes to EBP and barriers to its implementation. Although data indicate that practitioners welcome EBP, a number of significant barriers to its implementation have been identified:

- reasons relating to the *evidence base*, such as gaps in the evidence base, or the poor quality of evidence
- personal reasons relating to the *individual practitioner*, such as lack of skills to undertake EBP, or a lack of time
- reasons related to the *organisation*, such as inappropriate or inadequate support for EBP, a perceived threat posed by EBP, a lack of understanding of the process, economic constraints, access to evidence, resistance from colleagues (Gray 2009), competing agendas, lack of technical support, or lack of facilities (Brownson et al. 2010, Hall et al. 2010, Killoran & Kelly 2010).

Health practitioners might also face challenges relating to using evidence in a group situation, such as group-think syndrome, whereby, rather than the team approach enhancing performance, the quality of the group's performance and the participation of group members is reduced by group processes. Decisions may also be swayed by influential or vocal individuals, or competing agendas, such as professional rivalry, different perspectives, or distrust (Bali 2013, Fink 2013).

Studies suggest that apart from evidence-related reasons and personal barriers, organisational barriers are highly significant in preventing the implementation of EBP (Henderson et al. 2006, Smith 2013). Reasons seemingly related to the individual practitioner, such as a lack of time or motivation (consider the handwashing example) can also be influenced by organisational factors.

Why don't healthcare organisations use EBP? First, healthcare practice has evolved over a prolonged period of time, during which the role, expectations and environment of the health practitioner have changed dramatically (Dziegielewski & Roberts 2006, Hall et al. 2010). In particular, a shift to practice based on evidence rather than on experience and judgement represents a fundamental change (Steinberg & Luce 2005). Second, healthcare is a complex industry, with national, state and local political responsibilities, services and funding, and public and private industry divisions, all of which influence decisions (Gray 2009). Health-related organisations also frequently have multiple (sometimes conflicting) goals, such as improving health, gaining funding, reducing expenditure, fostering staff development, and influencing government and community stakeholders (Gray 2009, Smith 2013). This can mean that staff groups may have interests that are incompatible with those of others, so that each group becomes focused on achieving its narrow task and finds it difficult to achieve larger organisational objectives (e.g. EBP) (Gray 2009, Smith 2013). The nature of public health (and other allied health professions) also influences uptake of EBP. Public health is frequently described as a mixture of 'science, art and politics', in that its legitimacy and practice is based on factors such as ideological conviction (e.g. that every individual has a 'right' to health), as well as evidence (United Kingdom Public Health Association website). This can lead to debate regarding which practices are 'best', using non-scientific criteria (Killoran & Kelly 2010).

Aspects of organisations themselves also influence the uptake of EBP (see (the hypothetical) Examples 9.4 and 9.5).

Allison

EXAMPLE 9.4

Allison is a recent graduate who works as a dietician for a public hospital in community A. Allison was taught how to critically appraise research during her university course, and is keen to ensure that her practice is based on current evidence. The organisation Allison works for is very busy, and Allison finds she has little time to review journals and keep up-to-date during her work time. One day when she was reading abstracts online, her supervisor noticed and said, 'That's not your job; get back to work.' Allison also finds it difficult to follow EBP, as her organisation has limited information resources and has not subscribed to many journals electronically. After working at the hospital for a few months, Allison finds that, despite her best intentions, she is largely following the organisational line and basing her practice on what is standard practice in the hospital, even though she suspects that new research regarding dietetic practice is available.

Bianca

EXAMPLE 9.5

Bianca is another recent graduate who works as a dietician for a private hospital in community B. Although there are variable levels among staff of an understanding of EBP, the organisation's CEO believes that the ability to adapt to change is crucial for the organisation's future success, and ongoing training is mandatory. Thus, EBP is widely understood and valued. Groups of staff working in various areas also meet monthly to discuss the latest developments in their field, and how these developments can be applied in their practice. Bianca is expected to be familiar with the latest research, and has access to journals online at work. Although her job is very busy, Bianca schedules time in her diary during work hours each week to peruse the evidence and reflect on current practice. Bianca is currently working in conjunction with other hospital staff to identify and overcome potential barriers to changing an aspect of current practice, and feels confident that she will be able to implement this change to improve patient outcomes.

One way Allison's and Bianca's organisations clearly differ is in their organisational culture. Schein defines culture as the 'taken-for-granted, shared, tacit ways of perceiving, thinking and reacting' (1996 p 231). Although norms (common ways of behaving, interacting and so on) are visible manifestations of these underlying assumptions, the assumptions are generally never examined or questioned, making them difficult to change (Schein 1996).

Some cultural beliefs that operate in organisations which might make it difficult to introduce new practices include:

- a reluctance to change historical practices (e.g. 'this is how we've always done things')
- a belief that practice is already at a high level
- a lack of preparedness to ask questions (e.g. 'Why do we do things this way?') (Brownson et al. 2010, Henderson et al. 2006, Smith 2013).

A number of models have been developed to describe organisational cultures; four of the most common are highlighted in Box 9.3. As you examine these models, consider how different cultures will hinder or drive change.

From the example presented in Box 9.3, we might identify Allison's organisation as having a role culture, in that it is clearly focused on individual responsibilities, whereas Bianca's organisation might be considered a learning culture, where original thinking is valued.

This example also shows the need for organisational infrastructure, such as information resources. Mullen (2004) suggests that the following organisational and environmental support is required for practitioners to apply EBP:

- supportive organisational culture, policies and procedures (e.g. the organisation is open to change, provides information technology support, opportunities, incentives and funding for EBP)
- external environment of the organisation (e.g. funders, accreditation groups, national/regional/local authorities) must provide similar opportunities and incentives supporting EBP
- organisational procedures to ensure implementation of guidelines and other evidence-based prescriptions for practice
- methods for systematically evaluating the implementation of EBP and providing feedback to stakeholders on practice effectiveness
- staff trained as evidence-based practitioners capable of working in evidence-based organisations.

Another characteristic of organisations that governs, to some degree, the extent to which practitioners can implement EBP relates to organisational structures.

Organisational structures

One of the key features of an organisation's structure is whether the structure is centralised or decentralised. In centralised structures, decision-making occurs at the senior level while employees at lower levels implement the decisions. In decentralised structures, decisions are made by employees at the lowest possible level in the organisation (Carson 2005, Flitcroft et al. 2011, Head 2010). These are two extremes, and in reality, while most organisations will be more centralised or more decentralised, most will not be 'strictly' either.

There are differences in the distribution of power between these models. Practitioners require real power to change practices, so EBP may be easier to implement in a decentralised organisation, where individual practitioners make decisions influencing their practice. However, centralised structures may more easily be able to coordinate system-wide support, such as funding. Although neither approach is 'better' for EBP, an awareness of the limitations of each may assist you to identify barriers to implementing EBP in your organisation, and possibly advocate for change.

BOX 9.3

MODELS OF ORGANISATIONAL CULTURE

Mechanistic versus organic

This model presents two extremes of organisational structure and activities. In reality, most organisations tend to fall somewhere along the continuum between these two extremes. The *mechanistic organisation* is governed by rules and procedures, generally with extremely hierarchical structures. Communication is most likely to be top-down, and decision-making is centralised. The opposite organisation to this is the *organic organisation*, which is flexible, with few rules and decentralised decision-making. Communication can easily occur across the organisation.

Role versus task

This model again presents a dichotomy, while in reality most organisations fall somewhere between the two. *Role cultures* are secure and predictable, with a focus on individuals' roles and responsibilities. These organisations tend towards hierarchy and bureaucracy, as positions of authority are regarded as important. In contrast, *task-oriented cultures* are project- or job-oriented, enabling flexibility and creativity.

Club

This model emphasises personal power. The individual is conceptualised as an entrepreneur, with the organisation providing administrative resources. This can lead to tensions between professional and corporate entities. This model has been common within healthcare organisations.

Learning

The learning culture is characterised by enquiry, autonomy, creativity and entrepreneurship among employees. It most often occurs in flexible, open and pragmatic organisations.

(Source: Carson 2005)

Finally, although we may expect that as individuals with new ideas enter an organisation these ideas will diffuse through the organisation, organisations may display 'defensive routines', or resist new ideas as a way of 'protecting' the way everything has always been done (Flitcroft et al. 2011, Schein 1996). Conflict is particularly likely when a proposed change is at odds with existing values and assumptions (Flitcroft et al. 2011, Schein 1996).

Finding the evidence

Closing evidence–practice gaps requires recognising situations where EBP is not being practised, identifying and addressing barriers to new practices, challenging past beliefs and practices, and implementing new practices (Brownson et al. 2010). As a trained practitioner who keeps abreast of the latest developments and reflects on current practice, you should be able to recognise when practice is not evidence-based, and recognise many of the common barriers to change. The next step involves analysing the barriers to EBP in your particular setting, which is crucial for understanding how to change current practice.

A number of different techniques can be used to identify barriers, depending on the setting, available funding, expertise and time, and how rigorous the barrier identification process is designed to be (NICS 2006). Table 9.3 provides a brief outline of a number of techniques. The appropriate technique for a given situation will depend on the nature of the organisation or the work undertaken by the organisation, as well as the strengths and limitations of each technique. You should investigate techniques thoroughly before applying them, and seek help from relevant experts when required.

TABLE 9.3 Techniques to overcome bias in research			
Technique	Description	Advantages .... Disadvantages	Other considerations
Brainstorming	A group of participants is brought together to stimulate discussion around a specific idea	Relatively fast and easy Generates a wide range of ideas in a short time Involves future participants in change process Needs skilled moderator Participants may be inhibited in front of others May need incentives for participation	Not suitable when a group session cannot be organised, or when powerful group members may dominate
Case study	A comprehensive description and analysis of a specific past situation or event	Provides very detailed information May gain insights not seen using other techniques Requires multiple forms of data collection and analysis Can be time-consuming and expensive Findings may be subjectively interpreted, not generalisable	Not suitable when investigations may influence action, or when the group of interest is highly variable

		TABLE 9.3 Continued	
Technique	**Description**	**Advantages** / **Disadvantages**	**Other considerations**
Key informant	Seeking the views of individuals who have significant insights into a particular problem or situation	Can obtain detailed, in-depth information Can clarify ideas as the investigation continues Relatively fast and inexpensive Requires suitable informants Relationship between investigator and informants can influence information collected Informants' views may not be representative	Not suitable when strong evidence is required
Interview	Discussion between investigator and participants, or specific questions asked of participants	Can obtain detailed, in-depth information Participants can express their own views Can explore complex or unanticipated issues Interviewer bias may influence information gained Can be time-consuming and expensive Participants may be inhibited Can be difficult to summarise and compare responses	Not suitable when anonymity is required

		TABLE 9.3 Continued	
Technique	Description	Advantages .... Disadvantages	Other considerations
Focus group	A facilitated discussion among a group of people in which a moderator uses open-ended questions to encourage discussion of a particular topic or issue	Relatively fast and easy Generates a wide range of ideas in a short time Can obtain detailed, in-depth information Participants can express their own views Involves future participants in change process Participants may be inhibited in front of others Needs skilled moderator May need incentives for participation Planning and analysis can be time-consuming	Not suitable when the group is widely dispersed, when a group session cannot be organised, or when powerful group members may dominate
Direct observation	Observing interpersonal interactions, events or activities in a given setting	Can provide direct information and reveal unanticipated outcomes May be difficult to obtain agreement for observation Can be time-consuming Requires skilled observer	Observer presence may influence behaviour, not suitable when privacy is required

TABLE 9.3 Continued

Technique	Description	Advantages ················· Disadvantages	Other considerations
Survey	Assessment of participants' knowledge, attitudes and/or self-reported behaviour using a standardised set of questions, usually administered via mail	Can send surveys to practitioners or clients anywhere in the country Can gather data from a large number of people in a short amount of time Participants can remain anonymous Relatively inexpensive Development and testing of questionnaires may be time-consuming Cannot ask follow-up questions Individuals may not accurately report their behaviour or the factors influencing their behaviour Response rates may be low	Not suitable when responses prone to social desirability bias (practitioners report responses they consider will be judged favourably) Validated questionnaires of perceived barriers to change are available
Nominal group technique	Highly structured discussion where ideas of the group are pooled and prioritised	Generates a wide range of ideas in a short time All participants can have input Relatively fast and easy Group consensus can be sought Needs skilled moderator May need incentives for participation	Not suitable for addressing complex issues, or when a group session cannot be organised

		Advantages	Other
Technique	Description	Disadvantages	considerations
Delphi technique	Information is collected from a group of participants in an iterative process	Participants can remain anonymous Can send surveys to practitioners or clients anywhere in the country	Needs continued cooperation and involvement of participants
		Development and testing of questionnaires, and analysis of responses, may be time-consuming Response rates may be low	

TABLE 9.3 Continued

(Source: National Institute of Clinical Studies 2006)

The National Institute of Clinical Studies (NICS) also suggests five principles which should be followed when researching barriers, regardless of the technique that is utilised (NICS 2006). These principles are:

1   *Acceptability*—the degree to which the technique used is acceptable to participants. A technique that encourages participants to express their ideas openly in a manner they find appropriate may assist in increasing the enthusiasm of participants in future processes to change practice.
2   *Accuracy*—the extent to which the barriers you identify are the barriers influencing practice. For example, if you identify a lack of staff understanding of EBP as a key barrier, training of staff to enhance understanding of EBP should improve practice.
3   *Generalisability*—the extent to which your findings can be generalised to other contexts or settings. This is influenced strongly by the representativeness of your sample.
4   *Reliability*—the dependability or consistency of a research strategy (Flitcroft et al. 2011, Liamputtong & Ezzy 2005). For example, a survey of a participant group administered on two or more occasions should yield similar results.
5   *Cost-effectiveness*—you must weigh the cost of investigating barriers to EBP against the possible benefits you may obtain from the knowledge. Barrier analysis is only appropriate if the knowledge obtained can and does subsequently improve practice (NICS 2006).

Henderson et al. (2006) researched barriers to EBP by analysing reports by leaders of projects funded to adopt innovative strategies to close the evidence–practice gap in everyday clinical practice. This group identified eight barriers to the implementation of EBP common to all projects (see Table 9.4).

This example demonstrates both key common barriers and some suggestions for improving the change process in organisations.

You should now have a thorough understanding of the barriers to implementing EBP in a workplace and techniques for investigating specific barriers. The final part of this chapter discusses the role of evidence in policy development.

	TABLE 9.4 Barriers to implementing evidence-based practice		
Theme	Critical elements to successfully implementing evidence into practice	Barriers: example concepts	Lessons for others
Leadership support	Executives sponsor support within the organisation A steering committee that is committed to a change A 'champion' from the senior staff Support from senior staff	Lack of leadership	Obtain support of executive, professional organisations, influential leaders and senior managers Identify a champion to drive the project
Key stakeholder involvement	Staff acceptance and commitment Multidisciplinary team of major stakeholders Establishing a core group of interested and committed staff and managers to work together	Conflict of interest between different stakeholders Difficulties in gaining key stakeholder engagement or support	Involve key individuals affected by the change in practice Include a multidisciplinary team Invite stakeholders to participate in project prior to commencement of changes

	TABLE 9.4 Continued		
Theme	Critical elements to successfully implementing evidence into practice	Barriers: example concepts	Lessons for others
Practice changes	Should be simplified and incrementally implemented Incorporation of practice changes into current processes	Belief that current practice is at a high level Lack of uptake or compliance with project initiative by practitioners Difficulty in acceptance of new practices Resistance to changes in the status quo Lack of experience in uptake of new projects	Implement simple changes first
Communication	Oral presentations to all stakeholder groups Regular written communication A widespread campaign publicising the project to staff	Lack of awareness of project Restricted processes of communication between professional groups Poor intra-departmental communication	Convey the evidence clearly to key staff Use marketing or awareness-raising strategies, including regular updates on the progress of change

	TABLE 9.4 Continued		
Theme	Critical elements to successfully implementing evidence into practice	Barriers: example concepts	Lessons for others
Resources	Provide funding to initiate the application of research knowledge	Gaining funding when the project area does not easily fit into one speciality Competing demands of human resources Existing high workloads Time commitments to clinicians involved Insufficient funds to conduct projects Cost-effectiveness of project not initially able to be clarified	Provide funding to initiate project to apply the evidence Identify ways to measure multiplicity of effect Allocate a budget for a project officer Allocate a training budget
Staff education	Training of staff in the principles and practice Provide data and examples which demonstrate value of the project Training to know how to rank the quality and generalisability of evidence	Lack of appropriate training for health workers	Commence prior to practice changes being implemented Educate staff on the reasons for making changes

	TABLE 9.4 Continued		
Theme	Critical elements to successfully implementing evidence into practice	Barriers: example concepts	Lessons for others
Evaluating outcomes	Effectiveness of practice changes monitored Feedback to doctors by an opinion leader Inclusion of project in a broader quality-improvement framework	Weak grasp of the necessity of defining evaluation measures	Establishing continual evaluation of progress with feedback to stakeholders Support evaluation with external review, data audits Evaluate baseline practices
Consumers	Provision of adequate information at point of decision-making Ensuring consumer expectations and perceptions about practice are appropriate Experiences, beliefs and perception that are based on the available evidence and not obsolete knowledge or anecdote The involvement of patients and their family members in embracing the initiative through discussions about the rationale	Consumer demand for specific (other) options Social barriers to behaviour changes Media influences Multiple education brochures on the same topic	Involve patients and family in practice changes and as potential agents of change Educate patients about benefits of changes in practice

(Source: Henderson, A.J., Davies, J., Willet, M.R., 2006. The experience of Australian project leaders in encouraging practitioners to adopt research evidence in their clinical practice. Australian Health Review 30 (4), 474–484. Reproduced with the permission of the Australian Health Review. © Australian Healthcare and Hospitals Association 2006. Published by CSIRO PUBLISHING. Available: <http://www.publish.csiro.au/nid/ 270/paper/AH060474.htm>.)

Evidence and policy development

Although you may not believe that you currently are or will be a policymaker, you are likely to influence policy at some level. Policy (defined in Chapter 3) can be made within legislative, judicial or executive arenas, and within both large and small organisations (Cooper et al. 2006). Based on what you have read about the barriers to using evidence in organisations, do you believe that health policy is likely to be evidence-based?

Consider, for example, policy development regarding influenza vaccination. A review of evidence for influenza vaccination has identified three central problems in the data currently available. First, there are limitations to the methodological quality of the studies found (Jefferson 2006). For example, few randomised studies exist, limiting interpretations that could be drawn from the data, and many studies have suffered from selection bias. Secondly, evidence surrounding most of the effects promised by the vaccination campaign (e.g. a reduction in absenteeism and the number of cases) was absent or not convincing (as data sets were very small) (Jefferson 2006). Thirdly, although the review did not point to evidence that annual vaccination of healthy individuals is harmful, it found few studies that considered the safety of the vaccine (Jefferson 2006). The authors of the review thus concluded that there was a large gap between the policy and the evidence.

But why is policy not based on evidence? When you have the skills to find and evaluate evidence, you might expect every decision to be based on a careful consideration of the available data and application to the appropriate context. However, as the Institute of Medicine (IOM) noted in 1988, decisions regarding health may be based more on 'crises, hot issues, and concerns of organised interest groups' than on an appraisal of the evidence (IOM 1988 p 4). In the case of the influenza vaccination, policymakers may have fallen for 'availability creep'—the favouring of doing what is available over doing nothing, even if what is available is imperfect (Jefferson 2006). Policymakers may also have felt that it was better to do something than to wait for better data, although this approach may limit the resources that could be used elsewhere. This is particularly so in crisis management when the need for decisive action might not be able to await the compilation of evidence, particularly if primary research is required.

However, criticism of policymakers must be tempered by an understanding of the complexity of policymaking. Policymaking is not a linear process, and policymakers may be influenced by information from a variety of sources (not necessarily scientific evidence), other individuals, personal and political agendas, and long-standing practices (Ashford et al. 2006, Brownson et al. 2009b). The following model developed by the Population Reference Bureau (Ashford et al. 2006) describes policy change as a complex interaction of three spheres (see Figure 9.2).

As this model shows, a 'window of opportunity' for policymaking is created only when problems and viable solutions are identified *and* the political environment is favourable (Ashford et al. 2006, Head 2010). Activities that may assist in opening the window of opportunity include focusing attention on issues to get them on the political agenda (agenda setting), creating or strengthening coalitions to sustain attention on an issue (coalition building), and increasing policymakers' knowledge about an issue (policy learning). Capacity building, the circle surrounding all other activity spheres, is about providing partners with the tools for policy communication, which assists in the use of data and research for policy change (Ashford et al. 2006, Brownson et al. 2009b, Head 2010).

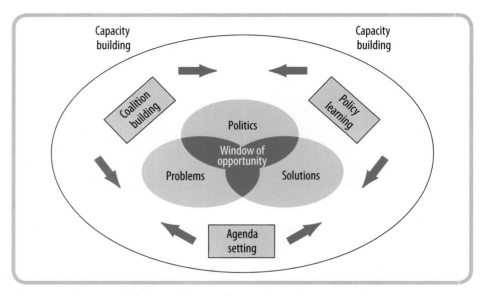

FIG. 9.2   Theoretical framework for transforming knowledge into policy actions.
(Source: Ashford et al. 2006, Bulletin of the World Health Organization 84(8):669–672)

This model explains why the release of new research findings alone is frequently insufficient to change policy on a health issue. However, if the research results are accompanied by attention-generating events to place the health issue on the policy agenda, and alliances that push for policy change are fostered, evidence regarding the problem and potential solutions may be used to reform or develop new policy (Ashford et al. 2006, Head 2010).

Lin (2003) suggests that health policy is influenced by a set of competing 'truths' that exist at the same time, based on one's viewpoint:

- *technical rationality*—the research evidence regarding the health issue, solutions, etc. (these may be difficult for policymakers to interpret, or to translate from the research setting to the local context)
- *cultural rationality*—values, ethics, perceived societal opinions and significance of an issue, which vary across place and time
- *political rationality*—the political imperative, such as the distribution of power, influence of lobbyists, accountability.

The influence of each of these rationalities will depend on the breadth of a policy (e.g. whether it is a broad strategic plan for a government or a program-level policy for a specific intervention), with research evidence becoming less important as policies become broader and more influenced by political imperatives (Brownson et al. 2009b, Head 2010, Sindall 2003). However, although cultural and political rationalities may be seen to compete with evidence in influencing policy, it must be noted that, from a health practitioner perspective, these rationalities are not necessarily to the detriment of the community receiving the policy. Ethical principles such as equity may ensure that a policy is written to favour those who are disadvantaged, and health practitioners frequently advocate to raise awareness of a health issue, and influence policy development (Brownson et al. 2009b, Head 2010, Sindall 2003).

A final word

This chapter has introduced you to the reality of evidence–practice gaps, and why policy is not always based on evidence. We have described the influence of organisational and other factors in influencing evidence uptake, and described techniques for identifying barriers to change in your workplace. The next chapter will provide guidance in ways to make personal and organisational change to reduce evidence–practice gaps.

REVIEW QUESTIONS

- What is 'evidence-based medicine', and how does this term differ from evidence-based practice (EBP)?
- What are the main elements of EBP, and how might it be useful to you in your day-to-day work?
- Why do you think evidence is not used consistently to guide practice?
- One of the issues you may have identified in the previous question was the organisational context in which a person works. What issues might arise in an organisation that might make it difficult to use EBP?
- What are the steps involved in identifying evidence that should guide practice?
- Is EBP only guided by high-quality quantitative evidence? What role might qualitative evidence play in making decisions about evidence?
- As a public health practitioner, how might you identify and use qualitative evidence to guide your practice?
- Outline a health issue in Australia where technical, cultural and political rationalities compete to influence policy.

Useful websites

- The Cochrane Collaboration: http://www.cochrane.org
- National Health and Medical Research Council website on the hierarchy of evidence: http://www.nhmrc.gov.au/publications/synopses/cp65syn.htm

References

Ashford, L.S., Smith, R.R., De Souza, R.-M., et al., 2006. Creating windows of opportunity for policy change: incorporating evidence into decentralized planning in Kenya. Bulletin of the World Health Organization 84 (8), 669–672.

Bali, R.K., 2013. Pervasive Health Knowledge Management. Springer, New York.

Brownson, R.C., Chriqui, J.F., Stamatakis, K.A., 2009a. Understanding evidence-based public health policy. American Journal of Public Health 99 (9), 1576–1583.

Brownson, R.C., Fielding, J.E., Maylahan, C.M., 2009b. Evidence-based public health: a fundamental concept of public health practice. Annual Review of Public Health 30, 175–201.

Brownson, R.C., Baker, E.A., Left, T.L., et al., 2010. Evidence-Based Public Health. Oxford, New York.

Carson, S., 2005. Organisational change. In: Hamer, S., Collinson, G. (Eds.), Achieving Evidence-Based Practice: A Handbook for Practitioners. Elsevier, Sydney, pp. 175–194.

Cooper, S.R., Trotter Betts, V., Butler, K., et al., 2006. Evidence-based practice and health policy: a match or a mismatch? In: Malloch, K., Porter-O'Grady, T. (Eds.), Introduction to Evidence-Based Practice in Nursing and Health Care. Jones and Bartlett Learning, Sudbury, MA, pp. 221–234.

Corcoran, K., Vandiver, V.L., 2004. Implementing best practice and expert consensus procedures. In: Roberts, A.R., Yeager, K.R. (Eds.), Evidence-Based Practice Manual: Research and Outcome Measures in Health and Human Services. Oxford University Press, New York, pp. 15–29.

Dawes, M., 2005. Evidence-based practice. In: Dawes, M., Davies, P., Gray, A., et al. (Eds.), Evidence-Based Practice: A Primer for Health Care Professionals. Elsevier, Sydney, pp. 1–10.

Dziegielewski, S.F., Roberts, A.R., 2006. Health care evidence-based practice. In: Roberts, A.R., Yeager, K.R. (Eds.), Foundations of Evidence-Based Social Work Practice. Oxford University Press, Melbourne, pp. 122–129.

Fink, A., 2013. Evidence-Based Public Health Practice. Sage, Thousand Oaks.

Flitcroft, K., Gillespie, J., Salkeld, G., et al., 2011. Getting evidence into policy: the need for deliberative strategies? Social Science and Medicine 72, 1039–1046.

Frommer, M., Rychetnik, L., 2003. From evidence-based medicine to evidence-based public health. In: Lin, V., Gibson, B. (Eds.), Evidence Based Health Policy: Problems and Possibilities. Oxford University Press, Melbourne, pp. 56–69.

Gerrish, K., 2006. Evidence-based practice. In: Gerrish, K., Lacey, A. (Eds.), The Research Process in Nursing. Blackwell, Carlton, pp. 491–505.

Gray, M., 2009. Evidence-Based Health Care and Public Health, third ed. Elsevier, Oxford.

Guillemin, M., Gillam, L., 2006. Telling Moments: Everyday Ethics in Health Care. East IP Communications, Hawthorn.

Hall, B.A., Armstrong, R., Francis, D., et al., 2010. Cochrane update: enhancing capacity for 'systematic' thinking in public health. Journal of Public Health 32 (4), 582–585.

Hamer, S., 2005. Evidence-based practice. In: Hamer, S., Collinson, G. (Eds.), Achieving Evidence-Based Practice. Elsevier, Sydney, pp. 3–14.

Head, B.W., 2010. Editorial. Reconsidering evidence-based policy: key issues and challenges. Policy and Society 29, 77–94.

Henderson, A.J., Davies, J., Willet, M.R., 2006. The experience of Australian project leaders in encouraging practitioners to adopt research evidence in their clinical practice. Australian Health Review 30 (4), 474–484. Reproduced with the permission of the Australian Health Review. © Australian Healthcare and Hospitals Association 2006. Published by CSIRO PUBLISHING. Available: <http://www.publish.csiro.au/nid/270/paper/AH060474.htm>.

Institute of Medicine, 1988. The Future of Public Health. Committee for the Study of the Future of Public Health; Division of Health Care Services. National Academy Press, Washington DC.

Jefferson, T., 2006. Influenza vaccination: policy versus evidence. British Medical Journal 333, 912–915.

Killoran, A., Kelly, M.P., 2010. Evidenced-Based Public Health Effectiveness and Efficiency. Oxford University Press, Oxford.

Kraaijenhagen, R.A., Haverkamp, D., Koopman, M.M.W., et al., 2000. Travel and risk of venous thrombosis. Lancet 356, 1492–1493.

Liamputtong, P., Ezzy, D., 2005. Qualitative Research Methods. Oxford University Press, Melbourne.

Lin, V., 2003. Competing rationalities: evidence-based health policy? In: Lin, V., Gibson, B. (Eds.), Evidence-Based Health Policy: Problems and Possibilities. Oxford University Press, Melbourne, pp. 3–17.

Mazurek Melnyk, B., Fineout-Overholt, E., 2005. Creating a vision: motivating a change to evidence based practice in individuals and organizations. In: Mazurek Melnyk, B., Fineout-Overholt, E. (Eds.), Evidence-Based Practice in Nursing and Healthcare: A Guide to Best Practice. Lippincott Williams & Wilkins, Sydney, pp. 443–456.

Michie, S., Johnston, M., Abraham, C., et al., 2005. Making psychological theory useful for implementing evidence based practice: a consensus approach. Quality and Safety in Health Care 14, 26–33.

Mozaffarian, D., 2012. Researchers identify evidence-based public health interventions for policymakers. Circulation 126, 1514–1563.

Mullen, E.J., 2004. Facilitating practitioner use of evidence-based practice. In: Roberts, A.R., Yeager, K.R. (Eds.), Evidence-Based Practice Manual: Research and Outcome Measures in Health and Human Services. Oxford University Press, New York, pp. 205–209.

Naidoo, J., Wills, J., 2005. Public Health and Health Promotion: Developing Practice. Baillière Tindall, Edinburgh.

National Institute of Clinical Studies, 2008. Evidence-Practice Gaps Report, Volume 1: A Review of Developments: 2004-2007. National Health and Medical Research Council, Canberra.

National Institute of Clinical Studies, 2006. Identifying Barriers to Evidence Uptake. NICS, Melbourne.

Oliver, A., McDaid, D., 2002. Evidence-based health care: benefits and barriers. Social Policy and Society 1 (3), 183–190.

Rosenthal, M., Sutcliffe, K.M. (Eds.), 2002. Medical Error. What Do We Know? What Do We Do. Jossey-Bass, San Francisco.

Rychetnik, L., Wise, M., 2004. Advocating evidence-based health promotion: reflections and a way forward. Health Promotion International 19 (2), 247–257.

Sackett, D.L., Rosenberg, W.M.C., Gray, J.A.M., et al., 1996. Evidence based medicine: what it is and what it isn't. British Medical Journal 312 (7023), 71–72.

Schardt, C., 2011. Health information literacy meets evidence-based practice. Editorial. Journal of the Medical Library Association 99 (1), 1–2.

Schein, E.H., 1996. Culture: the missing concept in organizational studies. Administrative Science Quarterly 41 (2), 229–240.

Scurr, J., Machin, S., Bailey-King, S., et al., 2001. Frequency and prevention of symptomless deep-vein thrombosis in long-haul flights: a randomised trial. Lancet 357 (9267), 1485–1489.

Sindall, C., 2003. Health policy and normative analysis: ethics, evidence and politics. In: Lin, V., Gibson, B. (Eds.), Evidence Based Health Policy: Problems and Possibilities. Oxford University Press, Melbourne, pp. 80–94.

Smith, K., 2013. Beyond Evidence Based Policy in Public Health: The Interplay of Ideas. Palgrave Macmillan, Basingstoke.

Steinberg, E.P., Luce, B.R., 2005. Evidence based? Caveat emptor! Health Affairs 24 (1), 80–92.

Taylor, B., Roberts, K., 2006. Research in nursing and health. In: Taylor, B., Kermode, S., Roberts, K. (Eds.), Research in Nursing and Health Care: Evidence for Practice, third ed. Thomson, South Melbourne, pp. 1–32.

Topping, A., 2006. The quantitative-qualitative continuum. In: Gerrish, K., Lacey, A. (Eds.), The Research Process in Nursing. Blackwell, Carlton, pp. 157–172.

United Kingdom Public Health Association (UKPHA) website. Definition of public health. Online. Available: <http://www.ukpha.org.uk/about-us/index.html> (14 May 2014).

CHAPTER 10

Planning and evaluation

Elizabeth Parker

Learning objectives

After reading this chapter, you should be able to:

- understand the importance of planning and evaluation in public health practice

- recognise the links between planning and evaluation

- identify the core concepts of needs assessment in public health

- describe the evaluation cycle, and the importance of an evaluation plan

- understand evaluation designs and their application in practice.

Introduction

This chapter builds on the analysis of public health policies in Chapter 3. Public health planning and evaluation are the means by which to maximise these policy aspirations. For example, integrated planning is in place to ensure that all emergency health services, hospitals and population/public health units are prepared for an efficient response to any major infectious disease outbreak, such as 'bird flu' (avian influenza). The emergency response to Australia's natural disasters, such as the New South Wales bushfires (2013) and the Queensland floods and cyclone Yasi in 2011, demonstrate the value of a coordinated, planned response by emergency health professionals, government officials, media and volunteers. You will develop an array of plans from community-based 'public health' programs, such as a physical activity or nutrition education programs, and media campaigns—for example, vaccinating children against infectious diseases, promoting dental health for school children, and screening programs for bowel cancer. And of course health professionals in clinical settings develop patient care plans.

All levels of government are involved in planning. Local governments (councils) create healthy environments to promote and protect the wellbeing of residents. They plan parks for recreation, construct traffic-calming devices near schools to prevent accidents, and build shade structures and walking paths. Environmental health officers ensure food safety in restaurants, and monitor water quality. Federal and state governments plan to protect and promote health through various policy and program initiatives (see Chapter 3).

How do we know whether many of these plans achieve their goals? Often it is difficult to measure with any confidence whether a program has achieved its goals and objectives, and it is only through a robust evaluation that a program can be deemed to be successful. The best way to do this is to integrate an evaluation plan into your program. Unfortunately, evaluation plans are often not integrated, as planning and evaluation tend to be seen as two distinct entities. This chapter introduces the concepts of public health program planning and evaluation, with models presented to help you integrate these two processes. Case studies, activities and reflections illustrate key points. As various authors use different terminology to describe 'planning' and 'evaluation', the glossary at the end of this book will clarify the terms used in this chapter.

Planning and evaluation in public health

As described in Chapter 2, the roots of public health planning go back to some of the earliest sanitary control measures. Without good planning, we would not be effective in preventing disease, and promoting and restoring health in the community. Lenihan (2005) has identified three models that have typified planning in public health practice. The first is problem/program planning and community assessment. These 'are well established components of health education with a focus on improving the health of defined population groups' (Lenihan 2005 p 382). The second is advocacy planning, where 'the planner becomes a change agent to raise awareness and mobilise a population group to solve a community problem or develop a program' (Lenihan 2005 p 382). Advocacy planning adds community participation to the planning process, but planners or health professionals often control the process through technical aspects of planning. The third is strategic planning, which connects public health planning practice to the current and potential partners needed to meet future challenges (Lenihan 2005). Often this happens through senior government officials and politicians— for example, planning for potential health emergencies and disasters. Other examples are the Municipal Public Health and Wellbeing Plans in Victoria, which outline public health actions to minimise public health dangers and to maximise health and wellbeing for residents in a municipality, and integrates other plans of community partners with an interest in health (Victorian Government Department of Health 2014). Common to each of these models is an identified public health need, and adequate financial and human resources, to ensure successful program

ACTIVITY 10.1 Types of planning

What form of planning are the following examples?

- A consultative process with Aboriginal and Torres Strait Islander health workers and community women, in a forum to discuss improved services for cervical cancer screening.

- The government commissioning a taskforce of experts to plan and implement a disaster management plan for rural areas in New South Wales at risk of floods and bushfires.

- A health education program designed after data revealed the need to improve nutrition education for young men.

REFLECTION 10.1

Are there any differences in your approaches and understanding of the models? Can changes in population health occur only through long-term strategic planning at the government level? What are the barriers to relying on government to plan specific programs to promote health?

development, implementation, evaluation and sustainability. The National Chronic Disease Strategy could be described as strategic planning from a policy perspective (see Chapter 3).

The next section will summarise some of the key developments in program planning.

Models of planning

Public health planning models help us to organise our thinking about the steps required to achieve our desired goals. They can be simple or sophisticated in design. Bartholomew et al. (2001) developed a detailed planning model called 'intervention mapping'. The word 'intervention' is sometimes used interchangeably with the term 'program'. Intervention mapping outlines the explicit steps you would use to plan a community-based public health program, particularly where your aim is to influence behaviour change. It considers the evidence and the use of behaviour change theories from previous successful 'interventions' as a basis, in order to increase the likelihood of success. Intervention mapping has been applied successfully to large-scale health promotion programs in communities, as has the next model.

Green and Kreuter (1991) developed the PRECEDE model (Predisposing, Reinforcing, Enabling Constructs in Educational/Environmental Diagnosis and Evaluation). This was expanded to PROCEED to include Policy, Regulatory and Organisational Constructs in Education and Environmental Development (Green & Kreuter 2005). Planners are encouraged to be systematic and analytical in identifying the cause of a community health problem, and the various influences that can assist or hinder solving the problem. This model diagnoses the influences of both behavioural and environmental factors on community health. Questions are asked, such as what are the *predisposing* factors that may facilitate or hinder behaviour change? For example, does the community lack knowledge about the impact of smoking on health? What can *reinforce* a behaviour change once it is adopted? And what can *enable* behavioural or community change? For instance, smoke-free environments may reinforce non-smoking behaviour. Both the intervention mapping and the PRECEDE/PROCEED models have a focus on planning that is well informed, addresses a well-defined problem, and has adequate resources. There are fundamental questions that begin the planning process.

- *What am I trying to achieve?* Here, you are identifying needs and priorities, and being clear about intended aims and objectives.
- *What am I going to do?* More specifically: what is the best approach to achieving your aims? Identify the resources needed. Establish a clear action plan of what people are going to do what and when.
- *How will I know whether I have been successful?* Again, integration of your evaluation plan at the outset of planning should set a clear direction for gathering the data you need to answer your questions (Scriven 2010).

Scriven (2010) proposes a seven-stage model that can be used as a template for program planning and action:

1 Identify needs and priorities.
2 Set (goals) and objectives.
3 Decide on the best way of achieving the aims or ultimate outcome (using evidence from the literature and/or focus groups/discussions with providers and the users of your program).

4   Identify the resources needed (staffing, space, transport, financial resources).

5   Plan evaluation methods.

6   Set an action plan.

7   ACTION—implement your plan, including your evaluation (modified from Scriven 2010).

Clearly, planning and evaluation are integrated. Each of the steps is cyclical, but can be worked on simultaneously. Hence, the evaluation plan should be developed simultaneously when building and progressing the program plan.

The first step in Scriven's (2010) model is to *identify needs and priorities*. So how do we identify needs and what kinds are there? Knowing various types of 'need' is important knowledge for all health professionals.

Identifying needs and priorities

Public health plans are based on identifying and assessing needs—existing or anticipated. For example, emergency and disaster plans to protect the public are developed in anticipation of events, or are quickly put into action if there is a sudden outbreak of an infectious disease, such as measles. Moreover, as public health information becomes more sophisticated and robust, policymakers may have already identified the health issues, as discussed in Chapter 3. Australia has excellent data sources, such as the Australian Institute of Health and Welfare (AIHW) and the Australian Bureau of Statistics (ABS), to assist health professionals to plan effective programs.

How are needs identified? Bradshaw (1972, in Katz et al. 2000) identified a 'taxonomy of needs'; a 'taxonomy' is simply a categorisation. There are commonly four types of need in public health: *normative, comparative, expressed* and *felt*. Additionally, there are other ways to gauge needs, such as *rapid appraisals* and the use of *epidemiological evidence*.

- *Normative needs*—These reflect the views of health professionals and their judgements and standards. For example, 'doctors may define some people's health or behaviour as falling within a "normal" range' (Katz et al. 2000 p 262). Normative standards may change. In nutrition, the norms of healthy food have altered—for example, consuming up to six eggs per week, once implicated in raised cholesterol, is no longer associated with an increased risk in healthy people (Dietitians Association of Australia website).

- *Comparative needs*—Decisions are based on comparing options for program development. If the prevalence of childhood obesity is higher in low socioeconomic areas, should investments and programs be targeted at those neighbourhoods or across the whole population? Should healthcare resources be moved to outer suburbs or should they remain in more central locations? Comparative needs are often the focus of planning decisions.

- *Expressed needs*—These are what can be inferred by assessing service use (Hawe et al. 1990), or by what people say they need (Katz et al. 2000). Long waiting lists are an expressed need that politicians often talk about. All the options regarding the provision of services need to be thoroughly considered. Could the long waiting lists be dealt with by community clinics? And are people using emergency services in hospitals because they cannot find a bulk-billing doctor?

- *Felt needs*—These are often the responses to community surveys, based on what people feel they want or identify as problems. Hawe et al. (1990 p 19) caution that people often report solutions to the need—for example, 'more nursing home beds'—rather than stating the need itself.

- *Rapid appraisals*—Rapid appraisals have increased in popularity in public health in local planning, in both developed and developing countries. They can involve qualitative interviews with healthcare providers and consumers or patients, focus group discussions, and interviews with key informants. Because rapid appraisals employ both quantitative and qualitative methods to gain insights into needs assessment, processes and gaps, or program use and utility, they are rich sources of information and can be done quickly.
- *Epidemiological evidence*—This is where there is sufficient evidence that an intervention is needed to improve the health of a population or subpopulation (see Case Study 10.1).

CASE STUDY 10.1

Defining food literacy and needs 2011

'Food literacy' is an emerging term used to describe what we know and understand about food and how to use it to meet our needs. The term is increasingly used in policies, plans and among the general public, despite the absence of an agreed meaning, shared understanding of its components, or the evidence-based need to invest in this area within multistrategic public-health nutrition work. A Delphi study of food experts was conducted in 2010/11 to help determine what these might be. This was the first of two studies which made up a research project that examined the concept of food literacy and whether it influences what we eat. Experts came from a range of professions nationally, from education, health, welfare (agriculture, gastronomy and the food industry) and work settings (research, policy, practice and advocacy) in government, non-government and private sector settings. All experts were passionate about food, but differed in what they thought were core components of food literacy. They also prioritised needs differently—for example, choosing ethically and sustainably produced foods, choosing foods to prevent chronic disease, choosing foods for an economically sustainable local food industry, choosing foods that support household harmony, and being food-secure enough to have a choice of foods. These results were reviewed by practitioners, and tested by using them to review a range of existing interventions.

The second study interviewed young people, aged 16–25 years, across a spectrum of disadvantage, about how they use food to meet their needs and what knowledge and skills they call on to do this. These findings were contrasted with the results of the first Delphi study. Results of these two studies were used to develop a definition of 'food literacy', identify its components, and develop a model for its relationship to food intake. These results were again presented to peers and practitioners to test their interpretation and understanding. This work has been used to inform investment and practice in food literacy in Australia and internationally.

This project illustrates how the starting point for a program and various assessments and layers of 'needs' can differ.

(Source: Vidgen, H., 2014. Case Study on Food Literacy and Needs. School of Public Health and Social Work, Queensland University of Technology, Brisbane)

Beginning your program plan

The second stage of Scriven's (2010) model is writing goals, objectives and strategies, identifying a target group (a population or subpopulation), identifying resources, and planning an evaluation. A program logic model is one way of doing this.

A *program logic model* is a diagrammatic representation of the logical connections among the elements of a program, including its goals and objectives, activities, impact and outcomes, and evaluation plan. All of those with a vested interest in the outcomes of the program would ideally be engaged in developing the model. Thus, a program logic model can be displayed in a flow chart, map or table, to portray the sequence of steps leading to program results (see Figure 10.1).

Be clear about defining your 'stakeholders'. These are the people who are often the funders of your program, but your stakeholders can be the community members or patients for whom the program is intended. They can be government or non-government officials, or staff from a granting body (Rootman et al. 2001).

It is wise to spend concentrated time at this stage of program development. Those involved in developing and funding your program have an interest in it, and they will want to see that you are achieving your intended outcomes. Understand that various stakeholders can have diverse views as to the goals (aims) and objectives of the program, and how to measure its success. It is vital that there is consensus among the program developers on this issue (see Activity 10.3).

> **ACTIVITY 10.2 Types of need**
>
> Write a sentence summarising each of *expressed*, *felt*, *normative* and *comparative* need. Choose a current public health issue (e.g. skin cancer) and consider how each of these types of need may have influenced a program of action for skin cancer prevention. How were the needs identified, and by whom? Were the needs based on evidence?

> **REFLECTION 10.2**
>
> Did you agree on who defined the need? In practice, planners can propose solutions and programs to inadequately defined needs through political pressure. Can you think of such a program? This means that you need to be aware of the complexities and competing agendas that may arise in planning programs when there are competing types of need.

WRITING GOALS AND OBJECTIVES

Goals and objectives need to be written specifically so they can be measured (Hawe et al. 1990). A goal is written to describe the desired change in the health or behaviour of a group—for example, the reduction in obesity in Year 9 teenagers by 20% over three years.

Objectives are specific, should be linked to the goals, and be realistic and evidence-based. This means that you can confidently predict that your objectives are logical and are linked to the evidence base. For example, a goal could be related to nutrition education—for instance, increase the number of children aged 5–15 who eat the recommended daily amount of fresh fruit and vegetables by 30% in 12 months (National Health and Medical Research Council, 2013). An aid to writing objectives is that they should be SMART—that is:

- S—specific
- M—measurable
- A—achievable
- R—realistic
- T—time-limited.

In the above example, a SMART objective could be 'Within six months, at least 80% of parents and carers of children aged 5–15 years will know how much fresh fruit and vegetables the children must eat to meet recommended daily requirements.' Writing

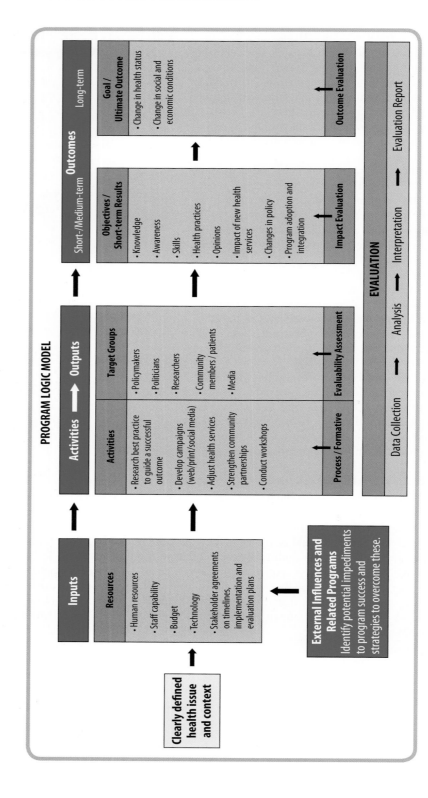

FIG. 10.1   Program logic model.

(Source: Adapted from McLaughlin, J.A. Jordan, G.B. 1999. Logic models: a tool for telling your program's performance story. Evaluation and Program Planning 22: 65–72)

objectives really specifically not only focuses the program goals, but also assists with the questions asked in an evaluation.

WRITING STRATEGIES

Strategies are the activities you are going to undertake to reach your objectives—in other words, *what* you are going to do. Examples of public health strategies include television campaigns, such as a national skin cancer prevention campaign, websites informing people about how to check their skin, development of new health services that offer skin-checks; and new policies, such as those in schools that enforce the 'no hat, no play' rule for students.

IDENTIFYING A TARGET GROUP

As public health is about populations, it is common to identify the target group as 'everyone', irrespective of age, socioeconomic status, income or education. Measuring the impact of such programs in large population groups is difficult, so being clear and precise about the profile of your population is important. There is evidence that modifying people's health status through the use of public health campaigns, especially those that use multiple methods (legislative, media campaigns, advocacy, group and individual education), can take up to five years (Green & Anderson 1986). See Chapter 14 for a discussion on tobacco control in Australia, and how diverse strategies, sustained over many years, were used to achieve the goals.

IDENTIFYING RESOURCES—OR PROGRAM 'INPUTS'

All programs require resources, and the answers to the following questions will assist in your planning. How many staff will be needed? Who will manage the program? Will there be a joint planning group that includes staff to manage the program, staff from another department within your organisation, staff from outside your department, and community members? What are the roles assigned to those on the planning group? Are they advisers, budget planners or web designers? It is critical to define the roles for each member of the planning group. Many programs flounder through unstructured 'networks' of people who are involved, with everyone wanting a say. This can mean that the program becomes disjointed and unfocused. Will a director or a project officer be hired specifically for the program? Has the development, implementation and evaluation of the program been built into the job description of the staff? Is there a contingency plan if staff resign, and sufficient money available in the budget for printing, computers, transport, telephones, evaluation and writing the evaluation report? Note that 10 per cent of the budget should be allocated for evaluating the program—these funds are often not factored into the development of the resources plan. A well-crafted budget is necessary for program sustainability. This is where your program logic plan is so important, as you will have gained consensus with all the players prior to program commencement.

We now turn our attention to the evaluation, an important element in program planning.

Planning the evaluation methods

'Evaluation is the process by which we judge the worth or value of something' (Suchman 1967, in

> ### ACTIVITY 10.3 The program logic model
>
> - Why is a program logic model useful in planning public health initiatives?
> - What are some of the pitfalls you see in writing goals and objectives for public health programs?
> - What sources of evidence could you use in planning a specific public health program?
> - Who would be some of the important stakeholders if you were designing a health program in your discipline? Write down the names, and compare with other students. Do you have stakeholders in common in different disciplines?

In your response to the first question, did you consider that program logic models could be useful in getting everyone to agree on the various components of the program? The 'map' is a useful way for moving a program forwards once the various stakeholders involved have reached agreement. For the second question, often objectives are not written specifically, so it becomes difficult to evaluate programs (this is discussed in the next section). There are many sources of health data available at national, state and local levels. We often don't include stakeholders from outside the health sector; yet professionals such as the police, or local service clubs, businesses and media can all be stakeholders in program planning.

Hawe et al. 1990 p 6). If you were buying a house, you would have some criteria against which you were judging its worth. Imagine you are house-hunting—you want a three-bedroom house, and the house you are looking at meets this criterion. Originally, you wanted a swimming pool; this house doesn't have one, and, if water restrictions are in force, this is now not a priority. In other words, you are prioritising the criteria against which you are making your decision. In public health evaluation, the principles are the same. You need criteria against which you would measure the worth or success of your program. 'Without a comparison of some kind, even if it is only comparison with an imaginary ideal or a subjective preference, there can be no evaluation' (Fleming & Parker 2007 p 112). Obviously, evaluation must be connected to the goals and objectives of your program, and the measurement of its strategies and activities needs to be appropriate.

PURPOSES OF EVALUATION

There are two purposes for completing an evaluation: to ensure accountability to stakeholders, especially those who have funded your program; and to make judgements about the program—for example, were the goals/objectives achieved? What worked? What could be improved? Because public accountability for health spending is a top priority for governments as the demand for health services increases, one of your responsibilities as a health professional is to consistently improve the quality of the programs you design. Through reflecting on the evaluations of our programs, we ensure that our program judgements are ethical and reinforce our professional values to make certain that our efforts continually strive to improve the health of our populations or patients. Evaluations also teach us, through reflecting on what has been achieved, how we can improve our practice. Different types of evaluation incrementally strengthen the evidence base of program effectiveness from 'small scale process evaluations through to hard-outcome random controlled trials' (Thorogood & Coombes 2010 p 9).

Evaluation focuses on systematically collecting and assessing data that provide useful feedback about a program/intervention, and is defined by Stufflebeam as a 'study designed and conducted to assist some audience to assess an object's merit or worth' (2001 p 11). It is about generating information to assist in making judgements about a program, service, policy or organisation. Owen (1999), in Fleming and Parker (2007 p 115), refines these points by providing a set of questions. Is the evaluation to: determine the way a program is to be implemented; synthesise information to aid program development; clarify a program; improve the implementation of a program; monitor its outcomes; or determine its worth? A clear set of questions about the purpose of the evaluation can set the course for your evaluation plan. Your program logic model will be helpful in this regard, as it sets out all of the components of program development and implementation, and thus assists you in clarifying your thinking about the kinds of question you want the evaluation to answer. Glasgow et al. (1999 p 1322) claimed that it was easier to measure medical interventions that produce immediate results, and that measuring results of interventions that address whole populations was much more difficult. Some evaluation progress had been made in health promotion evaluations, in particular, but that these advances were limited 'by the evaluation methods used'. We would also argue that behaviour change in populations can take a long time! Think about what has produced the decline in smoking rates in Australia. The decline has occurred through sustained campaigns over 30 years, and multiple evaluation strategies have been employed to measure these outcomes. Glasgow et al. (1999 p 1323) produced the RE-AIM framework to assist evaluators to be more systematic in their evaluation approach and in formulating questions. Five factors were involved: 'reach, efficacy, adoption, implementation and maintenance'.

- *Reach* captures the participation in a specific program (e.g. a patient counselling program at a clinic) or those in a community affected by a policy or program (e.g. a television campaign focused on healthy eating).
- *Efficacy* tests whether the design of our programs are likely to have an effect. For example, would the design of a media campaign be effective?
- *Adoption* measures the proportion of practices, or communities, that will adopt the program being planned.
- *Implementation* concerns whether the program is being delivered as it was intended.
- *Maintenance* asks to what extent the program is being sustained over time (adapted from Glasgow et al. 1999).

RE-AIM has been successfully utilised internationally to measure a range of public health programs—for example, an evaluation of a workplace intervention to promote commuter cycling in Amsterdam (Dubuy et al. 2013), and in Australia to measure the effectiveness of a community football training program (Finch et al. 2013).

You also need to think about the role of the decision-makers who are going to use the evaluation. Are the questions they want answered the same as yours? If not, how do you negotiate these differences? For example, you might be interested in finding out whether the program is reaching its intended participants, whereas your managers may want to know how effective the program is in improving participants' knowledge about the health problem. A useful start is to develop a list of the questions that each of you want answered. This way your evaluation process becomes a collaborative endeavour, although care has to be taken that the integrity of the evaluation is not compromised.

Now that you have decided on the overall purpose, it is time to put together your evaluation plan. Here is a summary of a framework developed by the US Centers for Disease Control and Prevention (CDC 1999). The steps in the framework (Fig. 10.2) are helpful for planning any public health evaluation.

- *Engage stakeholders (interested parties)*—This reinforces our previous discussion about the involvement of people or organisations that have something to gain or lose from what will be learned from the evaluation and what will be done with that knowledge.
- *Describe the program and its context*—Reflect on the dynamics of the program. Write a statement of expectations about the program—for example, what are the intended results and what will indicate success? What activities are being identified or implemented to bring about change, and what resources are needed? Importantly, identify the program's stage of development. How does the planning, implementation and maintenance of the program affect the goal of the evaluation? What are the dynamics of the program context that could potentially affect it? Will the political, social and economic conditions change during the course of the program? Will the organisational systems and dynamics that support a program influence a health program?

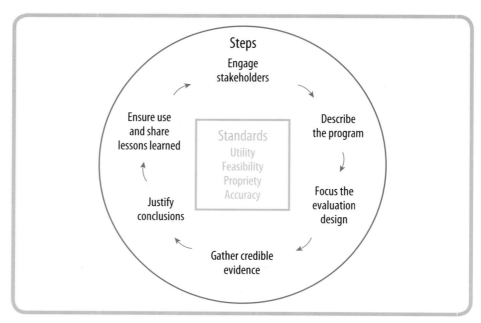

FIG. 10.2   Framework for program evaluation.
(Source: CDC 1999)

- *Focus the evaluation design*—What will the evaluation address, and how will it do so? How will the findings be used? Describe the goals of the evaluation (these are separate from the goals of the program), and what will be done to accomplish them. Evaluation goals may help you assess whether the program is working, how you could improve its quality, and determine the effects and impact of the program. What information is important to stakeholders? How well was the program planned and put into practice? How well has the program met its stated objectives? How much and/or what kind of difference has the program made in the community as a whole?

Methods

What study design will you use to evaluate the effects of the program? These designs include experimental, quasi-experimental, and descriptive case study designs. You can apply the knowledge you learned about study designs in Chapter 5 to select an appropriate evaluation design. What and how will you collect the data to help answer the evaluation questions? Some data collection methods are records, such as minutes that document the establishment and implementation of the program, surveys and interviews with program participants, and surveys to measure the impact of the program in the community.

- *Gather credible evidence*—Decide what the evidence is, and what features affect the credibility of the evidence. Specify the criteria used to judge the success of the program, and translate this into measures of indicators of success. For example, earlier in the chapter we presented an example of buying a house and the criteria you might use when buying a house—the number of rooms and whether it has a pool. In your health practice, the criteria could be the capacity to deliver a first-rate service, improved and increased participation in your program, levels of satisfaction, changes in behaviour, changes in community policies and practices, and improvements in community-level indicators. Sources of evidence can include interviews/ surveys with people, analysis of policy and procedure documents to gauge change, or direct observations. With respect to quality, this can be done by examining the reliability of the information, and how well it relates to the evaluation questions. With regard to the quantity of information, it is important not only to estimate the amount of data required to evaluate effectiveness, but also to know when to stop gathering data!

- *Justify conclusions*—Here, you analyse and synthesise the methods used to summarise the findings to see if there are any patterns in the evidence, interpret what the findings mean, and see how they translate into practical applications. Essentially, you are making judgements about the worth of your findings, and the recommendations for action to consider as a result of the evaluation.

- *Ensure the evaluation is used, and share the lessons learned*—The final step in the CDC framework for program evaluation (1999) is to ensure the use of the evaluation, and sharing lessons learned. This is called *disseminating the results* of the evaluation. Most often, you will write an evaluation report that documents all aspects of your evaluation and recommendations. The report should outline the program's features, particularly its goals and objectives, the strategies used, and whether the goals and objectives have been achieved. The report should delineate the evaluation design, methods of data collection and analysis, and outcomes and recommendations. The recommendations will provide assistance to decision-makers, other professionals, and policymakers with an interest in the health issue.

To disseminate the findings of the evaluation, a feedback report can be provided to the participants and stakeholders, describing the design of the evaluation, and the methods and processes used. Communicate the evaluation findings to your relevant audiences, and the lessons learned to the future users of your evaluation.

In Figure 10.2 (CDC 1999) you can see a set of standards as the basis for evaluation actions in the centre of the framework. These are *utility, accuracy, feasibility* and *propriety*. The CDC Evaluation website contains a comprehensive explanation of all of the standards. Each of the standards sets a foundation to guide the conduct of ethical and respectful evaluations. So why are they important? As you learned in Chapter 8, ethical practice is everybody's business, and evaluations rest on a foundation of ethical practice. These evaluation standards give you a guide to think about the conduct of your evaluation. You can use them as a checklist to tick off whether you have paid attention to each of the standards before you proceed with the evaluation actions.

- *Utility*—Utility standards ensure that an evaluation will serve the information needs of intended users. The evaluator should be both trustworthy and competent to perform the evaluation, so that findings achieve maximum credibility and acceptance. The information collected should be selected to address pertinent questions about the program and be responsive to the needs and interests of clients and specified stakeholders, and the interpretation of the findings should be carefully described. Evaluation reports should clearly describe the program being evaluated, including its context, and the purposes, procedures and findings of the evaluation, so that essential information is provided and easily understood. Evaluation reports should be disseminated to intended users in a timely manner.

- *Feasibility*—Feasibility standards ensure that an evaluation will be realistic, prudent, diplomatic and frugal. The evaluation should be practical to keep disruption to a minimum while needed information is obtained. One application of this standard in the real world is to make decisions about when to stop collecting data. The evaluation should be planned and conducted in anticipation of the different positions of various interest groups, so that their cooperation may be obtained, and so that possible attempts by these groups to stop aspects of the evaluation or to misapply the results can be averted or counteracted. Questions need to be asked and decisions made about cost-effectiveness. In summary, utility is about the practical considerations to be thought out prior to embarking on an evaluation.

- *Propriety*—Propriety standards make sure that an evaluation will be conducted legally, ethically, and with due regard for the welfare of those involved in the evaluation, as well as those affected by its results. In other words, propriety deals with correct and appropriate practices (some of which were introduced in Chapter 8); for example, evaluations should be designed and conducted in such a way as to respect and protect the rights and welfare of human subjects. Evaluators must respect the dignity and worth of others associated with an evaluation, so that participants are not threatened or harmed. Be familiar with your organisation's ethics committee prior to conducting any research or evaluation. Conflicts of interest should be dealt with openly and honestly, so that the evaluation is not compromised, and evaluations should be complete and unbiased in identifying and recording the strengths and weaknesses, so that the strengths of the program can be built upon and problem areas addressed.

- *Accuracy*—The evaluation should convey accurate information about the features that determine the program's merit. Describe and document clearly and accurately, so that the program is clearly identified. The program logic model will assist you in completing this task. Obviously, collecting and analysing valid and reliable information about the program is a given. The accuracy of this information assists in justifying conclusions. This standard also makes clear that when reporting the results you should guard against bias and distortion.

ACTIVITY 10.4 Standards for evaluation

Discuss with other students why the standards for evaluation are an important starting point in planning an evaluation. Write a definition of each of the standards to help you understand them. Next, review the first step in the CDC *Framework for program evaluation*. How would you go about engaging stakeholders in discussing the purpose and procedures in the evaluation? How would you resolve differences among stakeholders if there were any? Describe what you perceive to be the similarities and differences in program and evaluation planning.

REFLECTION 10.4

What, if any, were the differences of opinion among your fellow students about the importance of having a set of standards to guide evaluations? Were you able to understand the meaning of each of the standards? When you are undertaking an evaluation in practice, it is important, from the beginning, to be as explicit as possible about the standards of practice for the evaluation and the purpose of the evaluation, as agreement on these helps when and if any disputes arise during the evaluation. Did you have ideas about how you might resolve differences among stakeholders if the purpose and procedures in the evaluation vary?

The next section explores evaluation design, through the presentation of some basic designs and examples. This is the third step in the CDC framework.

Evaluation designs in practice

As you would have noted throughout the chapters in this book, the multiple and complex determinants of health indicate the need and possibilities for a wide range of actions for public health; therefore, conceptualising the design and measures in an evaluation cannot be rushed and requires reflection.

There are three commonly accepted levels of evaluation: *process*, *impact* and *outcome*. *Process evaluation* covers all aspects of program delivery, its quality and whom it is reaching. *Impact* evaluation measures the immediate effect of the program (whether it met its objectives). *Outcome* evaluation measures the long-term effect of the program (whether it met its goals) (Hawe et al. 1990 p 60).

Process evaluation to measure program strategies and activities

Process evaluation measures the activities of the program, program quality and target audience. It also measures program implementation, and participant satisfaction (whether the strategies that have been designed are successful).

You need to pay attention to the processes or strategies that have been developed to reach the final goal. Not paying attention to this can skew results, as it makes the assumption that all of the strategies chosen are successful, and that there is a logical connection between the process/impact and outcome evaluation. There are four components within a process evaluation: *reach, satisfaction, implementation* and *quality* (Hawe et al. 1990). How do we know whether the program is reaching its intended audience or target group? In a clinical setting, you could check attendance figures against the numbers you expected to attend. A telephone survey of the population is a method to assess whether a television campaign has reached its audience. To measure program satisfaction, use yes/no questionnaires or obtain feedback from participants about the convenience and comfort of the venue and the time of day; the cost and adequacy of the facilities; staff sincerity, empathy and approachability; and the content and relevance of the education materials. To assess program implementation, consider whether all aspects of the program are being conducted as planned, that all of the components of the program work, and that your messages were clearly understood by your target group.

Evaluability assessment

At the completion of a process evaluation, you will have an accurate picture of which strategies are working and which are not, and whether it is appropriate and necessary to make changes to the program. This is called an *evaluability assessment*. You can move to the next stage of the evaluation, and, because

---

ACTIVITY 10.5 Data collection

- Summarise the measures in a process evaluation. With classmates, jot down some tools you could use to gather data for each of these measures. For example, how would you gather data on the reach of a television campaign that informs the public about the risks of drink-driving? How could you gather data about the degree of satisfaction with a new service for diabetes patients in a super clinic? How could you gather data about the quality of the materials, such as brochures, or a website you have developed?

REFLECTION 10.5

Did you agree with your classmates on mechanisms for data collection? What web-based data collection tools could be available? Could you use online surveys, or chat rooms or blogs that the recipients of your program could use to indicate their levels of program satisfaction? Importantly, the analysis of your process evaluation can help you to change the program if necessary. See the following activity for an example.

ACTIVITY 10.6 Pilot-testing a campaign

- You are working in a non-government organisation that is producing a television campaign about sun safety, targeting people aged 18–25 years. A marketing company designed the campaign, but did not pilot-test it. You perform pilot-testing with young people through a series of focus groups to gauge their satisfaction with the design of the TV promotion and the accompanying website, the appropriate time of the day the promotion should be aired, and the website structure, content and interactivity. Feedback indicated low levels of satisfaction with the program components, and the planners realised that there were many limitations to the concept and the way the program was to be implemented, so it was adjusted to reach the intended target group more effectively.

REFLECTION 10.6

An effective process evaluation is very important, as it can identify and address problems prior to the program being launched on a large scale. It also becomes more likely that the program will be more cost-effective in reaching its goals and objectives, as refinements can be made once a process evaluation is undertaken. The program can then move to the next step, which is evaluability assessment.

ACTIVITY 10.7 Evaluability assessments

- Consider the following questions with several classmates. Why is an evaluability assessment significant as part of the evaluation process? What are the implications if an evaluability assessment is not conducted? Why would program logic models be useful in evaluability assessment?

the program is now more finely tuned, the evaluation itself will be more robust.

An evaluability assessment assists by eliminating common problems, and prepares you for the impact and outcome evaluation. It is a framework for making decisions about the shape of your evaluation and whether the objectives and goals (impact and outcome levels) of your program can be evaluated. For example, if your process evaluation revealed that patients attending an education program at your clinic had low levels of satisfaction with your self-management program, and one of the objectives of your program was to increase the self-management skills for monitoring their blood pressure, you would want to reassess your education methods prior to measuring the impact of this self-management program. Your evaluability assessment would make certain that your evaluation design is robust, your measurement tools—such as questionnaires—have been tested or reviewed, and your sample size is large enough for you to make valid judgements in your analysis. In using qualitative methods, your staff should be skilled in interviewing, conducting focus groups, transcribing and analysis. To assist your thinking about evaluability assessment, turn back to the program logic model and look at where the assessment sits in the model.

Stage 1 of the evaluability assessment makes certain that there are logical links between program planning, development and evaluation; it can reveal assumptions underlying the program by linking objectives (Macaskill et al. 2000). *Stage 2* involves refining and preparing the program for impact and outcome evaluation. Include a management plan to allow for contingencies, such as staff resignations, holidays and organisational change. An evaluable program has a rational fit between clearly defined strategies, objectives and goals. The program will be properly implemented with agreement on questions to be asked, how the evaluation should be conducted, and what should be measured. Once everything is in place, you will be ready to conduct an impact evaluation.

We now present a short discussion on impact evaluation.

Impact evaluation to measure program objectives

Impact evaluation measures the immediate observable effects of a program—specifically, whether the objectives of the program have been achieved, leading to the intended outcomes of the program goals (Green & Lewis 1986).

Impact evaluation can relate to the risk factors for the health problem you're trying to improve. For example, a risk factor for obesity is a lack of physical activity. An impact evaluation could measure the awareness, knowledge, attitudes and behaviour related to physical activity, and the policy, organisational and social factors that impact on the problem. An economic evaluation can measure the costs of a program. For example, are the program costs averaged for each life saved through your public health program? Impact evaluation is usually carried out after the program has been implemented, or shortly after its completion. If the program is ongoing, the evaluation should be conducted at a time when the program strategies have had time to have an effect on the key indicators identified in the objectives. The selection of impact evaluation instruments depends on the indicators being measured. If the risk factors usually include awareness, knowledge and attitudes, behaviour, or change to the policy, organisational, physical or social environment, then appropriate measurement tools need to be identified or developed for these factors.

Data collection measures include questionnaires, qualitative and quantitative surveys, face-to-face or telephone interviews, focus groups (e.g. a facilitated group discussion with participants on the effects of the program), self-completed questionnaires, journals, observations, and other data sources. Impact evaluation assesses whether objectives have been achieved.

> **REFLECTION 10.7**
>
> Did you come up with the same answers? Can you think of the messages in some current public health campaigns that you find confusing? How could you find out whether focus groups or other feedback mechanisms were considered in campaign development?

Outcome evaluation to measure program goals

Outcome evaluation measures the extent to which a program goal has been met. Often these goals are long-term and are about changes to indicators of health status, such as changes in morbidity or mortality statistics in a population. However, it may be possible to make some short-term gains on a health problem—for example, reducing personal violence outside nightclubs by closing clubs and pubs early, through an increased police presence, and having efficient and safe transport available. The next section outlines some evaluation designs that are commonly used to measure impact and outcome.

Evaluation designs for impact and outcome evaluation

Chapter 5 presents some of the designs used in public health research that can be applied to an evaluation. Evaluation design decisions need to be made at the outset of your program, and particularly during the evaluability assessment phase. The type of intervention you are proposing, and its goals and objectives, will influence the design. Some common designs include: a post-test, self-reported questionnaire for participants if no pre-evaluation test has been undertaken; a single group, pre-test/post-test design administered to the participants; and a time-series design.

Whether any changes have occurred in health status and quality of life could be determined by an outcome evaluation.

Evaluations can also be designed to measure broader aspects of a program—for example, measuring an organisation's system and its policies, and what impact these have on the delivery and outcomes of a program—as programs are not implemented in a vacuum.

Stufflebeam and Shinkfield's (2007) CIPP model is used for Case Study 10.2, as it is particularly useful when evaluating organisational systems and policy development. Four elements are proposed in this evaluation model: *context*, *input*, *process* and *product*.

Context evaluation defines the environment in which change is to occur. *Input evaluation* determines how one can utilise resources to meet program goals by identifying capabilities of the organisation in implementing a program. *Process evaluation* is an ongoing evaluation of the program's implementation, while *product evaluation* measures, interprets and judges the effectiveness of a program or policy (Fleming & Parker 2007 p 119). Case Study 10.2 demonstrates how CIPP was used by the authors to compare a diabetes prevention pilot initiative in two different health services.

Table 10.1 presents a checklist to guide your planning and evaluation.

A final word

This chapter introduced public health planning and evaluation, and its crucial role in addressing public health issues. Program logic models provide a graphic overview of all of the components of a program plan and its evaluation. Various aspects of needs assessment were introduced to ensure that your programs are based on evidence. The CDC framework is a starting point for developing an evaluation plan, and its standards set a foundation for ethical practice as an evaluator. Levels of evaluation and evaluability assessment were discussed. A model for assessing organisational dynamics and policy development was considered. The significance of a comprehensive evaluation report to disseminate evaluation findings concluded this chapter.

CASE STUDY 10.2

Evaluation of a diabetes prevention pilot initiative

Diabetes is a national health priority (see Chapter 3). It is estimated that 4.2% of the Australian population (nearly 1 million people) have diabetes (AIHW 2013), with 85% to 90% of these having type 2 diabetes (AIHW 2012). Studies show that type 2 diabetes can be prevented or delayed through pharmacological interventions and, more efficaciously, through lifestyle interventions. The *Diabetes Prevention Pilot Initiative* (DPPI) Evaluation Project aimed to evaluate two projects that were funded by the Commonwealth Department of Health and Ageing in 2003.

The projects needed to develop and conduct innovative community-based projects to test methods of implementing the National Health and Medical Research Council's *National Evidenced Based Guidelines for the Management of Type 2 Diabetes Mellitus: Primary Prevention* (NHMRC 2001). Projects were required to increase physical activity, improve diet, and achieve a healthy weight for people at risk of developing diabetes. One project was linked to a university department in a rural area where participants were recruited through general practitioners; the other project was conducted through a regional health service in a medium-sized town, where patients were recruited through the local community health service.

Stufflebeam's (2003) CIPP model was used to evaluate the program. It ensured that common aspects of both projects were considered. The similarities and differences between the two projects were able to be synthesised and analysed using the four constructs of the CIPP in a comparative analysis. Context evaluation assessed the needs, assets and problems within the defined environments. Input evaluation assessed the work plans and budgets of the selected approaches in the two trials. Process evaluations assessed the program's activities, and product evaluation included an impact evaluation of: (1) the program's engagement of the targeted audience as outlined in the NHMRC guidelines (2001) for case detection and assessment; (2) an effectiveness evaluation that assessed the quality and significance of the program's outcomes; and (3) a sustainability evaluation that included the extent to which the program's contributions could be successfully institutionalised and continued over time. Economic evaluation examined the costs and potential health benefits of the programs. Stufflebeam's CIPP model provided a lens through which the components of each of the programs could be analysed and compared.

(Source: Queensland University of Technology 2007. Case study approved November 2007)

TABLE 10.1 Planning and evaluation checklist: evaluation and dissemination

Stage	Action
Problem analysis and needs assessment	Getting started—what issues do I need to consider in the planning and evaluation cycle?
	Engage stakeholders—who are they, and what are their values/expectations/concerns?
	Determine program objectives/mission—hierarchy of outcomes to guide action, and to link strategies and evaluation
	Pilot testing – how many participants?
Program planning and implementation	Select/describe strategies and methods—selection is linked to objectives
	Implementation process—needs to be managed in detail; suggested implementation and evaluation plan
	Evaluation procedures—qualitative, quantitative, or elements of both
	Data collection—what, when, and how to measure (pre-intervention testing—otherwise there is no basis for doing a reasonable evaluation, and post-testing)
	Analysis of data—how much and what should be analysed

TABLE 10.1 Continued	
Stage	Action
	Costs, and what resources (human, financial, time) are available to meet the planned actions
	Using external evaluators—costs, expertise and independence of the evaluation
Evaluation and dissemination	Evaluation management
	Dealing with all of the players in the evaluation process and their individual expectations about program outcomes
	Participant burden—be aware of over-evaluating participants (the tyranny of evaluation)
	Process, impact, outcome levels—how do you make these judgements, and what are the implications for broader applications of the evaluation beyond the program?
	Investment in evaluation—money, time, personnel
	Evaluation outcomes—what did I learn, and how can I use that information for the future?
	Dissemination of the results—to whom and for what purpose

(Source: O'Connor-Fleming, M., Parker, E., Higgins, H., et al., 2006. A framework for evaluating health promotion programs. Health Promotion Journal of Australia 17 (1), 61–66. Reproduced with permission from Health Promotion Journal of Australia. Copyright © Australian Health Promotion Association 2006. Published by CSIRO PUBLISHING. Available: <http://www.publish.csiro.au/nid/292/paper/HE06061.htm>.)

REVIEW QUESTIONS

1. Why are planning and evaluation important practices in public health?
2. How are planning and evaluation linked, and why should these be integrated activities?
3. What are the types of needs assessments that can be used to build effective programs, and what are their differences?
4. What are the steps in the CDC *Framework for program evaluation*, and how can it be used?
5. What are three evaluation designs that could be used in an impact and outcome evaluation?
6. Why is it important to write SMART objectives?
7. Define a program logic model, and give three reasons for its use.
8. Glasgow et al. (1999) devised the RE-AIM framework to guide program evaluations. What does 'RE-AIM' stand for?
9. Using the RE-AIM framework, what methods of data gathering could you use to assess whether a statewide media campaign on eating healthier food is reaching its target audience of young adults?
10. Name the four standards for 'good evaluation' in the CDC framework.

Useful websites

- Australian Bureau of Statistics: http://www.abs.gov.au
- Australian Institute of Health and Welfare: http://www.aihw.gov.au
- Centers for Disease Control and Prevention: http://www.cdc.gov
- VicHealth, Victorian Health Promotion: http://www.vichealth.vic.gov.au/

References

Australian Institute of Health and Welfare, 2012. Australia's Health 2012. AIHW Cat. No. AUS 156. AIHW, Canberra.

Australian Institute of Health and Welfare, 2013. Prevalence of diabetes. Online. Available: <http://www.aihw.gov.au/diabetes-indicators/prevalence/> (10 Apr 2014).

Bartholomew, K., Parcel, G.S., Kok, G., et al., 2001. Intervention Mapping: Designing Theory and Evidence-Based Health Promotion Programs. Mayfield, Mountain View.

Bradshaw, J., 1972. The concept of social need. New Society 19: 640–643. In: Katz, J., Peberdy, A. (Eds.), 2000. Promoting Health: Knowledge and Practice. The Open University, London, p 263.

Centers for Disease Control and Prevention, 1999. Framework for program evaluation in public health. MMWR 48 (RR-11). Online. Available: <http://www.cdc.gov/mmwr/PDF/RR/RR4811.pdf>.

Dietitians Association of Australia website. Online. Available: <http://daa.asn.au/for-the-public/smart-eating-for-you/frequently-asked-questions/can-i-eat-eggs-if-i-want-to-be-healthy/> (5 Mar 2014).

Dubuy, V., De Cocker, K., De Bourdeaudhuij, I., et al., 2013. Evaluation of a workplace intervention to promote commuter cycling: A RE-AIM analysis. BMC Public Health 13, 587.

Finch, C.F., Diamantopoulou, K., Twomey, D.M., et al., 2013. The reach and adoption of a coach-led exercise training programme in community football. British Journal of Sports Medicine 48 (8), 718–723. doi:10.1136/bjsports-2012-091797.

Fleming, M.L., Parker, E., 2007. Health Promotion: Principles and Practice in the Australian Context, third ed. Allen and Unwin, Crows Nest.

Glasgow, R.E., Vogt, T.M., Boles, S.M., 1999. Evaluating the public health impact of health promotion interventions: the RE-AIM framework. American Journal of Public Health 89 (9), 1322–1327.

Green, L.W., Anderson, C.L., 1986. Community Health Planning. Times Mirror/Mosby College, St Louis.

Green, L.W., Lewis, F.M., 1986. Measurement and Evaluation in Health Education and Health Promotion. Mayfield, Palo Alto.

Green, L.W., Kreuter, M., 1991. Health Promotion Planning: An Educational and Environmental Approach, second ed. Mayfield, Mountain View.

Green, L.W., Kreuter, M., 2005. Health Promotion Planning: An Educational and Ecological Approach, fourth ed. McGraw-Hill, New York.

Hawe, P., Degeling, D., Hall, J., 1990. Evaluating Health Promotion. MacLennan and Petty, Sydney.

Katz, J., Peberdy, A., Douglas, J. (Eds.), 2000. Promoting Health: Knowledge and Practice, second ed. The Open University, London.

Lenihan, P., 2005. MAPP (mobilizing for action through planning and partnerships) and the evolution of planning in public health practice. Journal of Public Health Management and Practice 11 (5), 381–386.

Macaskill, L., Dwyer, J.M.J., Uetrecht, C., et al., 2000. An evaluability assessment to develop a restaurant health promotion program in Canada. Health Promotion International 15 (1), 57–69.

McLaughlin, J.A., Jordan, G.B., 1999. Logic models: a tool for telling your program's performance story. Evaluation and Program Planning 22, 65–72.

National Health and Medical Research Council (NHMRC), 2001. National Evidence Based Guidelines for the Management of Type 2 Diabetes Mellitus: Primary Prevention. NHMRC, Canberra.

National Health and Medical Research Council (NHMRC), 2013. Australian Dietary Guidelines (2013). NHMRC, Canberra. Online. Available: <https://www.nhmrc.gov.au/guidelines-publications/n55> (29 Apr 2015).

O'Connor-Fleming, M., Parker, E., Higgins, H., et al., 2006. A framework for evaluating health promotion programs. Health Promotion Journal of Australia 17 (1), 61–66. Copyright © Australian Health Promotion Association 2006. Published by CSIRO PUBLISHING. Available: <http://www.publish.csiro.au/nid/292/paper/HE06061.htm>.

Owen, J., 1999. Program Evaluation: Forms and Approaches. Allen and Unwin, Sydney.

Queensland University of Technology, 2007. Diabetes Prevention Pilot Initiative: Evaluation Project. Final Report for the Australian Government Department of Health and Ageing. Queensland University of Technology, Brisbane, p 6–13.

Rootman, I., Goodstadt, M., Hyndman, B., et al., 2001. Evaluation in Health Promotion: Principles and Perspectives. WHO Regional Publications, European Series No. 92. WHO, Copenhagen.

Scriven, A., 2010. (previous editions by Ewles L., Simnett, I.) Promoting Health: A Practical Guide, sixth ed. Baillière Tindall Elsevier, London.

Stufflebeam, D.L., 2001. Evaluation models. New Directions for Evaluation 89, 7–98.

Stufflebeam, D.L., 2003. The CIPP model for evaluation: an update, a review of the model's development, a checklist to guide implementation. Presented at the 2003 Annual Conference of the Oregon Program Evaluators Network (OPEN), Portland, Oregon. Online. Available: <http://goeroendeso.files.wordpress.com/2009/01/cipp-modeloregon10-031.pdf> (10 March 2001).

Stufflebeam, D.L., Shinkfield, A.J., 2007. Evaluation Theory, Models and Applications. Jossey-Bass, San Francisco.

Suchman, E.A., 1967. Evaluative Research. Russell Sage Foundation, New York.

Thorogood, M., Coombes, Y. (Eds.), 2010. Evaluating Health Promotion: Practice and Methods, third ed. Oxford University Press, Oxford. (Ebook.).

Victorian Government Department of Health, 2014. Municipal public health and wellbeing plans. Online. Available: <http://www.health.vic.gov.au/localgov/municipal-planning.htm> (1 Sep 2014).

Vidgen, H., 2014. Case study on Food Literacy and Needs. School of Public Health and Social Work. Queensland University of Technology, Brisbane.

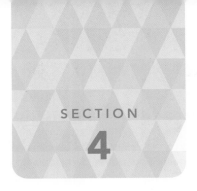

HEALTH PROTECTION AND PROMOTION

Introduction

- **The four chapters** that make up this section focus on a continuum of public health activity, from the always-present need for disease control and management, and through the important role of environmental health re-emerging in contemporary society and a timely examination of emergency planning and response, given the number of local and global disasters in recent years, to the promotion of health in the population.

- **Public health activity** has always focused on a continuum of care from promotion and prevention to treatment and rehabilitation. Along this continuum are a range of strategies and intervention activities that provide the population or subpopulations with appropriate interventions to meet their diverse needs.

- **The first of the four** chapters, Chapter 11, addresses public health's role in disease control and management. The chapter outlines the impact that infectious and chronic diseases have on the health of the community, the public health strategies that are used to reduce the burden of those diseases, and the historical and emerging risks to public health. It examines the comprehensive approaches implemented to prevent both chronic and infectious diseases, and to manage and care for people with these conditions. It analyses models of care in the context of need, service delivery options, and the potential to prevent or manage early intervention for chronic and infectious diseases.

- **The focus for public health** is clearly on chronic disease prevention in the first instance, and then the management and control of the condition once a chronic disease has developed. Over 3 million Australians, or nearly one in seven, suffer from chronic disease, and the problem is likely to be one of the great health challenges for Australia and the world in the twenty-first century.

- **Chronic diseases and conditions** are generally defined as those that are long-term (lasting more than six months), non-communicable, or long-lasting communicable conditions (e.g. HIV/AIDS), involving some functional impairment or disability, and are usually incurable. They can affect people of all ages, and contribute to the disease burden in our society.

- **Chronic diseases**, such as diabetes, cancer, cardiovascular disease, asthma and certain mental health conditions, are among the most significant contributors to morbidity and mortality in Australia, and thus are recognised as National Health Priority Areas. Public health has an important role to play in preventing and managing these conditions. Just as we discussed in the earlier section on risk and determinants, these health conditions are complex and multifaceted. Strategies to prevent and deal with the health consequences also need to be multidisciplinary and diverse. Chapter 11 presents you with a broad introduction to both chronic and infectious disease prevention and control. Infectious diseases are a common and significant contributor to ill health throughout the world, particularly in developing countries. Illness and death from infectious diseases can in most cases be avoided at an affordable cost. Chapter 11 examines examples of both infectious diseases and zoonotic diseases; it covers the concept of immunity, and explores the range of public health strategies that can be put into place to deal with infectious disease prevention and treatment.

- **Environmental impacts** on human health are the subject of Chapter 12. The chapter discusses the definition of 'environmental health' and how human health can be protected from environmental hazards, as well as exploring the key environmental health issues and how they might be managed through a range of public health strategies. The other fundamental issue facing the planet is the question of environmental sustainability and the importance of managing our environment to protect human health. Chapter 12 discusses the range of management tools, including legislation and risk assessment, as mechanisms for controlling environmental hazards and protecting the population's health.

- **Disaster preparedness and public health** is the focus for Chapter 13. In this chapter, issues such as how 'disaster' is defined, and the principles of disaster management, form the focus of the first part of our discussion. While there are many definitions of 'disaster', there is little agreement on what a disaster is. This chapter looks at the multiple factors that influence the challenges facing a community or communities, and the resources available to deal with disasters. The chapter concludes with an examination of the recovery, rehabilitation and redevelopment processes for restoring functionality, and, where possible, for development and improvement through reconstruction.

- **The final chapter** in this section, Chapter 14, looks at the concept of promoting health and protecting people from illness through health education and promotion strategies. Education and promotion are an important part of public health activity, as the future will need to see far more attention placed on promotion and prevention if governments are going to manage healthcare costs. The costs of living with chronic disease, as an example, far outweigh the costs of promoting health and preventing the development of such diseases. Chapter 14 briefly explores the history of health education and health promotion and the emergence of the 'new public health'. It discusses the *Ottawa Charter for Health Promotion* (World Health Organization 1986) as the seminal development in the discipline in the past half-century, and examines a range of health promotion strategies that can be utilised in a variety of settings. The chapter contains interesting new settings for health promotion, and concludes by considering the emerging challenges facing health promotion into the future.

Reference

World Health Organization, 1986. The Ottawa Charter for Health Promotion First International Conference on Health Promotion, Ottawa, 21 November 1986. Available: <http://www.who.int/healthpromotion/conferences/previous/ottawa/en/> (20 May 2014).

CHAPTER 11

Disease control and management

Thomas Tenkate, Mary Louise Fleming & Gerry FitzGerald

Learning objectives

After reading this chapter, you should be able to:

- define 'chronic condition' and 'chronic disease'

- understand the similarities and differences in definitions of 'non-communicable disease', 'chronic condition' and 'chronic disease'

- describe an integrated approach to chronic disease management, and what the elements of that approach might be

- understand the broad nature and causes of infectious diseases

- identify the public health principles used to prevent, treat and manage infectious diseases

- identify, by working through a number of case study examples, the principles of disease control and prevention.

Introduction

Globally, the main contributors to morbidity and mortality are chronic conditions, including cardiovascular disease and diabetes. Chronic disease is costly and partially avoidable, with around 60% of deaths and nearly 50% of the global disease burden attributable to these conditions. By 2020, chronic illnesses will likely be the leading cause of disability worldwide. Existing healthcare systems that focus on acute episodic health conditions, both national and international, cannot address the worldwide transition to chronic illness; nor are they appropriate for the ongoing care and management of those already dealing with chronic diseases. As such, chronic disease management requires integrated approaches that incorporate interventions targeted at both individuals and populations, and emphasise the shared risk factors of different conditions. International and Australian strategic planning documents articulate similar elements to manage chronic disease, including the need for aligning sectoral policies for health, forming partnerships, and engaging communities in decision-making.

Infectious diseases are also a common and significant contributor to ill health throughout the world. In many countries, this impact has been minimised by the combined efforts of preventative health measures and improved treatment methods. However, in low-income countries, infectious diseases remain the dominant cause of death and disability. The World Health Organization (WHO) estimates that infectious diseases (including respiratory infections) still account for around 23% (or around 14 million) of all deaths each year, and result in over 4.6 billion episodes of diarrhoeal disease and 243 million cases of malaria each year (Lozano et al. 2012, WHO 2009).

In addition to the high level of mortality, infectious diseases disable many hundreds of millions of people each year, mainly in developing countries, with the global burden of disease from infectious diseases estimated to be around 300 million DALYs (disability-adjusted life years) (WHO 2012).

The aim of this chapter is to outline the impact that infectious diseases and chronic diseases have on the health of the community, describe the public health strategies used to reduce the burden of those diseases, and discuss the historical and emerging disease risks to public health. This chapter examines the comprehensive approaches implemented to prevent both chronic and infectious diseases, and to manage and care for communities with these conditions.

Defining chronic condition and chronic disease

The terms 'non-communicable disease', 'chronic condition' and 'chronic disease' are sometimes used interchangeably. The term *non-communicable disease* is used by the WHO as an overarching definition for chronic disease (WHO 2013a). *Chronic condition* 'encompasses disability and disease conditions that people may "live with" over extended periods of time, for example more than six months' (Flinders Human Behaviour and Health Research Unit (FHBHRU) 2014). They are amenable to generic approaches because there are generic self-management tasks regardless of diagnosis (FHBHRU 2014). *Chronic disease* is a subset of chronic condition, and refers to a specific medical diagnosis. It may be more likely to have a progressively deteriorating path than other chronic conditions (FHBHRU 2014, WHO 2005c, WHO 2013a). In this chapter, the term 'chronic disease' will be used. Chronic diseases are those involving a long course in their development or their symptoms. They account for a high proportion of deaths, disability and illness, and are a major health problem worldwide. Yet many of these diseases are preventable, or their onset can be delayed, by relatively simple measures.

For a number of reasons, including the fact that people are living to older age, chronic diseases have increased in prevalence over the past century, and today they affect one in four Australians. Most chronic diseases are generally not curable. Some can be immediately life-threatening, such as heart attack and stroke; others are often serious, including various cancers, depression and diabetes. They all persist in an individual through his or her life. They are, however, not always the cause of death. Chronic

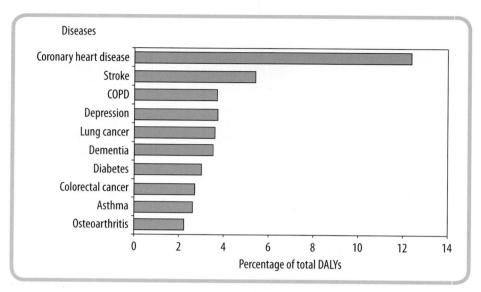

FIG. 11.1   Top 10 leading causes of disease burden in DALYs* terms, Australia, 1996.
Note: *DALYs—disability-adjusted life years—count equivalent years of 'healthy'
life lost due to poor health or disability and potential years of life lost due to
premature death. COPD—chronic obstructive pulmonary disease.
(Source: Mathers et al. 1999)

diseases are listed as the top 10 causes of the burden of disease in Australia (see
Figure 11.1). These diseases have accounted for an increasing total disease burden in
Australia (Australian Institute of Health and Welfare (AIHW) 2012a).

A number of behaviours can prevent or delay the development of many chronic
diseases, such as controlling body weight, eating nutritious foods, avoiding tobacco use,
controlling alcohol consumption, and increasing physical activity. Figure 11.2 illustrates
a number of risk factors that contribute to the onset, maintenance and prognosis of
many chronic diseases. In this figure, these are classified as 'behavioural risk factors',
'biomedical risk factors' and 'other factors'.

Most of the chronic diseases have multiple risk factors and are considered to be
'adult' behaviours and conditions; however, the situations that lead to their initiation
often begin early in life, or even in the womb. Therefore, it is important to have a lifecourse perspective of chronic diseases and their risk factors, one that recognises the
interactive and cumulative impact of social and biological influences throughout life.
Table 11.1 examines the relationship between risk factors and chronic diseases in Australia. It clearly points out the strong relationship between a range of behavioural and
biomedical risk factors and chronic diseases (AIHW 2002).

The success of public health initiatives, in part, means that people are living longer
(National Health Priority Action Council (NHPAC) 2006, WHO 2014a), and this
increased lifespan allows more time for chronic illness to develop (AIHW 2012a,
Centers for Disease Control and Prevention (CDC) 2013, NHPAC 2006). Chronic
diseases place an extra burden on healthcare systems, and it is predicted that by the
year 2020 chronic diseases will be the leading cause of disability in the world, with over

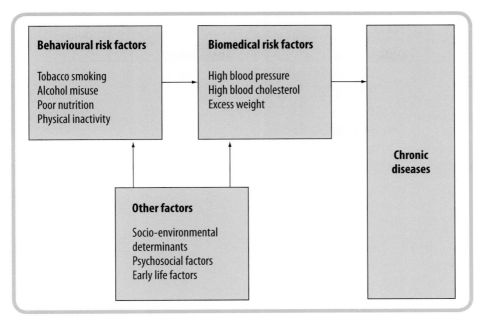

FIG. 11.2   Behavioural risk factors, biomedical risk factors, and other factors contributing to chronic disease.
(Source: Modified from AIHW 2002)

70% of the global burden of illness mainly attributable to CVD (cardiovascular disease—covering all diseases and conditions of the heart and blood vessels), cancer, diabetes and chronic respiratory diseases, as well as mental health problems, injuries and violence (AIHW 2012a, CDC 2013, NHPAC 2006). Similar to the WHO, Australia continues to acknowledge chronic disease as a major health challenge (AIHW 2012a).

Continuum of care/integrated approach to chronic disease

In 2005, the NHPAC (2006) reviewed the national and international evidence for strategies for preventing and managing chronic disease, and endorsed the *National Chronic Disease Strategy* (NCDS). The focus nationally was on four key areas for improving outcomes for people with chronic diseases: prevention across the continuum, early detection and treatment, integrated and coordinated care, and self-management (NHPAC 2006). Supporting this approach was the amendment, and relaxation, of qualification criteria for the *Chronic Disease Management Plan* (formerly the *Enhanced Primary Care Plan*), which provided funding for a more multidisciplinary management plan for patients with chronic conditions and/or complex care needs, and more preventive care for older Australians (Department of Health (DoH) 2014).

Chronic disease prevention is an approach to healthcare that emphasises the maintenance of independence and continuing health. Prevention of chronic diseases follows a continuum of care, ranging from prevention strategies directed at minimising or eliminating future chronic illnesses, with initiatives such as smoking cessation, healthy

TABLE 11.1 Relationships between various chronic diseases, conditions and risk factors

Disease/ condition	Behavioural			Biomedical			
	Poor diet	Physical inactivity	Tobacco use	Alcohol misuse	Excess weight	High blood pressure	High blood cholesterol
Coronary heart disease	✓	✓	✓	✓	✓	✓	✓
Stroke	✓	✓	✓	✓	✓	✓	✓
Lung cancer			✓				
Colorectal cancer	✓	✓		✓	✓		
Depression		✓		✓	✓		
Diabetes	✓	✓			✓		
Asthma			✓		✓		
Chronic obstructive pulmonary disease (COPD)			✓				
Chronic kidney disease	✓				✓	✓	
Oral diseases	✓		✓	✓			
Osteoarthritis		✓			✓		
Osteoporosis	✓	✓	✓	✓			
Excess weight	✓	✓					
High blood pressure	✓	✓		✓	✓		
High blood cholesterol	✓	✓			✓		

(Source: Modified from AIHW 2012a)

eating and physical activity programs (International Association for the Study of Obesity 2014). Furthermore, public health has a place in managing chronic diseases, as there are two main types of prevention: avoiding the development of chronic disease, and delaying the expected complications of existing chronic diseases through good-quality treatment and management (WHO 2009).

Public health and health promotion embrace an inclusive model, one that incorporates a population health perspective that views disease prevention and health promotion as a continuum (Pruitt & Epping-Jordan 2005). This position accentuates the whole scope of care, from primary prevention for healthy populations to early detection and intervention for subgroups considered at risk, through to management, tertiary prevention, rehabilitation and palliative care for people with established disease (AIHW 2012a, NHPAC 2006, Pruitt & Epping-Jordan 2005, WHO 2009).

Chronic disease management programs

Disease management programs are a comprehensive approach to enhancing the quality of care for people with chronic diseases (Velasco-Garrido et al. 2003). They use evidence-based criteria of care, coordinate care through multicomponent and multidisciplinary programs, and focus on the entire path of chronic conditions. Although there is no generic model suitable for all conditions, Velasco-Garrido et al. (2003, adapted from Kesteloot 1999) identify seven major components of chronic disease management:

1 comprehensive care (multiprofessional, multidisciplinary, acute care, prevention and health promotion)
2 integrated care, care continuum, coordination of the different components
3 population orientation (defined by a specific condition)
4 active client/patient management tools (health education, empowerment, self-care)
5 evidence-based guidelines, protocols, care pathways
6 information technology, system solutions
7 continuous quality improvement.

Within Australia, there have been a variety of programs addressing the management and prevention of chronic diseases, most recently discussed in the document *Australia: The Healthiest Country by 2020* (National Preventative Health Taskforce 2008). It should be noted that many of these interventions are multifaceted, and therefore could be categorised in two or more of the action areas that follow.

Early detection and early treatment

Early detection and treatment can reduce complications, comorbidities and mortality. Recently, the AIHW (2012a) stated that there are no current estimates of the numbers of Australians living with undiagnosed diabetes. There are two primary approaches to early detection and treatment: population-based screening, and opportunistic screening

ACTIVITY 11.1 Diabetes detection and care

- Go to the website for the Australian Government's work on diabetes (http://www.health.gov.au/internet/main/publishing.nsf/Content/chronic-diabetes#pro)—there is a detailed account of both prevention activities and support for people with diabetes (DoH 2012).
- Design a table that examines the two levels of care and the strategies that are discussed at each level.
- Then add to your table activities in your own state, including government and the not-for-profit sectors, which include prevention, early detection and ongoing care for people living with diabetes.

by health workers for risk factors and/or early signs and symptoms (NHPAC 2006). Examples of the former include mammography for women aged 50–69, and bowel cancer screening.

Integration and continuity of prevention and care

Integration and continuity of prevention and care includes care planning and coordination through a range of providers and settings (NHPAC 2006). An example is the chronic disease management items available through Medicare for patients with chronic conditions and complex care needs; these include diabetes, heart disease and other chronic conditions (DoH 2012). The chronic disease management items cover a range of allied health workers, including exercise physiologists, diabetes educators, nutritionists, Aboriginal health workers and podiatrists (DoH 2012).

Self-management

Self-management entails a person's active involvement in his or her own healthcare. An important component of self-management is cooperation between the person, their family, health service providers and the healthcare system (FHBHRU 2009, Lorig et al. 2001, NHPAC 2006, WHO 2005b) (see Case Study 11.1).

CASE STUDY 11.1

Example of self-management

One example of a self-management program is the federal Department of Health and Ageing's *Sharing Health Care Initiative* (SHCI) demonstration projects, aimed at evaluating different approaches to chronic disease self-management. Through grant funding, the SHCI aims to: enhance the quality of life for people with chronic diseases and their communities; improve care providers' appreciation of the advantages of self-management, and advance collaboration between care providers, people with chronic conditions and their families; and improve the effectiveness of health service utilisation. Initial outcomes include a decline in depression, pain and general distress, improved symptom management, and a fall in general practitioner visits and hospitalisations (Department of Health (DoH) 2005). An example of the SHCI is the *Pika Wiya Health Service* in South Australia, a chronic condition self-management project for diabetes. A camp for Aboriginal people introduced education on medication, nutrition, exercise, podiatry, renal disease and palliative care. Many Aboriginal people in this area also have other chronic diseases, such as heart disease, renal disease and asthma (DoH 2005).

Chronic disease prevention and management—some issues

As indicated previously, healthcare systems generally focus on responding to acute episodic health conditions, and consequently they are inadequate for the ongoing care and management of those with chronic health problems (NHMRC 2001, NHPAC 2006, National Public Health Partnership 2001, Weeramanthri et al. 2003, WHO 2009). Furthermore, a large proportion of funding for chronic disease management is directed at programs that target comparatively restricted categories of populations, diseases or risk factors; therefore, managers of comprehensive chronic disease programs need to ensure that programs are integrated to reduce unnecessary duplication (CDC 2013).

Clearly, it is essential to coordinate realistic and comprehensive strategies to advance the Australian health system's ability to provide comprehensive chronic disease prevention and management (AIHW 2012b).

> **REFLECTION 11.2**
>
> Think about the important aspects that should be included in a successful chronic condition self-management program. Why are they successful? What aspects of the program make them successful? How do the principles apply to the range of programs identified? Why are principles important to consider in developing a program, and how do they guide program development?

Defining infectious disease

Infectious diseases are a common and significant contributor to ill health throughout the world, particularly in developing countries. The importance of infectious diseases is summarised in the following quote from a previous Director General of WHO, Dr Gro Harlem Brundtland:

> One out of every two people in low-income countries dies at an early age from an infectious disease. Most of these deaths should have been prevented. How can families, communities and countries reach their dreams with this burden? Healthy development removes these obstacles and helps individuals and countries achieve their full potential. If the world invests in priority strategies to fight infectious diseases, much of this death and suffering could be prevented. (WHO 1999 p i)

Unfortunately there is some inconsistency in the language used in regard to infectious diseases, and there is value in using the following simple (plain-English) approach to describe the various key terms.

A *communicable (or contagious) disease* is one that can spread from one individual to another. In contrast, *infectious diseases* are diseases caused by pathogenic microorganisms (also known as pathogens), such as various species of bacteria, viruses, parasites or fungi. More specifically, *zoonotic diseases* are infectious diseases of animals that can cause disease when transmitted to humans (WHO 1999).

Most communicable diseases are infectious diseases, but not all. For example, some chemically induced diseases—such as organophosphate poisoning—can be spread from one individual to another and could be described as 'communicable', but are clearly not infectious. In contrast, most infectious diseases can be spread from one individual to another, but some can only be transmitted by an inert life stage (e.g. tetanus spores) or via a vector (e.g. malaria transmitted by mosquitoes). Given this overlap in terminology, in this section we will focus our discussion on 'infectious' diseases.

Infectious diseases are very common in developed countries, and generally do not cause significant health outcomes in these communities. Some of the most common

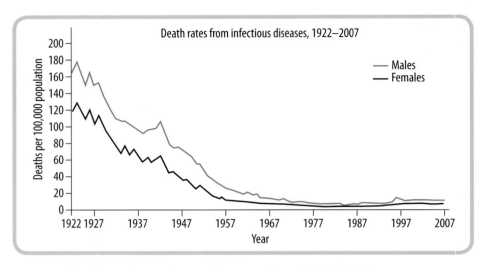

FIG. 11.3   Death rates from infectious diseases in Australia 1922–2007.
(Reproduced from Australian Institute of Health and Welfare, Australia's health 2010, p 205)

infectious diseases—such as the common cold, dental caries and acne vulgaris—have a highly significant economic and social impact, but do not have significant morbidity or mortality. For example, in Australia there are over 230,000 cases of infectious disease reported to health authorities each year (National Notifiable Diseases Surveillance System (NNDSS) Annual Report Writing Group 2013). Deaths from infectious diseases have, however, dramatically declined in Australia since the early part of the twentieth century, primarily due to improvements in sanitation and an improved quality of life. In 1922, deaths from infectious diseases accounted for 15% of all deaths, but by 2007 they accounted for a little over 1% (AIHW 2010) (see Figure 11.3). In contrast, infectious diseases continue to be a major cause of death and disability in developing countries. For example, in South East Asia infectious diseases account for 40% of deaths and 28% of illness and disability (WHO 2005a). Such countries often lack the economic capacity to provide the community with the public health infrastructure required to prevent or manage infectious diseases. Consequently, infectious diseases still account for 5 of the top 10 causes of death in low-income countries (WHO 2015b). Box 11.1 describes the challenges of some longstanding infectious diseases.

Models of infectious disease

The concept of human infectious disease is multidimensional, and includes our interaction with the pathogen, the impact within our body of contact with the pathogen, and the interaction between our body and the various environments in which we live. For any infectious disease to occur, there are always three elements (Hurster 1997):

1   a *person* or *host* who is the target of the disease, and who may be susceptible to it

2   an *agent*, which is either the direct cause of disease or a contributing or predisposing factor to its onset, and

3   the *environment*, which may influence the existence of the agent, the exposure of the host to the agent, or the susceptibility of the host.

BOX 11.1

THE OLD EPIDEMICS

Malaria is a major cause of the burden of infectious disease. Caused by the *Plasmodium* genus, it is transmitted from individual to individual by mosquitoes. Over 3 billion people are exposed to malarial risk, which is estimated to cause over 600,000 deaths each year (WHO 2014a), and has massive social and economic costs. Malaria is difficult to eliminate, although many countries, including Australia, have eliminated native malaria (Guinovart et al. 2006).

The term 'plague' is often used to describe any pandemic. However, the actual disease *The Plague* (or *Black Death*) is caused by *Pasteurella pestis* (or *Yersinia pestis*). The organism is spread by fleas directly from human to human, or via an intermediate host, typically rats. The Black Death is reputed to have caused the downfall of the Greek civilisation around 500BC, and to have contributed to the collapse of the Roman Empire 1000 years later. The Plague spread throughout Europe during the Middle Ages, where it is thought to have caused the death of one-third of Europe's population. Even today it causes small outbreaks around the world, but mostly in sub-equatorial Africa.

At the end of World War 1 (1918), a highly virulent form of *influenza* broke out, first in military camps in Europe, but then spreading to every continent and all countries. The disease, known as *Spanish flu*, was caused by the modification of a human influenza virus (H1N1), and was estimated to have caused up to 50 million deaths—in a world whose total population was approximately 1.7 billion. The epidemic had long-term economic consequences, and possibly contributed indirectly to the economic collapse of the 1930s and, thus, World War 2.

Smallpox is a human disease that caused epidemics in ancient Egypt, and continued to cause widespread disease until finally eradicated in 1980. Smallpox was reputed to have killed one in every five children at the height of its impact, and as recently as 1967 it caused 10 million to 15 million cases, and 2 million deaths, worldwide per year (Tucker 2001). The eradication of smallpox is significant not only because of its impact on human health, but also because it demonstrates that it is possible to eliminate a disease. Conquering smallpox was ultimately achieved through widespread vaccination programs.

These interactions are commonly described in terms of two models of infectious diseases: the *agent–host–environment triangle*, which is also known as the *epidemiological triad*, and the *chain of infection* model (see Figures 11.4 and 11.5).

For the chain model of infectious diseases, the following elements must apply, and these are illustrated in Table 11.2 (Weber & Rutala 2001):

- *Susceptible host*—Despite living in a sea of microbes, people are generally healthy due to intrinsic and specific host defences.

ACTIVITY 11.3 An outbreak of 'Spanish flu' today

- Write a paragraph about the possible effects of a new 'Spanish flu' outbreak today. What are the differences between the current social and structural conditions and those of 1918 that would alter the impact of the flu on the health and wellbeing of the community?

Susceptibility includes the host being immunocompromised, or other defects in the host's defences.

- *Infectious agent*—An agent must be present and capable of causing infection (e.g. virus, bacteria, fungi, protozoa).
- *Reservoir*—The agent needs a reservoir where it can propagate—that is, live, reproduce and die in the natural state. This includes humans, animals and the environment.
- *Portal of exit* from reservoir and *portal of entry* into a susceptible host—examples include the respiratory tract, the GI (gastrointestinal) tract, skin and mucous membranes.
- *Transmission*—The agent needs to be transmitted, directly or indirectly, from one place to another.

Mechanism of infectious disease

A pathogenic microorganism can cause disease via several mechanisms. Organisms can cause direct cellular injury when they invade healthy cells, resulting in cell death, with the consequences depending on the number of cells, body organs or systems affected. Microorganisms that invade and grow in the body can also cause symptoms or disease by releasing a toxin, which in turn causes injury to cells and resultant symptoms. For example, *Clostridium tetani* may invade small breaches in the skin and cause a minor infection, which may be unnoticed. However, the toxin released by the cells causes widespread neurological injury resulting in the characteristic symptoms and signs of tetanus.

Microorganisms can also cause disease by affecting the body's own protective responses. The human immunodeficiency virus (HIV) invades the body's immunological response mechanisms and leads to acquired immunodeficiency syndrome (AIDS). In this case, mortality and morbidity are related to the presence of other diseases that cannot be resisted. Microorganisms can also cause long-term, low-grade infections that can predispose the patient to other diseases. For example, human papillomavirus causes a low-grade (often asymptomatic) infection of the uterine cervix, which increases the rate of cervical cancer. Finally, organisms can act together to cause illness. For example,

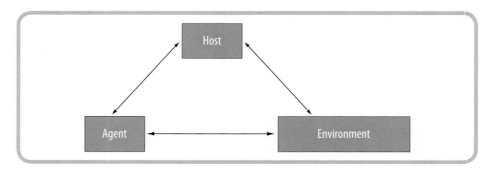

FIG. 11.4   The agent–host–environment triangle model of infectious diseases.
(Redrawn from: Weber & Rutala 2001 p 4, adapted from APIC 1996 p 12)

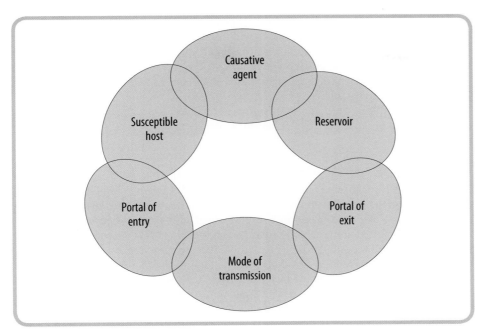

FIG. 11.5 Chain model of infectious diseases.
(Redrawn from: Weber & Rutala 2001 p 4, adapted from APIC 1996 p 18)

TABLE 11.2 Examples of the chain model of infection					
Pathogen	Disease	Portal of exit	Transmission	Portal of entry	Control
Influenza virus	Pneumonia	Respiratory secretions	Airborne	Respiratory tract (inhalation)	Vaccine, use of tissues
Cryptosporidium	Diarrhoea	Stool	Faecal–oral through water or food	Gastrointestinal tract (ingestion)	Separate faecal waste from water supply, filter water supply, pasteurise juice
Neisseria gonorrhoeae	Gonorrhoea	Genital secretions	Sexual	Genital tract	Screening of high-risk and symptomatic persons, followed by treatment

(Source: Weber & Rutala 2001)

the hepatitis viruses D and E have been shown to predispose people to infection by other hepatitis viruses, such as C and B, with more significant pathology.

Any particular pathogen can have a range of effects in any individual, from causing no disease, to mild disease or even severe illness. The extent of the impact of microorganisms on a host/patient is dependent on the organism itself, host factors (e.g. intact skin, immune status) or environmental factors (e.g. favourable moisture and pH conditions). For example, even if an organism has a relatively low pathogenicity, it can still cause severe illness in a host whose defences have been weakened by malnutrition or immunosuppression.

Infectious disease management

Managing infectious diseases in society is reliant on a range of complementary strategies, which together aim to prevent, monitor or treat disease. These strategies include those targeted at disease prevention, those involved with surveillance and early detection, and those aimed at managing disease when it occurs. This approach is equivalent to primary, secondary and tertiary prevention. This text focuses on the public health aspects of disease prevention and not on managing individual patients with disease, which is rightly the domain of medical practitioners. As such, we will focus our discussion on the following three key aspects of managing infectious diseases: disease prevention, through societal and environmental structures, immunisation, vector control, and personal protection; surveillance, early recognition and early intervention; and infection control.

Disease prevention

SOCIETAL AND ENVIRONMENTAL STRUCTURES

Because infectious diseases require close proximity in order to spread, one of the most important ways disease is prevented in developed countries is through the social isolation that results from increased living standards. In our high-income developed countries, we live in small population groups, often nuclear families at most, and in large, or at least separate, well-constructed homes that are often designed to exclude disease vectors (e.g. screens that keep out mosquitoes) and permit easy cleaning of surfaces to reduce person-to-person transmission.

Our societal systems and structures are also designed to minimise the risks of disease transmission. We have laws and regulations to provide access to safe drinking water, clean, safe food, and hygienic waste disposal. A long-established, but now rarely used, social prevention measure is that of quarantine (i.e. compulsory isolation of individuals).

In Australia we also value our personal space. Thus, we tend to maintain social separation, except with intimate contacts. We often travel alone in individual vehicles. We have rules and standards of social conduct which help limit disease transmission. We expect people to cover their noses and mouths when sneezing, not to spit in public, and to wash their hands after toileting. All of these aspects of our social norms contribute to reducing infectious diseases being easily transmitted.

IMMUNISATION

The primary aim of immunisation is to protect the individual who receives the vaccine. Additionally, vaccinated individuals are less likely to be a source of infection for others, thus also reducing the risk to unvaccinated individuals. This means that individuals who cannot be vaccinated will still benefit, and this concept is known as *population immunity* or *herd immunity*. When vaccination coverage is high enough to produce high levels of population immunity, infections can be eliminated from a community. However, if vaccination coverage is not maintained, it is possible for these diseases to return. Consequently, health agencies are extremely concerned with vaccine coverage levels in their community, and encourage the widespread uptake of immunisation through public and professional awareness campaigns and through free access to vaccines (see Box 11.2).

Immunisation is credited with dramatically reducing morbidity and mortality from infectious diseases during the twentieth century. The significant public health success of immunisation in the United States is clearly demonstrated in Table 11.3, and in Australia similar impacts have been seen with deaths from vaccine-preventable disease

---

BOX 11.2

HPV AND GARDASIL®

Human papillomavirus (HPV) is a common sexually transmitted infection, and is so common that nearly all sexually active men and women get it at some point. Most HPV infections occur without any symptoms, and go away without treatment over time. Our immune system is very effective in suppressing or eliminating HPV, but those HPV infections that are persistent can lead to genital warts and a range of cancers, particularly cervical cancer. To prevent infection with HPV, two vaccines are available—Gardasil® and Cervarix®. Gardasil® was developed by Australian researchers Jian Zhou and Ian Frazer, and was released onto the market in 2006. As nearly half a million women develop cervical cancer each year worldwide, and more than a quarter of a million die from it, widespread vaccination has the potential to reduce cervical cancer deaths by as much as two-thirds (National Cancer Institute 2011).

TABLE 11.3 Vaccine-preventable disease data for the United States

Disease	Baseline twentieth-century annual morbidity*	2003 morbidity	% decrease
Smallpox	48 164	0	100
Diphtheria	175 885	1	99.99
Pertussis	147 271	8067	94.52
Tetanus	1314	14	98.93
Poliomyelitis	16 316	0	100
Measles	503 282	42	99.99
Mumps	152 209	194	99.87
Rubella	47 745	8	99.98

(Source: Orenstein et al. 2005)
*These are representative figures; for example, for smallpox, this figure represents the average annual number of cases during 1900–1904, and for diphtheria, this figure represents the average annual number of reported cases during 1920–1922, three years before vaccine development. Also note that the decline in the absolute number of cases occurred despite considerable population growth.

CASE STUDY
11.2   *The internet and immunisation*

With more than 90% of young people in developed countries being regular internet users, and the worldwide web being an important source of health information for laypeople, the potential for the web to play an important role in providing accurate and up-to-date information on immunisation issues is clear. One concern for public health officials is the potential for the internet to be used to spread incorrect and potentially dangerous information on immunisation. The web is used extensively by the anti-vaccination movement to portray highly emotional messages that counter the messages inherent in public health campaigns. In order to help laypeople judge the quality of immunisation information on websites, the WHO has developed criteria for assessing website quality in terms of credibility, content, accessibility and design. These criteria are available at the WHO's Vaccine Safety Net website.

(Source: Amicizia et al. 2013)

ACTIVITY 11.4 Evaluating immunisation information on the internet

- Access the WHO Vaccine Safety Net website (http://www.who.int/vaccine_safety/initiative/communication/network/vaccine_safety_websites/en/index1.html) and review the Essential Criteria for web-based immunisation information.

- Use a search engine (e.g. Google) to do a search of the internet for information on immunisation, using the search terms 'vaccination' and then 'immunisation'.

- Use the WHO's Essential Criteria to review the information presented by the top two sites for each search (i.e. the top two sites for the 'vaccination' search, and then the 'immunisation' search).

- How does the quality of the information on these sites compare with the WHO criteria? How different were the sites retrieved using the search term 'vaccination' versus 'immunisation'?

---

substantially decreasing from 9292 deaths in 1926–1935 to 24 deaths in 1996–2005 (National Centre for Immunisation Research and Surveillance 2010).

Immunity is the ability of the human body to protect itself from infectious disease. Humans can *acquire* immunity through either natural or artificial means. The most common natural means of acquiring immunity is through exposure to the disease, either by contracting the disease personally or by coming into contact with someone who has the disease. In response, the body produces *antibodies* to the *antigens* that are contained in the organisms that produce the disease. Vaccination programs, however, aim to replicate this naturally acquired immunity through artificial means which avoid the risks of the disease itself. Unfortunately, no vaccine offers 100% protection, and so a small proportion of people get infected despite being vaccinated. In addition, any vaccine may cause an adverse event. Even though most vaccines cause minor adverse events such as fever, pain or redness at the site of injection (NHMRC 2013), the devastating impacts of more substantial adverse events for a small number of individuals, mainly young children, and their families should be remembered when considering the overall effectiveness of this public health measure (see Case Study 11.2).

VECTOR CONTROL

Vector-borne transmission of an infectious agent is generally caused by an arthropod (i.e. an insect), either by simple mechanical transfer of microorganisms from the external parts of the vector (e.g. on its legs), or through the vector ingesting and later

> ### CASE STUDY 11.3
>
> ## *Malaria and bed-nets*
>
> A key control measure for malaria is the supply and use of insecticide-treated mosquito nets. These nets are a core element of malaria control, and are distributed free-of-charge to all persons at risk of malaria in 88 countries around the world. The nets are impregnated with an insecticide, and so provide both a physical barrier and an insecticidal effect to reduce mosquito-to-human contact while sleeping. Even though at least 150 million new nets are needed each year to protect all at-risk populations in sub-Saharan Africa, the number of nets distributed and then used has been increasing dramatically. As such, the public health efforts to encourage the use of bed-nets are seen to have been successful, with continued difficulties in supply and distribution the main constraint to widespread use.
>
> *(Source: WHO 2013b)*

expelling the agent, often through penetration of the skin of a susceptible host, as is the case for mosquitoes (Weber & Rutala 2001).

A large range of arthropods is associated with transmitting disease (including cockroaches, ants, flies, biting midges, mosquitoes, fleas, bedbugs, lice, ticks, scabies, fabric pests, and stored product pests), as are rodents. Globally, vectors such as these are responsible for a substantial level of disease, disability and illness, accounting for about 17% of the estimated global burden of infectious diseases (WHO 2004). The most deadly vector-borne disease, malaria, results in over 200 million cases and over 600,000 deaths annually, mostly African children under the age of five (see Case Study 11.3) (WHO 2013b). In addition, dengue fever, together with its associated dengue haemorrhagic fever (DHF), is the world's fastest-growing vector-borne disease. Dengue is of particular concern for northern areas of Australia, which regularly have outbreaks due to the presence in these areas of the dengue mosquito, *Aedes aegypti* (see Case Study 11.4). In other parts of Australia, diseases such as Ross River virus infection and Barmah Forest virus infection are commonly associated with mosquito vectors. The environmental health links with vector-borne diseases are extremely strong (refer to Chapter 12), with poorly designed irrigation and water systems, inadequate housing, poor waste disposal and water storage, deforestation and loss of biodiversity all being contributing factors.

Even though well-planned vector control measures can significantly contribute to reducing the burden of vector-borne diseases, the preventative power of vector control is grossly under-utilised in public health (Townson et al. 2005). Rather than relying on a single method of vector control, the WHO recommends implementing integrated

> ### REFLECTION 11.4
>
> Immunisation is the cornerstone of the control of infectious diseases in our society, yet there remain significant scientific, ethical, social and economic issues that impact on the level of immunisation. For example, in many poor countries people simply cannot afford the vaccines. Further, some people object to vaccines as a form of mass medication, and others believe that vaccines have serious adverse side-effects in some people and do not wish to take the risk. With these factors in mind, reflect on the following questions.
>
> - What do you believe are the barriers for parents in immunising their children?
> - As a population health strategy, how effective is childhood immunisation?
> - As an emerging health professional, what are your views on compulsory immunisation for children prior to entry to daycare and school? Why have you taken that position?
> - How much of a responsibility do we all share for maintaining the 'herd immunity'?

CASE STUDY
11.4

Dengue risk when Australians travel

Dengue is an important cause of illness for Australians returning from overseas travel, particularly in South East Asia. The number of dengue cases reported in Australia has increased substantially in recent years, including an increase in the number of cases known to have been acquired overseas. These imported cases also pose a risk to local Australian communities, due to the potential for transmission of the virus from these cases to their neighbours in areas where the *Aedes aegypti* mosquito—the vector for the disease—is known to exist. Therefore, with the increased popularity of South East Asia as a travel destination, travellers to these areas need to take precautions to avoid being bitten by mosquitoes. These include ensuring that their sleeping areas are free of mosquitoes by closing window screens, using insecticide sprays and bed-nets, and wearing insect repellent and long-sleeved clothing to minimise skin exposure to day-biting mosquitoes.

(Source: Knope et al. 2013)

vector management (IVM), which stresses the importance of first understanding the local vector ecology and local patterns of disease transmission, then choosing the appropriate vector control tools from the range of options available (WHO 2004). In Australia, most of the vector control activities are carried out by local governments in consultation with state health and environmental agencies.

PERSONAL PROTECTION

Actions can also be taken to protect individuals on a personal level. These include:

- encouraging behaviours that ensure safe practices, such as handwashing and covering your mouth when coughing
- encouraging 'safe sex' to reduce disease transmission, particularly sexually transmitted diseases, including HIV/AIDS
- encouraging the safe use of clean needles for drug addicts to reduce risks associated with cross-infection from dirty needles
- encouraging the use of personal protective barriers—for example, condoms for safe sex, and mosquito netting
- encouraging and supporting the use of prophylactic medication in circumstances where exposure is possible—for example, malaria prophylaxis for travellers to malaria-prone areas
- actively managing secondary (post-exposure) prophylaxis—for example, in the event of needlestick injuries to health workers.

Surveillance, early recognition and early intervention

We also ensure that systems and structures are in place to screen for the presence of disease and to investigate and manage outbreaks. Early warning functions are fundamental for national, regional and global health security. Outbreaks, such as the severe acute respiratory syndrome (SARS) and avian influenza, and potential threats from biological and chemical agents, demonstrate the importance of effective national surveillance and response systems (WHO 2006). There are a range of sources of public health surveillance, including vital statistics (e.g. birth and death certificates), sentinel surveillance/early warning systems for key health indicators, and registries such as those maintained for cancer and birth defects (Stroup et al. 1994). Public health officials also maintain a system of compulsory reporting of particular infectious diseases to facilitate early recognition and intervention. In Australia, surveillance of infectious disease is through the *National Notifiable Diseases Surveillance System* (NNDSS) (NNDSS Annual Report Writing Group 2013). Diseases are reported by diagnostic laboratories or by clinicians to state health agencies, who then forward the information to the NNDSS. The reports are made to state health agencies so that immediate outbreak investigation, contact tracing and public health interventions can occur. Part of this response is analysing the incoming data. The basic analytic approaches used in surveillance systems involve describing and analysing data in terms of:

- *time*—patterns of disease incidence, which may generate hypotheses, or may reflect patterns in reporting
- *place*—geographical distribution of disease or of its causative exposures or risk-associated behaviour
- *person*—characteristics of people or groups who develop disease or sustain injury, which helps in understanding the risk factors for disease or injury, and targeting interventions.

The most common method of displaying the results of such analysis is with frequencies (counts) of the health problem in simple tables and graphs. Rates and frequencies are also useful for comparing the occurrence of disease for different geographical areas or periods, because they take into account the size of the population from which the cases arose (CDC 2006). (Refer to Chapter 5 for further details on the use of epidemiological methods for disease surveillance and control.)

Infection control

The third level of management is considered to be tertiary prevention, and involves attention to infection control in environments of special risk, such as health facilities or services, and the appropriate management of infected patients. Infection control describes the systems, behaviours and structures that are designed to break the transmission of microorganisms from infected patients to unaffected people (see Box 11.3).

Infection control practice is an evolving discipline and, by the mid-1980s, the HIV/AIDS epidemic created an urgent need for new strategies to protect healthcare workers from blood-borne infections. Therefore, health authorities adopted a new approach in which all blood and body substances were to be considered potentially infectious, and introduced the principle of *standard precautions*. This level of care was applied to all people, regardless of their perceived or confirmed infectious status, as a strategy for minimising healthcare-associated infections in both asymptomatic and symptomatic people. The scope of this approach has evolved to our current multi-tier approach to infection control that consists primarily of standard precautions and *transmission-based precautions* (NHMRC 2010).

Standard precautions include handwashing between tending to different patients, wearing appropriate clothing to reduce cross-infection, wearing gloves where necessary, and wearing masks to reduce respiratory transmission. Transmission-based precautions are recommended for patients known or suspected to be infected with a pathogen that may not be contained by standard precautions alone. They include the highest standard of respiratory protection, isolation and barrier nursing, and care in a positive-pressure environment with closed-circuit air control.

BOX 11.3

TATTOOS AND BODY-PIERCING

Even though the infection control principles and practices have been developed for use in hospitals, there is a range of activities undertaken in non-medical settings that present the potential to transmit infectious diseases. Such activities include hairdressing, body-piercing, tattooing, hair replacements/implants, and permanent makeup. Therefore, appropriate infection control practices are equally important for these activities.

Tattooing and body-piercing are a worldwide fashion craze; however, this craze has also coincided with the emergence of blood-borne viral diseases such as hepatitis B and C, and HIV/AIDS. With the prevalence of tattooing and body-piercing being considerably higher among injecting drug users and youth, there is a high potential for transmitting blood-borne viral diseases (Makkai & McAllister 2001).

Surprisingly, there appears to be a very low medical complication rate with tattoos, with only sporadic reports of the transmission of blood-borne viruses. However, plastic surgeons report that much of the tattoo-related medical issues they encounter are concerned with treating patients who are dissatisfied with their tattoos. In contrast, there is strong evidence for a range of health-related complications from body-piercing. These range in severity from simple infections around the piercing site to the more serious systemic infections. There are also complications that occur in some specific piercings, such as chipped teeth, aspiration of the device, and speech impediments for oral piercings. In extreme cases, for oral piercing there may be permanent scarring that can cause problems with eating or drinking (Parliament of South Australia 2005).

ACTIVITY 11.5 Tattoos and body-piercing

- Do you or any friends have either a tattoo or a body-piercing? When deciding on getting a tattoo or piercing, did you (or your friends) consider the associated infection risks? If so, what sort of information was available to help with decision-making, and was the tattooist or body-piercer able to supply information on the risks? Finally, what sort of post-procedure care instructions were given in order to minimise infection?

Outbreak investigation and contact tracing

The public health strategies implemented to investigate a disease outbreak are an essential part of infectious disease management. These strategies involve:

- *identifying the disease and the causative agent*—this requires specimens from the infected patient(s) and the collection and testing of specimens for any possible or likely causes; for example, during an outbreak of a food-borne illness, specimens from food sources, food-handlers, and environmental contaminants may assist with tracking the cause
- *investigating the circumstances of the infection*—this may involve taking a detailed history of exposure and contacts

- *identifying and testing others who may have been the source of the infection*
- *identifying others who may be at risk* from similar exposure, and who may knowingly or unwittingly be a source of further transmission
- *timely implementation of appropriate control measures* to minimise further illness.

The choice and type of control measure should be guided by the results of the epidemiological and environmental investigations. However, any delay in implementing control measures may expose the public to unacceptable risks, and so sometimes controls are implemented based on limited information. Control measures for food-related outbreaks, for example, include food recalls, restaurant closures, excluding food-handlers, decommissioning food-processing equipment, and revising maintenance and operating procedures. The selection criteria for the most appropriate measures for the situation are based on their effectiveness for interrupting transmission, as well as their ease of implementation, expense and safety (see Case Study 11.5).

> ## REFLECTION 11.5
>
> It is clear that the infection risks for body-piercings are substantial—the procedure creates a wound and the body often rejects the foreign material inserted in the pierced area. Accordingly, infection control focuses on: appropriately trained and licensed operators; using sterile instruments and appropriate piercing techniques; and suitable post-procedure care.

Barriers to effectively managing infectious diseases

Despite the wide range of control measures available, there are many barriers to effective disease control (see Box 11.4). These generally relate to the failure of systems

---

CASE STUDY 11.5

Outbreak investigation

In June 2009, an outbreak of gastroenteritis occurred among participants of a car rally in the Northern Territory. The rally is an annual fund-raising event in which participants drive over 5000 km across the outback. This outbreak investigation was challenging, because there were a large number of participants (over 350) from all over Australia, and it commenced once the rally was completed. To make it easy for participants to respond, an online survey using SurveyMonkey was undertaken. Stool samples were also collected from five participants, and *Salmonella litchfield*—a reasonably common serotype of *Salmonella* in the Northern Territory—was found. This serotype, however, is not commonly found in other parts of Australia.

A total of 76 cases were identified, with the consumption of barramundi fillets at a dinner being the only food item showing an association with illness. Given the incubation period for *S. litchfield*, consumption of this food item was consistent with it being the cause of the illness. In addition, *S. litchfield* is known to be regularly isolated from barramundi. Unfortunately, the food safety practices of the caterers were not able to be assessed, but, given the nature of the rally, it is conceivable that they would have been working under quite unusual and difficult conditions. Overall, this outbreak highlights the difficulties that can be faced by investigators, and shows the importance of using online methods for data collection.

(Source: Wallace et al. 2010)

BOX 11.4

THE ONGOING CHALLENGE

While many in the developed world perceive that infectious diseases have been largely controlled, this chapter has illustrated the impact that infectious diseases still have throughout the world, and particularly in low-income countries. The following are ongoing challenges:

- *Tuberculosis* (TB) continues to cause more than 1 million deaths each year, principally in poorly nourished, poor and overcrowded communities, and the emergence of multiple-drug-resistant TB is challenging our capacity to prevent or treat infection.

- *Antibiotic-resistant organisms* are of significant concern to hospitals around the world, as they expose vulnerable people (often with surgical implants or undergoing surgical procedures) to infection with an agent that is largely untreatable.

- *Malaria* continues to cause over 600,000 deaths per year in countries where public health strategies for vector control, personal protection and prophylactic agents are unavailable because of poverty or social disruption.

- The ability of the common *influenza* virus to mutate has seen the emergence of both 'bird flu' (H5N1) and 'swine flu' (H1N1) in recent years. This potentially presents the highest risk of any organism for a major pandemic.

- *HIV*, which causes AIDS, is now the most common cause of death by infectious disease, causing 1.5 million deaths per year (WHO 2015b), with sub-Saharan Africa severely affected, with nearly 1 in every 20 adults living with HIV and accounting for nearly 71% of the people living with HIV worldwide (WHO 2015a). Vaccines remain ineffective, and personal protective strategies, such as safe sexual practices, are the only effective preventative measures.

- The outbreaks of novel diseases such as *SARS* and *Ebola* threaten widespread epidemics. SARS (severe acute respiratory syndrome), for example, spread rapidly to five continents and caused over 800 deaths. The outbreak had immeasurable economic and social impact before it was brought under control through public health controls. It led to enhanced international precautions and preparedness (Wong & Yuen 2005). Ebola first appeared in Africa in 1976, and there have been many outbreaks over the years since, with the largest outbreak occurring in 2014. Ebola is a severe illness that has a very high case fatality rate (up to 90%). The Ebola virus is transmitted to people from close contact with the body fluids of wild animals, and then spreads through the human population through human-to-human contact with the body fluids of infected people. Healthcare workers are particularly at risk of infection, and there is no specific vaccine or treatment available, although there are promising vaccine trials underway. Therefore, control measures rely on effective public health education and infection control (WHO 2014b).

and structures, which in turn relate to general societal problems. Some examples include:

- poverty and its associated failure of infrastructure, education and awareness, and resources
- community ignorance associated with poor education standards
- ideological views—in some circumstances individuals or communities hold ideological views that are contrary to known infectious disease management strategies; for example, some individuals believe on religious or personal grounds that vaccination is 'unnatural', whereas others believe that vaccines sourced from Western countries are an attempt to subjugate the people of developing nations
- failure of communication either about the importance and value of prevention strategies or about the particular circumstances and risks—this failure may simply reflect poverty and associated poor educational standards, or it may be due to the impediments associated with conflict whereby communities are deliberately deprived of information for the purposes of exercising political control
- lack of infrastructure related either to poverty or to the failure of appropriate investment in necessary systems and structures required to deliver on the public health measures
- lack of resources such as equipment, personnel or consumables.

A final word

This chapter has covered a wide range of issues related to the development, prevention, management and care of chronic and infectious diseases. We have defined both chronic and infectious diseases, and discussed models and mechanisms for disease development. We have also examined various approaches for managing and preventing disease, as well as outlining the importance of public health throughout the continuum of care for both chronic and infectious diseases.

REVIEW QUESTIONS

1   How would you define a 'chronic disease'?

2   What is an 'infectious disease'? Is this definition different to the definition of a 'communicable disease'? What is a 'zoonotic disease'?

3   How is chronic disease managed at state/territory and federal government levels?

4   The Australian Government's National Chronic Disease Strategy concentrates on four key areas for improving outcomes. In a table, identify the four key areas, and describe the contribution of each to the prevention and management of chronic disease.

5   What is the range of ways in which microorganisms can cause disease?

6   What protective mechanisms does the body use to prevent infection?

7   How might we prevent and/or manage infectious diseases?

8   What are the major strategies you would use to manage a disease outbreak?

Useful websites

- Australian Government Department of Health: http://www.health.gov.au/internet/main/publishing.nsf/Content/chronic-diabetes#pro
- Blue Book—Guidelines for the control of infectious diseases (Department of Human Services, Victoria): http://ideas.health.vic.gov.au/bluebook.asp
- Centers for Disease Control and Prevention: http://www.cdc.gov
- Centre for Healthcare Related Infection Surveillance and Prevention (CHRISP): http://www.health.qld.gov.au/chrisp
- Flinders University, Faculty of Medicine. The Flinders Program (2014): https://www.flinders.edu.au/medicine/sites/fhbhru/self-management.cfm
- Health Protection and Surveillance Branch, Department of Health (Australia): http://www.health.gov.au/internet/main/publishing.nsf/Content/cda-about.htm
- Immunise Australia Program: http://www.immunise.health.gov.au
- WHO Global Alert and Response: http://www.who.int/csr/en/

References

Amicizia, D., Domnich, A., Gasparini, R., et al., 2013. An overview of current and potential use of information and communication technologies for immunization promotion among adolescents. Human Vaccines and Immunotherapeutics 9 (12), 2634–2642.

Association for Professionals in Infection Control and Epidemiology (APIC), 1996. Infection Control and Applied Epidemiology: Principles and Practice. Mosby, St. Louis.

Australian Institute of Health and Welfare, 2002. Chronic diseases and associated risk factors in Australia, 2001. Online. Available: <http://www.aihw.gov.au/publication-detail/?id=6442467343> (1 May 2014).

Australian Institute of Health and Welfare, 2010. Australia's Health 2010. AIHW Cat. No. AUS 122. AIHW, Canberra.

Australian Institute of Health and Welfare, 2012a. Chronic diseases and associated risk factors in Australia, 2012. Online. Available: <http://www.aihw.gov.au/WorkArea/DownloadAsset.aspx?id=10737422169> (30 Apr 2014).

Australian Institute of Health and Welfare, 2012b. Australia's Health 2012. AIHW Cat. No. AUS 156. AIHW, Canberra.

Centers for Disease Control and Prevention, 2006. Principles of Epidemiology in Public Health Practice, third ed. Self-Study Course SS1000, CDC, Atlanta.

Centers for Disease Control and Prevention, 2013. National Center for Chronic Disease Prevention and Health Promotion (NCCDPHP). Department of Health and Human Services, Atlanta. Online. Available: <http://www.cdc.gov/chronicdisease/about/> (30 Apr 2014).

Department of Health, 2005. National evaluation of the Sharing Health Care Initiative demonstration projects. Online. Available: <http://www.health.gov.au/internet/main/publishing.nsf/Content/chronicdisease-nateval> (6 May 2014).

Department of Health, 2012. Chronic disease. Online. Available: <http://www.health.gov.au/internet/main/publishing.nsf/Content/chronic> (30 Apr 2014).

Department of Health, 2014. Chronic Disease Management (formerly Enhanced Primary Care or EPC)—GP services. Online. Available: <http://www.health.gov.au/internet/main/publishing.nsf/Content/mbsprimarycare-chronicdiseasemanagement> (6 May 2014).

Flinders Human Behaviour and Health Research Unit, 2009. Capabilities for supporting prevention and chronic condition self-management: a resource for educators of primary health care professionals. Online. Available: <http://www.gpscbc.ca/system/files/Capabilities%20Self-Management%20Resource.pdf> (30 Apr 2014).

Flinders Human Behaviour and Health Research Unit, 2014. Flinders University, Adelaide. Online. Available: <https://www.flinders.edu.au/medicine/sites/fhbhru/> (30 Apr 2014).

Flinders University, Faculty of Medicine. The Flinders Program, 2014. Online. Available: <https://www.flinders.edu.au/medicine/sites/fhbhru/self-management.cfm> (29 Apr 2014).

Guinovart, C., Navia, N.M., Tanner, M., et al., 2006. Malaria: burden of disease. Current Molecular Medicine 6 (2), 137–140.

Hurster, M.M., 1997. Communicable and Non-Communicable Disease Basics: a Primer. Bergin and Garvey, Westport.

International Association for the Study of Obesity, 2014. The Prevention of Obesity and NCDs: Challenges and Opportunities for Governments. IASO Policy Briefing January 2014. International Association for the Study of Obesity, London.

Kesteloot, K., 1999. Disease management: a new technology in need of critical assessment. International Journal of Technology Assessment in Health Care 15 (3), 506–519.

Knope, K., National Arbovirus and Malaria Advisory Committee, Giele, C., 2013. Increasing notifications of dengue in Australia related to overseas travel, 1991 to 2012. Communicable Diseases Intelligence 37 (1), E55–E59.

Lorig, K., Sobel, D., Ritter, P., et al., 2001. Effect of a self-management program on patients with chronic disease. Effective Clinical Practice (Nov./Dec.). Online. Available: <http://www.acponline.org/journals/ecp/novdec01/lorig.htm> (1 May 2014).

Lozano, R., Naghavi, M., Foreman, K., et al., 2012. Global and regional mortality from 235 causes of death for 20 age groups in 1990 and 2010: a systematic analysis for the Global Burden of Disease Study 2010. Lancet 380 (9859), 2095–2128.

Makkai, T., McAllister, I., 2001. Prevalence of tattooing and body piercing in the Australian community. Communicable Diseases Intelligence 25 (2), 67–72.

Mathers, C., Vos, T., Stevenson, C., 1999. The Burden of Disease and Injury in Australia. AIHW Cat. No. PHE 17. Australian Institute of Health and Welfare, Canberra.

National Cancer Institute, 2011. Human papillomavirus (HPV) vaccines—fact sheet. Online. Available: <http://www.cancer.gov/cancertopics/factsheet/prevention/HPV-vaccine/> (16 Aug 2014).

National Centre for Immunisation Research and Surveillance, 2010. Vaccine preventable diseases in Australia, 2005 to 2007. Communicable Diseases Intelligence 34 (Suppl.), S1–S167.

National Health and Medical Research Council, 2001. Tackling Chronic Disease: Exploration of Key Research Dimensions, Synopsis of Workshop, 5–6 July, 2001. NHMRC and Commonwealth Department of Health and Aged Care, Canberra.

National Health and Medical Research Council, 2010. Australian Guidelines for the Prevention and Control of Infection in Healthcare. NHMRC, Canberra.

National Health and Medical Research Council, 2013. The Australian Immunisation Handbook, tenth ed. NHMRC, Canberra.

National Health Priority Action Council, 2006. National Chronic Disease Strategy. Australian Government Department of Health and Ageing, Canberra. Online. Available: <http://www.health.gov.au/internet/main/publishing.nsf/Content/pq-ncds> (2 May 2014).

National Notifiable Diseases Surveillance System Annual Report Writing Group, 2013. Australia's notifiable disease status, 2011: annual report of the National Notifiable Diseases Surveillance System. Online. Available: <www.health.gov.au/internet/main/publishing.nsf/Content/cda-surveil-nndss-2011-annual-report.htm> (31 Mar 2014).

National Preventative Health Taskforce, 2008. Australia: the healthiest country by 2020. A discussion paper. Online. Available: <http://www.health.gov.au/internet/main/publishing.nsf/Content/cda-cdi3704b.htm> (2 May 2014).

National Public Health Partnership, 2001. Preventing chronic disease: a strategic framework background paper. Online. Available: <http://www.nphp.gov.au/publications/strategies/chrondis-bgpaper.pdf> (1 May 2014).

Orenstein, W.A., Wharton, M., Bart, K.J., et al., 2005. Immunization. In: Mandell, G.L., Bennett, J.E.Dolin, R. (Eds.), Principles and Practice of Infectious Diseases, sixth ed. Elsevier Churchill Livingstone, Philadelphia, pp. 3557–3589.

Parliament of South Australia, 2005. Report of the Select Committee on the Tattooing and Body Piercing Industries PP228. Parliament of South Australia, Adelaide.

Pruitt, S., Epping-Jordan, J., 2005. Preparing the 21st century global healthcare workforce. BMJ 330, 637–639.

Stroup, N.E., Zack, M.M., Wharton, M., 1994. Sources of routinely collected data for surveillance. In: Teutsch, S.M., Churchill, R.E. (Eds.), Principles and Practice of Public Health Surveillance. Oxford University Press, New York, pp. 31–85.

Townson, H., Nathan, M.B., Zaim, M., et al., 2005. Exploiting the potential of vector control for disease prevention. Bulletin of the World Health Organization 83 (12), 942–947.

Tucker, J.B., 2001. Scourge: The Once and Future Threat of Smallpox. Grove Press, New York.

Velasco-Garrido, M., Busse, R., Hisashige, A., 2003. Are Disease Management Programmes (DMPs) Effective in Improving Quality of Care for People with Chronic Conditions? WHO Regional Office for Europe (Health Evidence Network report), Copenhagen. Online. Available: <http://www.euro.who.int/document/e82974.pdf> (1 May 2014).

Wallace, P., Kirk, M.D., Munnoch, S.A., et al., 2010. An outbreak of *Salmonella litchfield* on a car rally, Northern Territory, 2009. Communicable Diseases Intelligence 34 (2), 124–126.

Weber, D.J., Rutala, W.A., 2001. Biological basis of infectious disease epidemiology. In: Thomas, J.C., Weber, D.J. (Eds.), Epidemiologic Methods for the Study of Infectious Diseases. Oxford University Press, New York, pp. 3–27.

Weeramanthri, T., Hendy, S., Connors, C., et al., 2003. The Northern Territory Preventable Chronic Disease Strategy—promoting an integrated and life course approach to chronic disease in Australia. Australian Health Review 26, 31–42.

Wong, S., Yuen, K., 2005. The severe acute respiratory syndrome (SARS). Journal of Neurovirology 11, 455–465.

World Health Organization, 1999. Removing Obstacles to Healthy Development. WHO, Geneva.

World Health Organization, 2004. Global Strategic Framework for Integrated Vector Management. WHO, Geneva.

World Health Organization, 2005a. Combating Emerging Infectious Diseases. WHO South East Asia. WHO, New Delhi.

World Health Organization, 2005b. Preparing a Workforce for the 21st Century: The Challenge of Chronic Conditions. WHO, Geneva.

World Health Organization, 2005c. Preventing Chronic Diseases—A Vital Investment: WHO Global Report. WHO, Geneva. Online. Available: <http://www.who.int/chp/chronic_disease_report/full_report.pdf> (10 Apr 2014).

World Health Organization, 2006. Communicable Disease Surveillance and Response Systems: Guide to Monitoring and Evaluating WHO/CDS/EPR/LYO/2006.2. WHO, Geneva.

World Health Organization, 2009. Global Health Risks: Mortality and Burden of Disease Attributable to Selected Major Risks. WHO, Geneva.

World Health Organisation, 2012. World Health Statistics 2012. WHO, Geneva.

World Health Organisation, 2013a. Global Action Plan for the Prevention and Control of NCDs 2013–2020. WHO, Geneva.

World Health Organization, 2013b. World Malaria Report 2013. WHO Global Malaria Programme, WHO, Geneva. Online. Available: <http://www.who.int/malaria/publications/world_malaria_report_2013/en/>.

World Health Organization, 2014a. World Health Statistics. WHO, Geneva.

World Health Organization, 2014b. Ebola virus disease. Fact Sheet No. 103. Updated September 2014. Online. Available: <http://www.who.int/mediacentre/factsheets/fs103/en/> (3 Nov 2014).

World Health Organization, 2015a. Global health observatory data. Online. Available: <http://www.who.int/gho/hiv/en/> (22 Apr 2015).

World Health Organization, 2015b. The top 10 causes of death. Online. Available: <http://www.who.int/mediacentre/factsheets/fs310/en/> (21 Apr 2015).

CHAPTER 12

Environmental health

Thomas Tenkate

Learning objectives

After reading this chapter, you should be able to:

- describe environmental health, and how human health can be protected from environmental hazards

- identify key environmental health issues, and how they are managed

- understand the importance of managing our environment in a sustainable manner so as to protect human health.

Introduction

Our understanding of how the environment can impact on human health has evolved and expanded over the centuries, with concern and interest dating back to ancient times. For example, over 4000 years ago a civilisation in northern India tried to protect the health of its citizens by constructing and positioning buildings according to strict building laws, having bathrooms and drains, and having paved streets with a sewerage system (Rosen 1993).

In more recent times, the Industrial Revolution played a key role in shaping the modern world, and with it the modern public health system. This era was marked by rapid progress in technology, the growth of transportation, and the expansion of the market economy, which led to the organisation of industry into a factory system. This meant that labour had to be brought to the factories, and by the 1820s poverty and social distress (e.g. overcrowding, and infrequent sewage and garbage disposal) was more widespread than ever. These circumstances led to the rise of the 'sanitary revolution' and the birth of modern public health (Rosen 1993).

This chapter will define 'environmental health', and discuss a number of significant environmental health issues and how they are managed.

What is 'environmental health'?

Many people think that 'environmental health' refers to the health of the environment. This view conjures images of wilderness, rivers and oceans, and is a term that is synonymous with environmental protection. For others, environmental health is recognised as human health issues associated with poor living conditions, contaminated water and vermin infestation, all 'old' battles that were fought—and generally won—over the past century. Unfortunately, both views are not entirely correct (however, the second view could be considered the 'old' view of environmental health). The easiest way to describe environmental health is to say that it is 'concerned with creating and maintaining environments which promote good public health' (enHealth Council 1999 p 1). *Environmental health* therefore is an integral component of the broad field of *public health*, but also has some overlap with the field of *environmental protection*. The relationship between these areas is shown in Figure 12.1.

Environmental health hazards

There is a range of environmental threats/hazards that affect human health, and these can either *result from human activity* in the environment (e.g. nitrogen oxides and particulates that come from fossil fuel combustion and can result in air pollution) or are *independent of human activity* (e.g. radon, ultraviolet radiation, disease-carrying mosquitoes); however, many of these so-called independent hazards are exacerbated by human activity. These threats can be further divided into traditional hazards and modern hazards. *Traditional hazards* are often associated with poverty and a lack of development, and include:

- lack of access to safe drinking water
- inadequate basic sanitation in the household and the community
- contamination of food with pathogens

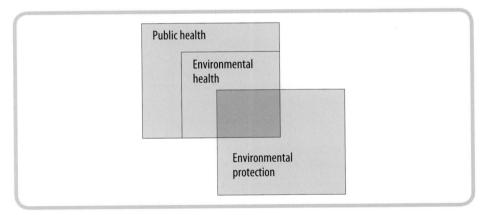

FIG. 12.1   Relationships between the fields of public health, environmental health and environmental protection.
(Adapted from: Environmental Health Standing Committee 1999, used by permission of the Australian Government)

- indoor air pollution from cooking and heating using coal or biomass fuel
- inadequate solid waste disposal
- occupational injury hazards in agriculture and cottage industries
- natural disasters, including floods, droughts and earthquakes
- disease vectors, mainly insects and rodents (World Health Organization (WHO) 1997).

Modern hazards are related to any rapid development that lacks health and environment safeguards, and also to the unsustainable consumption of natural resources. These include:

- water pollution from populated areas, industry and intensive agriculture
- urban air pollution from motor vehicles, coal power stations and industry
- accumulation of solid and hazardous waste
- chemical and radiation hazards following the introduction of industrial and agricultural technologies
- emerging and re-emerging infectious diseases
- deforestation, land degradation and other major ecological change at local and regional levels
- climate change, stratospheric ozone depletion, and trans-boundary pollution (WHO 1997).

One of the main differences between traditional and modern hazards is that the adverse health outcomes from traditional hazards often occur quickly, whereas modern hazards often have a long latency period before the adverse health effect is realised. This means that a range of management approaches is required to adequately address such a variety of issues.

An important concept associated with managing the risks posed by these hazards is *risk transition*. This term is used to describe the reduction in risk from traditional hazards and the increase in risk from modern hazards that take place with advances in economic development. However, when environmental health risks are poorly managed, both traditional and modern hazards threaten the health of the community; whereas when environmental health risks are well managed, the traditional hazards can be almost completely eliminated and the modern hazards can be reduced through effective prevention programs (WHO 1997).

Despite the wide range of potential environmental health hazards, the following are considered to be the basic requirements for a healthy environment: clean air; safe and sufficient water; adequate and safe food; safe and peaceful settlements; safe workplaces; and a stable global environment. Each of these environmental health issues, and some of their current management approaches, will now be discussed.

Air pollution

Air pollution is 'the result of emission into the air of hazardous substances at a rate that exceeds the capacity of natural processes in the atmosphere (e.g. rain and wind) to convert, deposit or dilute them' (Yassi et al. 2001 p 180). Air pollution can have the following effects:

- *human health effects*—acute respiratory illness, aggravation of pre-existing illnesses (e.g. cardiac or respiratory conditions, asthma), cancers (triggered by pollutants), eye or nose irritation, stress or loss of general wellbeing
- *loss of amenity*—odour, poor visibility, dust and residue deposits on surfaces (e.g. clothes, vehicles)

CASE STUDY
12.1

China's Huai River policy

Air quality in China is notoriously poor, with an inadvertent 'natural experiment' illustrating the health effects of coal-burning on human health. In the period 1950 to 1980, the Huai River policy provided free coal for heating to cities north of the Huai River, but did not provide free coal to cities south of the river. The use of coal for heating results in the release of a number of air pollutants, particularly particulates. A recent analysis of health and environmental data has shown that airborne concentrations of particulates in cities north of the Huai River were 55% higher than those south of the river, with this linked to northern residents suffering the loss of a staggering 2.5 billion life-years during the 1990s and having a reduction in life expectancy of 5.5 years compared with residents in the south (Chen et al. 2013).

- *damage to property*—acidic pollutants, deposition of soot and particles
- *effect on the environment*—death or injury to sensitive species, loss of biological diversity, excess nutrient loads in waterways, loss of specific ecosystems, acid rain
- *economic impact*—reduced property values, deterrent to new industries or residents, reduced crop production, loss of tourism, loss of productivity due to illness.

From an environmental health perspective, we are mainly interested in the human health effects of air pollution. The WHO estimates that nearly 4 million people die prematurely each year from indoor and outdoor air pollution (WHO 2014a), with many more people suffering from disabling or restrictive health conditions (e.g. asthma and other respiratory conditions). Of particular concern is the widespread use of biomass fuels and coal by over half of the world's population (see Case Study 12.1). These fuels are used for cooking and heating in homes across the developing world, and produce substantial quantities of particulate air pollution that are often trapped within the homes due to poor ventilation. This causes over 4 million deaths a year from indoor air pollution-related illnesses (WHO 2014b). In contrast, developed countries are more concerned about outdoor air pollution. For Australia, it is estimated that outdoor air pollution is responsible for around 3000 deaths each year (roughly 2.3% of all deaths); costing New South Wales alone around $4.7 billion a year in health costs (NSW Department of Environment and Conservation, 2005) (see Case Study 12.2).

Air quality in Australia is managed by all levels of government. At the national level, there are uniform air quality standards under the *National Environment Protection Measure for Ambient Air Quality* (Air NEPM). This sets goals for six pollutants (carbon monoxide, nitrogen dioxide, ozone, sulphur dioxide, lead and particles) and their long-term management. The Commonwealth government also has other programs that directly address air pollution, and these include motor vehicle emissions standards and national fuel quality standards.

At a state level, air pollution is mainly regulated through environmental protection legislation, which generally adopts or refers to the Air NEPM. At a local level, many councils protect air quality by: banning backyard burning/incinerators and requiring developers to minimise burning of land for clearing; effective town planning to keep

CASE STUDY
12.2   *Benefits of the US Clean Air Act*

In 1970 the United States introduced the *Clean Air Act*. This set standards for specific air pollutants (in a similar way to the Australian Air National Environment Protection Measure (NEPM)) and provided a range of programs for protecting public health and the environment. In 2011 the US Environmental Protection Agency (EPA) released a report describing the health and economic benefits of amendments made to the *Clean Air Act* in 1990. The improved standards of the *Clean Air Act* were attributed to have prevented more than 160,000 premature deaths, 130,000 heart attacks, and millions of cases of respiratory problems in one year (2010) alone. It was further estimated that the economic benefits of the air pollution reduction programs exceeded the costs by a factor of more than 30 to 1 (as a central estimate), with the high estimate showing benefits outweighing costs by more than 90 to 1 (US EPA, 2011).

ACTIVITY 12.1 Air quality

In Australia, air quality is monitored in each state and reported against the standards in the Air NEPM. Access the following websites, and compare the current air quality of our capital cities:

- Adelaide: http://www.epa.sa.gov.au/ environmental_info/air_quality/ current_air_quality
- Brisbane: http://www.ehp.qld.gov.au/air/data/ search.php
- Melbourne: http://www.epa.vic.gov.au/air/ bulletins/aqbhour.asp
- Perth: http://www.der.wa.gov.au/your -environment/air
- Sydney: http://www.environment.nsw.gov.au/ aqms/dailydata.htm

industry separate from residential areas, with appropriate areas of vegetation buffer zones; and encouraging public transport and bicycle use to reduce the use of private cars.

Safe water

The importance of water quality and sanitation for public health has been summarised by a former Director General of the WHO, Dr Lee Jong-wook:

> Water and sanitation is one of the primary drivers of public health. I often refer to it as 'Health 101', which means that once we can secure access to clean water and to adequate sanitation facilities for all people, irrespective of the difference in their living conditions, a huge battle against all kinds of diseases will be won. (WHO 2004)

As a resource, water is our most important. However, despite the large amount of water that makes up our planet, only a small amount is suitable and available for drinking. For example, only 2.5% of water is freshwater, and of this only 0.5% is accessible for drinking because the rest of it is frozen in glaciers or the polar ice caps, or is unavailable in the soil (National Health and Medical Research Council (NHMRC) 2004).

For Australia, water is a particularly fragile resource. We are one of the driest continents, and are highly dependent on rainfall to supply our drinking water. However, our rainfall is extremely variable from year to year and season to season. In Australia, agriculture is by far the biggest user of water (approximately 50%), while households use about 12% of the total water supply (Australian Bureau of Statistics (ABS) 2010). Despite all of the water supplied to homes being of a drinkable quality, only 1% is used

BOX 12.1

THE GLOBAL WATER CRISIS

The 2006 *Human Development Report* from the *United Nations Development Programme* (UNDP) focused on the 'global water crisis'. It identified access to water as a basic human need and a fundamental human right; however, more than 1 billion people are denied access to clean water, and 2.6 billion people access to adequate sanitation. The gulf between rich and poor countries also exacerbates the 'global water crisis', and is illustrated in the following statements: 'while basic needs vary, the minimum threshold is about 20 litres a day. Most of the 1.1 billion people categorised as lacking access to clean water use about five litres a day—one-tenth of the average daily amount used in rich countries to flush toilets'; and 'dripping taps in rich countries lose more water than is available each day to more than 1 billion people' (UNDP 2006).

for drinking. The rest is used on the garden, for cooking, washing clothes, showering and flushing the toilet. Thankfully, water consumption has decreased substantially over the past decade, with some users such as agriculture cutting their usage by over 50%, and households reducing usage by about 25% (ABS 2010). Clearly, sustainable water usage should be an ongoing priority for governments, industry and consumers alike (see Box 12.1).

Water can be contaminated with pathogenic microorganisms and a range of chemicals and other substances (see Case Study 12.3). Water provides the vehicle for spreading a range of infectious diseases, and these can be classified as follows:

- *Water-borne diseases*—Occur from water being contaminated by human/animal faeces or urine that is infected by pathogenic viruses or bacteria. They are directly transmitted when water is consumed or used in preparing food (e.g. cholera, typhoid).
- *Water-washed diseases*—A lack of access to safe water supplies leads to infrequent washing or inadequate personal hygiene, which then results in disease/illness (e.g. diarrhoeal diseases, eye infections).
- *Water-based diseases*—Water provides the habitat for the intermediate stages of the lifecycle of particular pathogens (e.g. the genus *Schistosoma*, worms carried by snails living in the water, which cause schistosomiasis).
- *Water-related diseases*—Water provides the habitat for vectors of disease (e.g. mosquito breeding, leading to malaria and dengue fever).
- *Water-dispersed infections*—Infections can proliferate in water and enter the body through the respiratory tract (e.g. *Legionella* spp.) (WHO 1992).

Water quality is managed in Australia under a framework established by the National Water Quality Management Strategy (NWQMS). Its objective is the sustainable use of water resources by protecting and enhancing water quality while maintaining economic and social development. Although managing water resources is a state and territorial government responsibility, the NWQMS emphasises the important role of the community in setting and achieving water quality objectives and developing

CASE STUDY 12.3

Chemical contamination of drinking water

Groundwater contamination by arsenic is a global health problem of enormous significance. Long-term exposure to arsenic in drinking water is associated with painful and debilitating skin lesions, and cancers of the skin, lungs and bladder. Many developing countries rely almost entirely on drinking water from bores and tube-wells; however, in many of these countries the groundwater is contaminated with naturally occurring inorganic arsenic. The country most affected by this is Bangladesh.

Historically, the surface water in Bangladesh has been highly contaminated with microorganisms that have caused a significant burden of disease and mortality. To overcome this problem, during the 1970s and 1980s a large number of tube-wells were installed across the country. However, at this time arsenic was not recognised as a problem in water supplies, and so the water from the wells was never tested. In the 1990s arsenic contamination of water from tube-wells was confirmed, and it is now estimated that up to 77 million people are at risk of drinking this contaminated water. Unfortunately, the cost of removing or capping the wells is prohibitive, and the options for sourcing other safe water are limited (Smith et al. 2000).

ACTIVITY 12.2 Paying for water

A contentious issue for some consumers relates to the price they pay for the water they use. Politicians across the country have warned that continual price rises for water are inevitable. Water is a precious resource and should be valued appropriately. For the household you currently live in, locate the water bills for at least the past year and review these to assess both the water usage patterns and the costs.

- What is the daily cost for the water that you use, and how much has this cost increased recently?
- Do you think this cost is too cheap or too expensive, and, given how precious a resource water is, how much would you be prepared to pay for the water you use?

management plans. Guidance on what constitutes good-quality drinking water is provided by the Australian Drinking Water Guidelines (ADWG). The ADWG incorporate a preventive risk management approach, and apply it to any water intended for drinking, irrespective of its source (e.g. municipal supplies, rainwater tanks) or where it is to be used (e.g. in homes or restaurants).

Safe food

Food is a fundamental human need, a basic right and a prerequisite to good health. While Australia has one of the safest food supplies in the world, it is estimated that contaminated food still causes between 4 million and 7 million cases of gastroenteritis each year (Hall et al. 2005). The costs to the community of illness from contaminated food is estimated to be around $1.2 billion in Australia (Abelson et al. 2006) and $77 billion in the United States (Scharff 2012). There are a number of factors that are influencing food safety to an increasing extent, including:

- *Centralisation and globalisation*—Food is increasingly being produced by larger and larger firms, is being processed by more industrial and mechanical means, and is being sold in supermarkets by multinational companies. These factors result in decreased cost per item and an increased variety of food items, but present an increased opportunity to impact large numbers of people if the food is contaminated (see Example 12.1).

The cost of supplying prawns to Scots

EXAMPLE 12.1

A total of 19,000 km is the round-trip journey planned for prawns caught in Scottish waters before they reach British stores. The seafood firm that catches the prawns calculates that hand-peeling in Thailand will be cheaper than machine-peeling in Scotland, with 50 cents being the hourly wage paid to Thai prawn-peelers. The move will mean the loss of 120 jobs in Scotland, where workers are paid $11 per hour (Time Magazine 2006).

CASE STUDY
12.4

International Salmonella outbreak

In July 2001, health agencies in Australia and Canada noticed an increase in locally acquired *Salmonella stanley* infections. Australian investigators interviewed the initial cases, who recalled eating 'dry-flavoured Asian-style' peanuts during the incubation period of their illness. Subsequently, *S. stanley* was isolated from samples of a particular brand of peanuts. As the supplier of the peanuts was located in an Asian country, information about the outbreak was publicised on an international electronic mailing list, ProMed. This prompted health agencies in other countries to investigate, and cases of *S. stanley* infection were identified in England, Wales and Scotland. An international outbreak was declared, and health agencies around the world shared information and investigated local cases. Even though 109 cases were identified across a number of countries, the source of the original contamination of the peanuts could not be identified. Supplies of the peanuts were, however, recalled, and this helped to prevent additional cases. This case study illustrates the potential for global food-borne disease outbreaks, and highlights the role of international surveillance systems in recognising and investigating such epidemics.

(Source: Kirk et al 2004)

- *National and trans-national FBI outbreaks*—There is an increasing trend for food-borne illness (FBI) outbreaks to have national and international impacts, particularly due to the centralisation and globalisation of the food supply process (see Case Study 12.4).
- A widening gap between first and third world countries—This impacts on food supply, nutrition and safety.
- An increasing number of emerging pathogens being identified—Some of these have drug-resistant strains that present difficulties for control and treatment.
- New production technologies being developed—These technologies (e.g. genetic modification, antibiotics) help improve efficiencies in the centralisation and globalisation of the food supply, and help to increase production, but the long-term impacts of these technologies are not well understood.
- Increasing pressures on food supply—With the world's population predicted to double over the next 50 years, food production will need to be undertaken in a more sustainable manner.

In Australia, all levels of government are responsible for food safety. At a national level, Food Standards Australia New Zealand (FSANZ) is a statutory body tasked to develop

ACTIVITY 12.3 OzFoodNet

In Australia, the Commonwealth and state governments operate OzFoodNet, an enhanced food-borne illness surveillance system. Each year they release an annual report that describes the incidence and causes of food-related diseases. Access the OzFoodNet website (www.ozfoodnet.gov.au), review the latest annual report, and answer the following questions:

- What food-related diseases does OzFoodNet keep track of?

- How many cases of these diseases were notified in the latest annual report?

- What are the most frequently notified food-related infections?

- How many outbreaks of gastrointestinal illness were reported for this year, and how many people were affected, hospitalised and died due to these outbreaks?

- What was the most common setting for food-borne outbreaks?

- What food items were most often implicated as causing the outbreaks?

food standards, which are generally consistent with international standards. These food standards are then administered federally, by the states and by local government, including food safety standards at local restaurants and takeaway stores.

The built environment

The built environment is 'part of the overall ecosystem of our earth. It encompasses all of the buildings, spaces and products that are created, or at least significantly modified by people. It includes our homes, schools and workplaces, parks, business areas and roads. It extends overhead in the form of electric transmission lines, underground in the form of waste disposal sites and subway trains and the country in the form of highways' (Health Canada 1997 p 141).

The built environment is arguably our main 'environment', because a large proportion of the world's population lives in cities (e.g. over 75% of the population in developed countries) (UN-Habitat 2011), and because we spend most of our time indoors—for example, in the United States people spend nearly 90% of their time indoors and around 5% of their time in vehicles (Klepeis et al. 2001). Therefore, modifying the built environment will have significant impacts on the health of the public. For example, some of the direct positive health effects are the availability of shelter, water and food, whereas direct negative impacts include indoor and outdoor air pollution, as well as traffic accidents. Indirect health effects result from changes in the natural environment that are due to human modification of, or by, the built environment. These include the predicted rise in some infectious diseases due to global warming, which is due to an increase in greenhouse gas emissions that are a result of urban human activity.

Urbanisation is the process by which an increasing proportion of the population comes to live in urban areas. In 2007, the number of urban dwellers passed the number living in rural areas for the first time in history, and this trend is predicted to continue at a rapid rate. By 2050 the world's urban population is expected to be double that of the rural population (United Nations 2010). Future urbanisation is expected to be greatest in developing countries, and this brings with it substantial public health challenges, as much of the growth is in large informal settlements or shanty towns where residents have limited access to the benefits that urban areas can provide (e.g. good shelter, safe food and water, access to health services and education).

It is also important to view a city or town as consisting of a network of interdependent human systems (e.g. transportation, energy, water supply and waste management) to meet our needs for raw materials, finished goods and services, and to dispose of the waste we generate. It is generally acknowledged that our current urban systems are unsustainable because they produce waste and pollution in excess of the Earth's capacity to absorb them, thereby poisoning humans and other species, resulting in climate change, and depleting resources (both renewable and non-renewable). The challenge,

Urban design, transport and health

Cities are largely shaped by their transport systems, and this is primarily due to the *Marchetti constant*—people do not want to travel more than one hour each day to and from work. In Australian cities, the current urban design and land use patterns mean that many people have no choice but to use a car, with the more sustainable options (e.g. efficient public transport, walking or cycling) often being too difficult to access. In 2006 it was estimated that there were 14.4 million motor vehicles in Australia, with an estimated 209,405 million km each year travelled in these vehicles. This heavy dependence on the car has a range of public health impacts: *road accidents*—there are around 1600 deaths and 22,000 serious injuries associated with motor vehicles each year in Australia; *air pollution*, particularly particulate matter which is thought to result in a disease burden similar to that caused by road accidents; *physical inactivity*—car dependency encourages sedentary lifestyles that are associated with increased risk of cardiovascular disease, diabetes and certain cancers (e.g. colon and breast cancer); and a lack of *social connectedness* within the community.

Significant changes are therefore required in the way we travel within our cities, with some available options including: more fuel-efficient vehicles; a better public transport system (particularly a substantial increase in light rail infrastructure); active transport strategies; workplace incentives to reduce car travel, such as public transport vouchers instead of company cars, and changing rooms and showers for cyclists; removing economic subsidies that hide the true costs of roads and parking facilities; and, most importantly, creative and sustainable approaches to land use planning that help people to access public transport and to live closer to their work, shopping and recreational activities.

(Sources: Australian Bureau of Statistics 2006, Australian Transport Safety Bureau 2005, Davis et al. 2005, Newman 2004, Woodward et al. 2002)

therefore, is to revamp the existing infrastructures and build new sustainable infrastructures (see Case Study 12.5).

The occupational environment

The workplace can be thought of as a localised subset of the larger environment, a setting in which people become exposed to environmental hazards while they earn their living. The occupational environment is particularly complex and important because:

- Work remains the central activity in which most people throughout the world spend most of their time outside of the home.
- Many hazardous substances are experienced at their highest level in the workplace.
- The workplace represents a broad range of exposures, from acute chemical poisoning to catastrophic injuries, from long-term chemical effects to psychological stress.

ACTIVITY 12.4 Cycle routes

Cycling is encouraged in many cities to help improve the physical activity of residents and to provide an alternative to using motor vehicles or public transport. Construct a cycle route from your home to either your university or workplace that will maximise the use of bike paths/cycle lanes and minimise the use of roads, particularly main roads. Based on the cycling route constructed, how easy is it for you to get to your destination, and would this be an option you would consider for regular travel? There is a range of websites that can assist with cycling maps, such as:

- http://www.bikely.com
- http://www.bikepaths.com.au/map
- http://www.brisbane.qld.gov.au/facilities-recreation/sports-and-leisure/cycling/bikeway-and-shared-pathway-maps/

REFLECTION 12.4

The built environment is an important environmental health setting, because we are exposed to a range of environmental health hazards (e.g. air and water pollution, contaminated food, traffic accidents) while conducting our daily lives within this setting. In what ways do you feel that your health is impacted both positively and negatively by the urban environment you live in? Following on from Activity 12.4, what do you think are some of the positive and negative health impacts of cycling within an urban setting? Overall, the influence of the built environment on human health is nicely summarised as follows: 'the health of a city's people is strongly determined by physical, social, economic, political and cultural factors in the urban environment, including the process of social aggregation, migration, modernization and industrialization, and the circumstances of urban living … the impact of urban process on health is not just the sum of the effects of the various factors taken individually, since they interact synergistically with each other' (WHO 1991, p 10).

- Occupational health is not only a subset of public health, it is also a subset of industrial relations, which consists of complex interrelationships between politics, power, history, justice and law.
- The workplace setting provides many opportunities for health interventions, from health education to medical screening (Perry & Hu 2005).

Some of the key public health aspects of the occupational environment are:

- The workforce of a country is the backbone of its development. Therefore, a healthy workforce increases productivity and generates wealth that is necessary for the good health of the community at large.

- Health concerns in workplace and community settings often have the same or similar sources of hazard. Therefore, a coordinated approach to addressing particular issues may be needed, and may also be the most effective way of dealing with the issue (see Case Study 12.6).

- Workplace exposures are generally much higher than similar exposures in the community; thus, workplaces can provide an early indication of broader public health impacts. For example, exposure to new products/materials such as nanoparticles can be monitored more easily in the workplace, as can the impacts of shift work and various mental and behavioural disorders.

As people spend a significant amount of their life at work, exposures in the workplace, as well as at their home and in the community, need to be considered together when investigating health impacts. These impacts may not only be on the workers themselves, but also on family members due to secondary exposure at home (Guo 2014, Yassi et al. 2001).

Globally, there are an estimated 2.3 million work-related deaths each year, exceeding the death toll from traffic crashes and war combined. In addition, there are around 337 million occupational accidents and 160 million new cases of occupational disease each year, resulting in economic losses in the order of US$2.8 trillion (International Labour Organization (ILO) 2010, 2013). Unfortunately, a disturbing development of globalisation is the continuing transfer/export of hazards from developed countries to developing countries that have inadequate safeguards for workers (Perry & Hu 2005).

Port Pirie and lead exposure

Port Pirie in South Australia provides an important example of the complex relationship that can exist between a workplace and its community. Port Pirie is a small town that is dependent on its lead smelter, which has been operating for over 100 years and is the third largest in the world. In the 1980s, a number of studies concluded that environmental lead contamination due to the emissions from the smelter presented a public health problem. This lead contamination was the likely cause of elevated blood lead levels in the Port Pirie children, with high blood levels linked to effects on mental development. Since this time, intensive lead reduction, remediation and decontamination activities have been undertaken within the community and by the smelter, with the blood lead levels of children dramatically decreasing (i.e. improving). Despite these efforts, elevated levels of environmental lead remain, and these present an ongoing health hazard for the community. The owner of the lead smelter has recently announced that the smelter will undergo a major redevelopment that will transform the operation and provide significant reductions in lead air emissions (refer to: www.portpirietransformation.com). This case illustrates how both the history and the future of an industry and its community can be intertwined and inseparable, particularly when it comes to workplace hazards.

(Source: Heyworth et al. 2009, Taylor et al. 2013)

The global environment

Throughout this chapter, we have discussed the dependence of human health on the environment in which we live. Unfortunately, we are currently experiencing the early stages of a global ecological crisis, the outcomes of which are predicted to have a significant impact on our way of life in the coming centuries. Some of the fundamental reasons for this crisis are:

- Rapid technological development in the developed world is introducing new potential hazards.
- Rapid population growth and industrial development, based largely on obsolete technologies in the developing world, is accelerating existing environmental degradation.
- Environmental degradation is being aggravated by poverty, urbanisation without adequate infrastructure, rural development policies that do not strengthen local economies, and a limited economic base that is dependent on commodity prices (Yassi et al. 2001).

The global nature of this environmental degradation is a new phenomenon for humans to deal with. Previously localised environmental problems (e.g. air pollution) are now becoming widespread, regional and global, and are affecting areas that are not the sources of the pollution. In addition, the economic and political systems that create and sustain these problems are now influenced by the global marketplace, which is beyond the capacity of individual governments to regulate effectively.

In the past, the ecological systems of the planet (particularly local systems) have been capable of adapting to the changes forced onto them by human development.

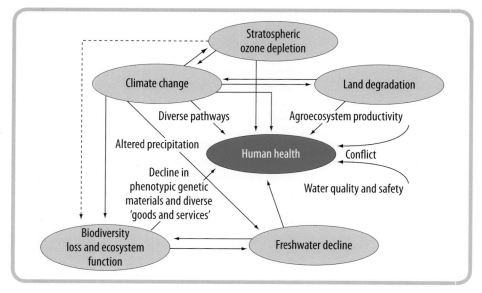

FIG. 12.2   Interrelationships between major types of global environmental change.
(Source: McMichael et al. 2003)

However, these changes are now producing an imbalance in global systems (e.g. climate), and the actual long-term outcomes of these changes are hard to predict.

Global environmental change is being observed in a range of systems, with the main systems affected being climate, stratospheric ozone, land, freshwater, biodiversity and the general functioning of the world's ecosystems. Unfortunately for humans, we are at the centre of all of these systems, and so the adverse impacts on each of these systems will affect us directly and synergistically. The interrelationships between the major types of environmental change are shown in Figure 12.2.

This issue is too broad and complex to cover in great detail in this component of the chapter; therefore, we will focus on climate change, as it is the issue that attracts most of the political and public attention.

GLOBAL CLIMATE CHANGE

Global climate change has been defined as 'a change of climate which is attributed directly or indirectly to human activity that alters the composition of the global atmosphere and which is in addition to natural climate variability observed over comparable time periods' (United Nations 1992b p 3).

This definition highlights that human activity is considered to be altering the world's climate, primarily through the production of 'greenhouse gases' that amplify the natural greenhouse effect that makes Earth habitable. Greenhouse gases—such as carbon dioxide, methane and nitrous oxide—are naturally present at low concentrations in the lower atmosphere and help to keep Earth's mean surface temperature at around 15°C. Without this trapping of heat, the mean air temperature would be −18°C. However, greenhouse gas concentrations have been increasing rapidly due to increased combustion of fossil fuels, increased deforestation, irrigated agriculture, and a range of other human activities. Unfortunately, the warming effects of these gases are much larger than the natural atmospheric cooling processes. This

CASE STUDY
12.7

Ocean acidification

The world's oceans readily absorb carbon dioxide from the atmosphere, having absorbed a quarter of all man-made CO_2 emissions since the Industrial Revolution. This CO_2 absorption results in an increase in the acidity of the seawater, known as ocean acidification. Ocean acidification causes ecosystems and marine biodiversity to change (e.g. coral reef growth is affected, and many shellfish are highly sensitive to changes in pH), and it has the potential to affect food security, particularly for those nations dependent on fishing. Also, as the acidity of seawater increases, the capacity of our oceans to absorb CO_2 from the atmosphere decreases. This will have significant impacts on the ocean's role in moderating climate change. Therefore, reducing CO_2 emissions is considered to be the only way to minimise long-term, large-scale risks to marine ecosystems and the climate more broadly.

(Source: International Geosphere-Biosphere Programme, Intergovernmental Oceanographic Commission, Scientific Committee on Oceanic Research 2013)

has resulted in Earth's climate now being warmer than at any time since records were kept.

The *Intergovernmental Panel on Climate Change* (IPCC) is the leading international body for the assessment of climate change. In its fifth and latest assessment report, it concluded that 'warming of the climate system is unequivocal, and since the 1950s, many of the observed changes are unprecedented over decades to millennia. The atmosphere and ocean have warmed, the amounts of snow and ice have diminished, sea level has risen, and the concentrations of greenhouse gases have increased' (IPCC 2013 p 4) (see Case Study 12.7). They also concluded that by the end of the twenty-first century the global average surface temperature is likely to exceed 1.5°C relative to 1850–1900 levels under all climate models, apart from those where it is likely to exceed 2°C (IPCC 2013) (see Figure 12.3).

> **ACTIVITY 12.5 Ocean acidification**
>
> Visit the website http://www.abc.net.au/catalyst/stories/s2029333.htm to view an important story on ocean acidification from ABC TV's *Catalyst* program.

Such a small temperature rise may not seem to be too significant; however, such an increase is likely to have disastrous consequences for ecosystems and our way of life. It is also important to realise that: (1) this increase in temperature is a global average, and so it masks extremes in temperature that will be experienced in particular locations; and (2) the greenhouse gases emitted will remain in the atmosphere for hundreds or thousands of years, and that, because of this 'inertia' in the climate system, climate change will continue to occur for centuries even if greenhouse gas concentrations have been reduced and stabilised. Therefore, to minimise the temperature rise by 2100, global emissions (which are still rising) will need to peak within the next decade and then decline rapidly, despite the world's population continuing to increase rapidly (Australian Academy of Science 2010). The IPCC reiterate this by stating that 'continued emissions of greenhouse gases will cause further warming and changes in all components of the climate system. Limiting climate change will require substantial and sustained reductions of greenhouse gases' (IPCC 2013 p 19).

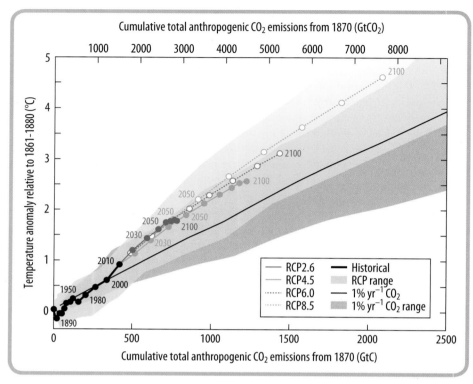

FIG. 12.3   Predicted increase in global mean surface temperature as a function of CO_2 emissions from various lines of evidence. This graph displays historical data from 1860 to 2010, along with predictions from various climate models taking account of differing scenarios. The models predict that by 2100 there will be an increase in the global mean surface temperature of between 1.5°C and 4.5°C, depending on the rate of future CO_2 emissions.
(Source: Intergovernmental Panel on Climate Change 2013)

HEALTH AND SOCIAL IMPACTS OF CLIMATE CHANGE

The impacts of climate change are currently causing, and will continue to cause, widespread harm to human health, with children suffering the most. Impacts include food shortages, polluted air, contamination of or a reduction in water supplies, and an expansion in the distribution of vectors of infectious disease. More extreme weather events also cause physical and psychological impacts within the communities affected (Hansen et al. 2013). The IPCC predicts the following human health impacts: (1) increased malnutrition and consequent disorders, including those related to child growth and development; (2) increased death, disease and injuries from heat waves, floods, storms, fires and droughts; and (3) increased cardio-respiratory morbidity and mortality associated with ground-level ozone (IPCC 2007).

As mentioned, due to the inertia in the climate system, if large-scale climate change of the order predicted is allowed to occur, it will last for many centuries. Therefore, climate change will have 'substantial intergenerational effects, with young people and future generations inheriting a situation in which grave consequences are assured, practically out of their control, but not of their doing. The possibility of such intergenerational injustice is not remote—it is at our doorstep now' (Hansen et al. 2013). Therefore, human-caused climate change is ultimately a moral issue, where the actions we take now will determine what future we will deliver to the generations to follow.

Sustainable environmental health

It is clear from the preceding sections that human activity, particularly over the past half-century, has had a significant impact on our environment (i.e. on both local and global ecosystems, including the climate system), and that the current level of human activity/consumption is unsustainable for both the environment and human survival. Further, 'maintaining sustainable ecosystems as essential prerequisites for human health is now beginning to be accepted as part of the responsibility of public health' (Brown et al. 2005 p 5). It is therefore important to understand what 'ecological sustainability' is, and what it means for public health policy and practice. A good definition of *ecological sustainability* is 'a balance that integrates—protection of ecological processes and natural systems at local, regional, State and wider levels; and economic development; and maintenance of the cultural, economic, physical and social wellbeing of people and communities' (Government of Queensland 2009).

Often the economic development aspect of sustainability is emphasised, whereas the health needs of current and future generations is of primary importance. For example, the first principle of the *Rio Declaration on Environment and Development* (known as Agenda 21) states that human beings are at the centre of concerns for sustainable development and are entitled to a healthy and productive life in harmony with Nature. It goes onto emphasise the need to protect and promote human health, particularly by: addressing primary care needs, specifically in rural areas; controlling infectious diseases; protecting vulnerable groups within the community; meeting urban health needs; and reducing health risks from environmental pollution and hazards (United Nations 1992a). The Rio Declaration still serves as a pillar for action, with the *Earth Charter* as an example of a more recent international covenant to help guide us on a path of justice, sustainability and peace (Soskolne et al. 2008) (see Box 12.2).

BOX 12.2

THE EARTH CHARTER

The *Earth Charter* is a declaration of fundamental ethical principles for building a just, sustainable and peaceful global society. It is primarily concerned with encouraging a transition to sustainable ways of living and sustainable human development. It emphasises that the key themes of ecological integrity, eradication of poverty, equitable economic development, respect for human rights, democracy and peace are interdependent and indivisible. The Earth Charter began as a United Nations initiative, but was completed (and is overseen) by the Earth Charter Commission, an independent international entity. It has been endorsed by over 4,500 organisations, including many governments. At a time when the sustainability of our planet is in question, the Earth Charter challenges us to examine our values and to choose a better way.

(Source: Earth Charter International: www.earthcharterinaction.org)

Risk assessment and risk perception

The appropriate assessment of risk, in its many and varied forms, is an essential component of human survival, and is fundamental to the management of environmental health hazards. Each day we make decisions on what actions to take based on an assessment of risk. For example, whether to jay-walk or not is based on an assessment of how risky it is to do so. However, the concept of risk is more complicated than whether a 'bad' outcome will occur if a particular action is taken. The following key elements are considered to determine risk (Ropeik & Grey 2002):

- *Probability*—This is the statistical element of risk and conveys the notion of 'chance'. It describes the likelihood that something will happen (e.g. the chance of getting cancer from exposure to chemical X is 1 in 1 million).
- *Consequences*—This describes the severity of the potential outcomes of an action or event (e.g. the potential consequences of a nuclear plant meltdown are significant).
- *Hazard*—This is the capacity or potential of an agent/thing to produce an adverse effect (e.g. asbestos is known to cause asbestosis and mesothelioma).
- *Exposure*—This is contact between the agent and the target (e.g. if a worker comes into contact with asbestos through breathing fibres that have been released into the air).

Given these elements, a more complete definition of risk is: 'the probability that exposure to a hazard will lead to a negative consequence' (Ropeik & Grey 2002 p 4). This definition highlights an important aspect of environmental health risk—that risk is significantly influenced by exposure; therefore even if a hazard exists (e.g. a particular chemical may cause cancer), if there is no exposure then the level of risk posed in this circumstance will be minimal. An example of the application of these risk principles is described in Chapter 13.

Despite a range of technical and scientific approaches that are used to assess human health risk from exposure to environmental agents, much of the social science literature argues that risk is inherently subjective and based on the perceptions held by the individuals involved or affected (Slovic 1997). Therefore, a key issue for risk perception is definition: how each of us defines risk and establishes our own risk priorities. In addition to the scientific elements that underpin the definition of risk, there are many qualitative aspects of risk that include values, emotions, power relations, and the need for action (Sandman 1987). These qualitative aspects of risk have been described in terms of 'outrage factors'. These factors influence a person's perception of the level of risk, and include whether the risk is imposed or voluntary, whether the person feels they have some level of control over the risk, and whether the risk is familiar or unfamiliar. Ten of the most common outrage factors in environmental health are listed in Table 12.1.

TABLE 12.1 Outrage factors for individual risk perception

Factors that decrease risk	Factors that increase risk
Voluntary	Imposed
Control	Lack of control
Fair	Unfair
Ordinary	Memorable
Not dreaded	Dreaded
Natural	Technological, artificial
Certain	Uncertain
Familiar	Unfamiliar
Morally acceptable	Morally unacceptable
Trustworthy source	Untrustworthy source

(Source: Blake 1995)

The influence of the outrage factors can result in very different definitions of risk being held by scientific/technical experts versus those held by the public (Fischhoff et al. 1984, Slovic 1987) (see Example 12.2). Appropriate risk communication therefore plays an important role in environmental health management, and provides a way of bridging the gap between the 'experts'' and the public's definitions of risk. Risk communication is more than just disseminating risk information; it involves elements of conflict resolution, public participation and two-way messages. Aakko (2004) states that in the 'traditional' communication model, the risk messages flow in one direction—from regulator to public—but risk communication has to be a two-way process with active participation from both the sender and the audience.

ACTIVITY 12.7 Risk assessment

- Consider the following scenario: you work for a public health agency and a major chemical fire takes place in your area. Shortly after the fire is extinguished, the local residents start to complain of a range of adverse health effects. A health risk assessment is conducted, and this indicates that the health risk posed to the residents is minimal. For this scenario, what are the perceptions of risk likely to be held by the residents and the experts, and what outrage factors might influence the perception of risk?

Risk perception of 'experts' versus the 'public'

EXAMPLE 12.2

In a study by Kraus et al. (1992), members of the public and a group of toxicologists were asked to express their attitude and beliefs about chemicals and chemical risk assessment. Examples of the differences in views can be seen in the responses to the following statement: *'If you are exposed to a toxic chemical substance, then you are likely to suffer adverse health effects'*—32.3% of toxicologists agreed with this statement, whereas 85.5% of the public agreed. In response to the statement *'There is no safe level of exposure to a cancer-causing agent'*—25.3% of toxicologists agreed with this statement, whereas 53.9% of lay respondents agreed.

Scenarios like the one described in Activity 12.7 are regularly faced by public health agencies. For example, in Sydney a contaminated and disused gasworks site was being cleaned up, and some of the perceptions of the risk held by various stakeholders were:

- 'There are no real emissions leaving the site, so there are no real risks to health' (environmental engineers).
- 'People are experiencing health effects, but they can be reassured that these will not cause long-term damage' (health agency).
- 'It is okay for the professionals to think that there is no health risk, because they don't have to live here' (residents).
- 'We are experiencing significant effects on our health and no one is taking our complaints seriously' (residents).

This case highlights the challenge for environmental health practitioners to combine scientific information from a risk assessment with qualitative approaches that recognise the differing perceptions of risk held by the various stakeholders (Rutherford 2003).

A final word

This chapter has provided an introduction to environmental health, some of the key environmental health issues faced in Australia and in other countries, and various approaches to managing these issues. This chapter has reinforced how dependent human life and wellbeing is on our environment, with the implications of the current global ecological crisis arguably being the greatest challenge faced by the world today. However, history has shown that when there is a will to do so, we have been able to develop effective strategies to address the issues of the time. We should therefore be optimistic that solutions to the enormous and complex challenges that we now face are possible, but this relies on enhanced and sustained community and political support, and an emphasis to 'think globally, act locally'. Overall, the importance of environmental health is nicely summarised in the following quotation:

> Human health ultimately depends on society's capacity to manage the interaction between human activities and the physical and biological environment in ways that safeguard and promote health but do not threaten the integrity of the natural systems on which the physical and biological environment depends. (WHO 1992)

REVIEW QUESTIONS

1. If someone said to you that environmental health related only to the health of the environment, are they correct and what would you say to them in response?

2. Can you describe the concept of risk transition as it relates to environmental health hazards?

3. What are the adverse effects of air pollution?

4. How is water quality and quantity related to human health?

5. For the city you live in, can you identify the various human systems that have been established, and are there any examples of 'urban sprawl'?

6. What impacts do you think global climate change will have on your lifestyle during your lifetime, and what actions can you take to promote sustainability?

Useful websites

- Australian Drinking Water Guidelines: http://www.nhmrc.gov.au/guidelines/publications/eh52
- Department of the Environment (Australia): http://www.environment.gov.au

- Environmental Health (free access journal): http://www.ehjournal.net
- Environmental Health Australia (professional association): http://www.eh.org.au
- Environmental Health Perspectives (journal): http://ehp.niehs.nih.gov/
- Environmental Health Standing Committee (enHealth): https://www.health.gov.au/internet/main/publishing.nsf/Content/ohp-environ-enhealth-committee.htm
- Environmental Protection Agency (United States): http://www.epa.gov
- Food Standards Australia New Zealand: http://www.foodstandards.gov.au
- Garnaut Climate Change Review: http://www.garnautreview.org.au
- Global Footprint Network: http://www.footprintnetwork.org
- Human Development Reports: http://http://hdr.undp.org/en/
- Intergovernmental Panel on Climate Change: http://www.ipcc.ch
- National Center for Environmental Health (USA): http://www.cdc.gov/nceh
- National Institute of Environmental Health Sciences (USA): http://www.niehs.nih.gov
- Smart Growth Online: http://www.smartgrowth.org
- Sustainable Development Gateway (Australian Broadcasting Commission): http://www.abc.net.au/science/sustainable
- United Nations Sustainable Development Knowledge Platform: http://sustainabledevelopment.un.org/
- World Health Organization—Public Health, Social and Environmental Determinants of Health homepage: http://www.who.int/phe/en/

References

Aakko, E., 2004. Risk communication, risk perception, and public health. Wisconsin Medical Journal 103 (1), 25–27.

Abelson, P., Potter Forbes, M., Hall, G., 2006. The Annual Cost of Foodborne Illness in Australia. Australian Government Department of Health, Canberra.

Australian Academy of Science, 2010. The Science of Climate Change: Questions and Answers. AAS, Canberra.

Australian Bureau of Statistics, 2006. 2006 Survey of Motor Vehicle Use. ABS, Canberra.

Australian Bureau of Statistics, 2010. Water Account Australia 2008–09. ABS Cat. No. 4610.0, ABS, Canberra.

Australian Transport Safety Bureau, 2005. Road Crash Casualties and Rates, Australia, 1925 to Latest Year. ATSB, Canberra.

Blake, E.R., 1995. Understanding outrage: how scientists can help bridge the risk perception gap. Environmental Health Perspectives Supps 103 (Suppl. 6), 123–125.

Brown, V.A., Ritchie, J., Grootjans, J., et al., 2005. Public health and the future of life on the planet. In: Brown, V.A., Grootjens, J., Ritchie, J., et al. (Eds.), Sustainability and Health: Supporting Global Ecological Integrity in Public Health. Allen and Unwin, Crows Nest, pp. 1–37.

Chen, Y., Ebenstein, A., Greenstone, M., et al., 2013. Evidence of the impact of sustained exposure to air pollution on life expectancy from China's Huai River policy. Proceedings of the National Academy of Sciences 110 (32), 12936–12941.

Davis, A., Cavill, N., Rytler, H., et al., 2005. Making the Case: Improving Health Through Transport. Health Development Agency, London.

Earth Charter International website. Available: <www.earthcharterinaction.org> (31 Oct 2014).

enHealth Council, 1999. National Environmental Health Strategy. enHealth Council, Commonwealth Department of Health and Aged Care, Canberra.

Environmental Health Standing Committee (previously the Environmental Health Council), 1999. The National Environmental Health Strategy. Commonwealth Department of Health, Canberra.

Fischhoff, B., Watson, S., Hope, C., 1984. Defining risk. Policy Sciences 17, 123–139.

Government of Queensland, 2009. Sustainable Planning Act 2009. Government Printer, Brisbane.

Guo, H.-R., 2014. Frontiers and challenges in occupational safety and health. Frontiers in Public Health 2, Article 85, 1–3. doi:10.3389/fpubh.2014.00085.

Hall, G., Kirk, M.D., Becker, N., et al., 2005. Estimating foodborne gastroenteritis. Emerging Infectious Diseases 11 (8), 1257–1264. Online. Available: <http://www.cdc.gov/ncidod/EID/vol11no08/pdfs/04-1367.pdf> (7 Mar 2014).

Hansen, J., Kharecha, P., Sato, M., et al., 2013. Assessing 'dangerous climate change': required reduction of carbon emissions to protect young people, future generations and Nature. PLoS ONE 8 (12), e81648, 1–26. Online. Available: <http://www.plosone.org/article/info%3Adoi%2F10.1371%2Fjournal.pone.0081648> (11 Mar 2014).

Health Canada, 1997. Health and Environment: Partners for Life. Health Canada, Ottawa.

Heyworth, J.S., Reynolds, C., Jones, A.L., 2009. A tale of two towns: observations on risk perception of environmental lead exposure in Port Pirie and Esperance, Australia. Environmental Health 9 (1&2), 60–73.

International Geosphere-Biosphere Programme (IGBP), Intergovernmental Oceanographic Commission (IOC), Scientific Committee on Oceanic Research (SCOR), 2013. Ocean Acidification Summary for Policymakers—Third Symposium on the Ocean in a High-CO_2 World. International Geosphere-Biosphere Programme, Stockholm, Sweden.

Intergovernmental Panel on Climate Change, 2007. Climate change 2007: impacts, adaptation and vulnerability. In: Contribution of Working Group II to the Fourth Assessment Report of the Intergovernmental Panel on Climate Change. Cambridge University Press, Cambridge.

Intergovernmental Panel on Climate Change, 2013. Climate change 2013: the physical science basis—summary for policymakers. In: Contribution of Working Group I to the Fifth Assessment Report of the Intergovernmental Panel on Climate Change. IPCC, Geneva. Online. Available: <http://www.climatechange2013.org/images/report/WG1AR5_SPM_FINAL.pdf> (28 Aug 2014).

International Labour Organization, 2010. Linking Safety and Health at Work to Sustainable Economic Development: Project Outline. ILO, Geneva.

International Labour Organization, 2013. Safety and Health in the Use of Chemicals at Work. ILO, Geneva.

Kirk, M.D., Little, C.L., Lem, M., et al., 2004. An outbreak due to peanuts in their shell caused by *Salmonella enterica* serotypes Stanley and Newport—sharing molecular information to solve international outbreaks. Epidemiology and Infection 132, 571–577.

Klepeis, N.E., Nelson, W.C., Ott, W.R., et al., 2001. The National Human Activity Pattern Survey (NHAPS): a resource for assessing exposure to environmental pollutants. Journal of Exposure Analysis and Environmental Epidemiology 11, 231–252.

Kraus, N., Malmfors, T., Slovic, P., 1992. Intuitive toxicology: expert and lay judgements of chemical risks. Risk Analysis 12, 215–232.

McMichael, A.J., Campbell-Lendrum, D.H., Corvalan, C.F. (Eds.), 2003. Climate Change and Human Health: Risks and Responses. World Health Organization, Geneva.

National Health and Medical Research Council, 2004. Water Made Clear: a Consumer Guide to Accompany the Australian Drinking Water Guidelines 2004. Australian Government, Canberra.

New South Wales Department of Environment and Conservation, 2005. Air Pollution Economics: Health Costs of Air Pollution in the Greater Sydney Metropolitan Region. NSW Department of Environment and Conservation, South Sydney. Online. Available: <http://environment.nsw.gov.au/resources/air/airpollution05623.pdf> (30 Mar 2015).

Newman, P., 2004. Sustainable transport for sustainable cities. In: United Nations Asia-Pacific Leadership Forum. Sustainable Development for Cities, Hong Kong. Online. Available: <http://planning.cityenergy.org.za/Pdf_files/planning/sustainable_transport/Sustainable%20 Transport%20for%20Cities.pdf> (16 Mar 2014).

Perry, M., Hu, H., 2005. Workplace health and safety. In: Frumkin, H. (Ed.), Environmental Health: From Global to Local. Jossey-Bass, San Francisco, pp. 648–682.

Ropeik, D., Gray, G., 2002. Risk: A Practical Guide for Deciding What's Really Safe and What's Really Dangerous in the World Around You. Houghton Mifflin, Boston.

Rosen, G., 1993. A History of Public Health (Expanded Edition). Johns Hopkins University Press, Baltimore.

Rutherford, A., 2003. But you don't have to live here! Risk assessment and contaminated sites: a case study. NSW Public Health Bulletin 14 (8), 171–173.

Sandman, P., 1987. Risk communication: facing public outrage. EPA Journal 13 (9), 21–22. Online. Available: <http://www.psandman.com/articles/facing.htm> (6 Mar 2014).

Scharff, R.L., 2012. Economic burden from health losses due to foodborne illness in the United States. Journal of Food Protection 75 (1), 123–131.

Slovic, P., 1987. Perceptions of risk. Science 236, 280–285.

Slovic, P., 1997. Public perception of risk. Journal of Environmental Health 59 (9), 22–24.

Smith, A.H., Lingas, E.O., Rahman, M., 2000. Contamination of drinking-water by arsenic in Bangladesh: a public health emergency. Bulletin of the World Health Organization 78 (9), 1093–1103.

Soskolne, C.L., Westra, L., Kotzé, L.J., et al., 2008. Sustaining Life on Earth: Environmental and Human Health Through Global Governance. Lexington Books, Lanham, MD.

Taylor, M.P., Camenzuli, D., Kristensen, L.J., et al., 2013. Environmental lead exposure risks associated with children's outdoor playgrounds. Environmental Pollution 178, 447–454.

Time Magazine, 2006. Numbers. 27 Nov 2006, p. 32

UN-Habitat, 2011. Cities and Climate Change: Global Report on Human Settlements 2011. Earthscan, London. Online. Available: <http://unhabitat.org/?wpdmact=process&did =NDM0LmhvdGxpbms=> (10 Mar 2014).

United Nations, 1992a. United Nations Conference on Environment and Development—Agenda 21. United Nations Division for Sustainable Development, New York. Online. Available: <http://sustainabledevelopment.un.org/content/documents/Agenda21.pdf> (11 Mar 2014).

United Nations, 1992b. United Nations Framework Convention on Climate Change. United Nations, New York.

United Nations, 2010. World Urbanization Prospectus: The 2009 Revision. UN Department of Economic and Social Affairs, New York.

United Nations Development Programme, 2006. Human Development Report 2006. UNDP, New York.

US Environmental Protection Agency, 2011. The Benefits and Costs of the Clean Air Act from 1990 to 2020: Final Report. US Environmental Protection Agency, Office of Air and Radiation, Washington, DC.

Woodward, A.J., Hales, S., Hill, S.E., 2002. The motor car and public health: are we exhausting the environment? Medical Journal of Australia 177, 592–593.

World Health Organization, 1991. Environmental Health in Urban Development. WHO Technical Report Series 807. WHO, Geneva. Online. Available: <http://apps.who.int/iris/bitstream/10665/40612/1/WHO_TRS_807.pdf?ua=1> (10 Mar 2014).

World Health Organization, 1992. Our Planet, Our Health. WHO, Geneva. Online. Available: <http://www.ciesin.org/docs/001-232/chpt1.html> (19 Mar 2014).

World Health Organization, 1997. Health and Environment in Sustainable Development: Five Years After the Earth Summit. WHO, Geneva.

World Health Organization, 2004. Water, Sanitation and Hygiene Links to Health: Facts and Figures Updated November 2004. WHO, Geneva. Online. Available: <http://www.who.int/water_sanitation_health/publications/facts2004/en/print.html> (6 Mar 2014).

World Health Organization, 2014a. Ambient (Outdoor) Air Quality and Health. Fact Sheet 313. WHO Media Centre, Geneva. Online. Available: <http://www.who.int/mediacentre/factsheets/fs313/en/> (16 Apr 2015).

World Health Organization, 2014b. Household Air Quality and Health. Fact Sheet 292. WHO Media Centre, Geneva. Online. Available: <http://www.who.int/mediacentre/factsheets/fs292/en/> (16 Apr 2015).

Yassi, A., Kjellstrom, T., de Kok, T., et al., 2001. Basic Environmental Health. Oxford University Press, New York.

CHAPTER 13

Disaster preparedness and public health

Gerry FitzGerald

Learning objectives

After reading this chapter, you should be able to:

- define 'disasters'
- explain the principles of disaster management
- describe trends in disasters and their impact
- describe the particular impact of special disaster types
- explain the role of public health practitioners in disaster management.

Introduction

Effective disaster management can reduce the health consequences of both natural and man-made disasters. The aim of this chapter is to outline the principles and practice of disaster health management with a view to providing public health practitioners with an understanding sufficient to enable them to participate in disaster preparation and response management, and thus to reduce the health consequences of disasters on the community.

Defining 'disasters'

There are many definitions of 'disasters', but little agreement on what is a disaster. In reality, it depends on a range of factors. Events or health challenges range from a single emergency or a single patient through to catastrophes, and, while we may be able to define the ends of the continuum, there is no single defining point at which this transition to a disaster occurs, but rather a gradient whereby the challenge and the resources available to deal with that challenge are influenced by multiple factors.

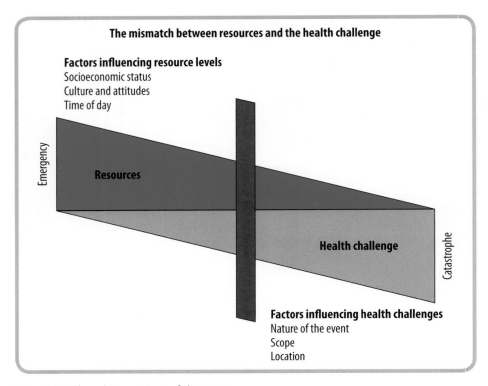

FIG. 13.1   The relative nature of disasters.

The extent of the challenge to the health and wellbeing of the community is determined by the nature of the event, its location, spread and impact, and by the characteristics and size of the affected community. The resources available to deal with the event are defined by the location, culture and socioeconomic status of the community, and such variables as the time of day or day of the week. Thus, whether any single event or challenge to health and wellbeing is a disaster or not depends on the influence and interaction of many factors. Figure 13.1 seeks to demonstrate the variable nature of this relationship. The slide on the scale marks a particular event, but its position on the scale is determined by those factors that influence the mismatch of resources and challenges to health.

Some have distinguished between emergencies and disasters based on the number of patients affected. However, the extent of the impact will depend not only on the numbers affected but also on the nature of the effect, and the resources available to deal with the impact.

Emergency Management Australia (EMA) defines a disaster as:

A *serious disruption* to community life which *threatens or causes death or injury* in that community, and *damage to property* which is *beyond the day-to-day capacity* of the prescribed statutory authorities and which *requires special mobilisation and organisation* of resources other than those normally available to those authorities [emphasis added]. (Emergency Management Australia 1998 pp 32–33)

This definition seeks to capture the special nature of events at the extreme end of the continuum. We use the term 'disaster health' as a working term for the focus of this chapter and for the special consideration of policymakers and service planners. The term 'disaster health' is used on the grounds that the principles and management practice outlined in this chapter are most necessary when the event stretches available resources sufficiently to require special mobilisation and organisation. In addition, we use the term 'disaster health' as a means of drawing focus to both the health consequences of disasters and the burden the event may impose on health services. Thus, public health authorities must have in place scalable arrangements whereby emergency responses may be escalated on the basis of standard principles and practices to such a level as to meet the particular challenge at that particular time.

Notwithstanding these definitional issues and the need for scalable arrangements, there is a time when the event reaches a stage where the approach of the authorities changes from a focus on the individual patients to the greater good of the whole community. This occurs because of the absolute or relative mismatch between the demands made on the system and its resources, or because the resources and health infrastructure have been degraded by the event. There is also a time when the approach changes from treating the sick to preserving the infrastructure, including the people who have a key role to play in the community. There are no rules related to when this occurs. It depends on the relative and absolute resources available and the level of mismatch between those resources and the demands being placed on them.

Some disasters are associated with single events such as a crash, explosion or earthquake. Some may be highly localised, while others are widespread. Some may be relatively silent, such as the HIV/AIDS pandemic, and others develop more slowly and less dramatically, such as influenza pandemics.

Sundnes and Birnbaum (2003) have described the context of disaster health as involving three essential domains: public health; emergency and risk management; and clinical and psychological care. Their conceptual map describes the interrelationship between these domains within a broader framework defined by community preparedness, response capability and resilience, political and social structures, and the support resources available. The focus of this discussion is mostly on the public health domain.

Context

Epidemiology

The number of recorded natural events and the number of people affected by those events continues to increase (World Health Organization CRED 2009). Figure 13.2 demonstrates the number of events and the number of people killed in disasters over the past century. What this figure demonstrates is that, while the number of events has increased, the recorded number of people killed has declined.

Why are the events increasing? It is unclear whether the apparent increase is merely an increased level of recording. It is difficult to understand why the number of natural events would be increasing, except where the effect of human intervention may be contributing to an increase in the frequency or severity of events. In particular, it has been suggested that global warming is contributing to the increased frequency and severity of cyclones (Intergovernmental Panel on Climate Change 2007), and deforestation may be contributing to the frequency of mudslides and forest fires.

However, at the same time, improvements in the relative safety of transportation, and in occupational health and safety, and reductions in the level of major conflict have reduced the exposure of the community to man-made risks, although increased

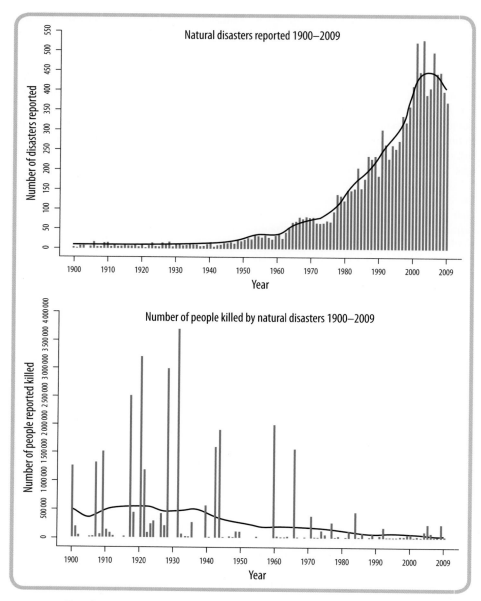

FIG. 13.2 Trends in incidents and deaths.
(Source: D. Guha-Sapir, R. Below, Ph. Hoyois, EM-DAT: Interantional Disaster Database (www.emdat.be), Université Catholique de Louvain, Brussels, Belgium)

population and levels of human activity may increase the frequency of such adverse events. The vulnerability of the community has been increased by demographic changes. Population growth and urbanisation has resulted in the growth of megacities, often in areas that are particularly vulnerable to natural disasters, because they are built on flood plains or in seismic areas. In addition, the social consequences of rapid urbanisation, including poverty and congestion, may lead to outbreaks of violence. Either way, this social change has increased the vulnerability of the community and the potential health consequences.

Each day over 20,000 people attend hospital emergency departments (EDs) in Australia (Steering Committee for the Review of Government Service Provision 2011). Australia has never had a single event with 20,000 casualties, yet every day we manage those numbers in our EDs. The difference between a quiet day and a busy day would exceed any major event to have confronted Australia. Thus, the cornerstone of our emergency health response arrangements should be the systems and structure that characterise and respond to the daily burden of emergency health.

Health impacts

The health impacts of disasters may be categorised into two dimensions:

- timeliness of the consequences—immediate, medium-term and long-term
- relationship of the consequences to the hazard—direct consequences are those related to direct contact of humans with the hazard, and indirect consequences are those in which the human impact is a consequence of damage to something else.

For example, the health impact of floods has been categorised into immediate, mid-term and long-term by Du et al. (2010). Direct effects of floods are those related to exposure to the water or the debris contained within the water. Thus, drowning and injury are direct immediate consequences. In addition, floods often disrupt transportation or industry, leading to longer-term economic constraints and the health consequences of poverty. Finally, the loss and grief that may accompany the flood, or the impact that the flood has on society, can have a long-term effect on an individual's mental health.

The health consequences of any particular event can be mapped. The strategies designed to reduce health consequences are then matched against those particular risks. Thus, reduction in immediate direct effects would involve prevention and mitigation, along with immediate rescue or evacuation. Strategies aimed at preventing long-term mental health consequences include psychological first aid, follow-up and dealing with the economic and social uncertainties that often characterise a poorly managed recovery phase.

Health is involved in such events in two ways:

- Any event is likely to cause adverse impact on the health and wellbeing of people, and health services have a key role to play in the provision of healthcare or the protection of life.
- Health services are part of the community's critical infrastructure, which needs protection to maintain services. Health infrastructure may be subject to the same risks as those that have caused the incident in the first place (see Case Study 13.1, Activity 13.1 and Reflection 13.1.).

Principles of disaster management

As outlined earlier, effective disaster health management can reduce the health consequences of serious events. Effective disaster health management is complex and multifactorial, so there is potential for complexity to paralyse any action. However, a number of core principles have been identified that may govern the approach to disaster health management, and these principles should form the core of any management strategies.

Evacuating health services

Health services are a critical component of any community's infrastructure, and during disasters health services are called upon to meet the increased demands associated with disasters. However, what happens when those facilities themselves are in danger, or are damaged, and patients have to be evacuated?

In February 2011, tropical cyclone Yasi, a category five cyclone, struck the north-east coast of Australia. As the cyclone approached the coast, a very real danger threatened the 330-bed Cairns Hospital, which is situated on the foreshore. The danger was posed by a combination of cyclonic conditions and storm surge. The decision was made to evacuate the patients to the state capital, Brisbane, an estimated 1700 km away. Thus, 356 patients, staff and family members were evacuated by ambulance from the hospital and taken to the airport, where they were loaded on a number of military and civilian aircraft.

It is not common that health facilitates require evacuation, but in this circumstance the physical threat from the cyclonic winds and the storm surge forced the decision. Because of the very broad nature of the physical threat, evacuation was only sensible to a location well outside the danger zone, and one with sufficient resources to absorb the patients. No significant adverse events were observed in the patients' health.

ACTIVITY 13.1 Decision to evacuate a hospital

- What are some of the possible consequences of evacuating an acute-care hospital?
- What factors would influence your decision to evacuate?
- What are the factors that would influence where you would evacuate the patients to?

REFLECTION 13.1

Consider the impact on families of a decision to evacuate patients from one hospital to another hospital some considerable distance away. How could you provide support to those families? Consider how you would re-establish emergency health services once the immediate danger had passed.

An engaged and prepared community

All disaster management is ultimately local disaster management. It is not possible for governments or external agencies to do everything without the direct involvement of the community in its own protection and recovery. This local engagement is critical. In major events, particularly those associated with the destruction of major infrastructure, the community will be on its own until help can be organised. The initial response will be from local agencies, local resources and bystanders, as the destruction of roads and other means of access may reduce the capacity for outside assistance.

Critical to an engaged community is the concept of *community resilience*, which, while ill-defined, implies the capacity of the community to withstand challenges to its wellbeing and to 'bounce back', taking control of its own destiny and restoring functionality. This concept places an emphasis on the partnership required between the community and government and non-government agencies. An engaged, resilient community helps governments and other agencies to obtain support for the investments required and the strategies necessary to facilitate preparedness, and efficient response and recovery. Such a community also participates directly in the planning and preparedness required to protect the community from the hazards that place it at risk. A resilient community is able to respond immediately to render initial aid and act quickly to restore community functionality.

RISK-BASED APPROACH

Defining 'risk' is difficult in this context. The terms 'risk' and 'hazard' are often used with little variation in meaning or understanding. A *hazard* is something that may cause damage. Thus, a volcano is a hazard. The *risk* to the community arising from that hazard is a combination of the nature of the hazard and the vulnerability of the community (risk = hazard × vulnerability). The vulnerability of the community is determined by the size, location and socioeconomic characteristics of the community. For example, the risk associated with Vesuvius in southern Italy is a combination of the risk posed by the presence of the volcano and the millions of people who now live within its potential impact zone.

Hazards have been categorised by the World Association for Disaster and Emergency Medicine (WADEM) into natural, man-made and mixed hazards (Sundnes & Bimbaum 2003).

Natural hazards are those arising from the natural environment:

- biological—pandemics, etc.
- geophysical—volcanos, landslides, earthquakes
- hydrological—floods and mudslides
- meteorological—storms and cyclones
- climatological—heat waves and droughts.

Manmade hazards are those derived from the human environment:

- technological—including transport and industrial technology
- conflict—including armed and unarmed conflict (e.g. sanctions).

Mixed hazards are those derived from the interaction of human development with the natural environment. Examples include desertification from land-clearing, and erosion and landslides from deforestation. In addition, the consequences of climate change on meteorological and climatological hazards may be classed as the ultimate mixed hazard.

A risk-based approach involves the identification of likely hazards and their impact, and the development of a risk profile or register for the community. The identified risks need to be evaluated for their likelihood and impact, and management strategies put in place to prevent, moderate or offset the risk.

Risk identification is informed by history; thus a history of floods or cyclones in a particular area, or earthquake-prone areas, will identify those risks. But it may also be informed by research or by creative and analytical thought. The possibility of a particular risk may be informed by thoughtful analysis of potential problems, even when there is no history of such an event to inform planning.

ALL-HAZARDS APPROACH

Because of the diversity of risks, and because of the initial confusion that characterises major incidents, it is not possible, and is potentially confusing, to plan or prepare for individual hazards. The all-hazards approach seeks common approaches to preparation and response, regardless of the hazard. Put simply, communities should respond in a standard way (at least initially), regardless of the challenge. This allows for standardised training and awareness, and for a relatively automated immediate response, even when the full extent or even the nature of the event may not be known. For example, the first information available may not identify the source of an explosion (accidental or deliberate). It is necessary to develop and implement safe and consistent initial responses that take into consideration the possible risks.

ALL-AGENCIES APPROACH

There is a risk that different agencies, or different levels within individual agencies, may react to a major incident in different ways. The consequence could be confusion, gaps in response, or overlap and wasted effort.

A more effective approach is for all agencies involved in preparation and response to major incidents to operate on the basis of similar and standard approaches. Approaches such as those outlined in the *Major Incident Management System* (MIMS) (Hodgetts & Porter 2002) help with the definition of roles and responsibilities, and the determination of the standard principles of action. In addition, the efforts of national standard-setting bodies such as Emergency Management Australia (EMA), and its interaction with similar international bodies, allows for consistency in approach.

FAMILIARITY

The principle of familiarity describes the understanding that the most effective response to major incidents is achieved when those responding are familiar with their roles and responsibilities. This is best achieved if the response arrangements are based on those that people undertake on a daily basis. An emergency is not the time to learn new tasks, but rather to utilise the expertise present within the community. Accordingly, task allocation should, wherever possible, reinforce normal practice. Surgeons should do the surgery, and fire-fighters should rescue people and put out fires. Organised responses should reflect normal practice wherever possible. For example, pre-hospital management should be undertaken by those who normally undertake this role, rather than placing individuals in new and challenging environments.

This principle not only reflects reality, but also ensures that the definitional issues discussed earlier become irrelevant. Response agencies will initiate the response on the basis of their familiar practice, then enhance that response until such time as resources appear sufficient to the particular challenge. This approach minimises the aspects of disaster response that require unusual responses, and therefore reduces the training needs of the community. Those additional areas should be the subject of special training that is reinforced by regular exercises, so as to build into the community's familiarity the special actions required.

COMPREHENSIVE APPROACH

The principle of a comprehensive approach is based on the cycle of disaster management, which seeks to ensure consistency throughout the lifecycle of *prevention, preparation, response* and *recovery* (PPRR).

Prevention and mitigation

Some hazards can be prevented, or at least reduced in likelihood. For example, road traffic management strategies are aimed at preventing or reducing the frequency of major transportation incidents, and land use policies may reduce the impact of desertification.

Other hazards are not preventable, but their impact can be mitigated by a combination of infrastructure investment and behavioural modification. Thus, while we cannot prevent cyclones, we can reduce their impact by imposing higher standards of building construction in cyclone-prone areas, and evacuating people at risk into secure shelters. Equally, we may not be able to prevent floods, but we can reduce their impact by investing in dams and high-level bridges over waterways, or by reducing the risk to people by constructing shelters above flood height, and by building flood-resistant community infrastructure, such as dams and bridges. However, while the principle of preparedness is straightforward, the balance between risk and community values remains difficult to deliver. People living in rural areas wish to preserve their natural environment, even though it poses a significance bushfire risk.

Preparedness and planning

Preparing the community for major incidents is part of building community resilience.

The most significant aspect of preparedness is planning. *Planning* describes the process of identification, evaluation and management of risks, and the development of strategies to mitigate or respond to those risks, should they cause an adverse impact on the community.

It is often considered that the process of planning is more significant than the plan itself. The process of formulating a plan engages the key agencies and leading individuals of the community, ensures their interaction, and helps identify the potential problems associated with the management of response and recovery. The planning process is educational in itself, and allows for the sharing of expertise. It also ensures that the key players know each other and are familiar with the capability of other individuals and agencies.

The planning process is further complicated by the need to ensure that plans are consistent with those of other agencies, and with other levels of government or community. For example, an agency's pandemic plan should be consistent not only with those of other agencies, but also with national and international pandemic preparedness plans. There is a need to avoid confusion in the planning process by ensuring that any plan is consistent with international principles, national standards and the response arrangements of other agencies.

Sensible construction of plans needs to follow some basic principles:

- Develop a hierarchy of plans which are consistent with each other but allow maximum flexibility.
- Develop a standardised approach to the content of the plan that includes risks, roles and responsibilities, and the sources of resources required to respond.

Figure 13.3 identifies a possible structure for a complex organisation, whereby the core plan is supported by operational plans for subunits of the organisation, by functional plans which summarise the roles of key functions, and by special plans which articulate the special requirements of particular hazards. Thus the core plan would

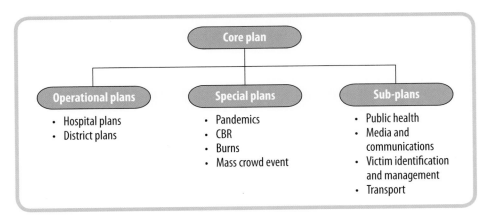

FIG. 13.3 Hierarchy of plans. CBR = Chemical, biological and radiological.

REFLECTION 13.2 Heatwaves

Heatwaves are the most significant risks to Australia. We need to respond on a whole-of-community
basis to heatwaves, caring for friends and neighbours; particularly the elderly and children who
are at most risk.

articulate the core principles, roles and responsibilities, while a special plan may identify how that core
plan would vary in the particular circumstance of a
flood, for example.

While planning is an essential component of
preparedness, there is more to it than planning. Preparedness also includes surveillance and early
warning. This is most obvious in pandemic surveillance, where close monitoring of infectious disease
outbreaks is an essential component of the prepared-
ness for disasters. However, surveillance as a concept is equally appropriate for other
hazards, such as the early warning system for tsunamis, or the activities of security and
protection agencies (see Reflection 13.2).

Preparedness is also about the resources required to respond. People need to be
prepared through appropriate education and training, and the testing of that familiarity
through exercises. Appropriate physical resources, including capital infrastructure and
consumables, need to be identified to ensure their availability in a time of need. The
concept of stockpiles of resources is a critical element of disaster preparedness, ranging
from pre-positioned flood boats to stockpiles of clinical consumables and drugs, such
as antiviral medications. When considering the stockpiles, it is important to take into
consideration the 'embedded' stockpiles. Many drugs and other consumables required
in disasters are in everyday clinical use. At the same time, drugs and other consumables
with a short shelf-life are very costly to stockpile, as they will often pass their use-by
date before ever being required for disaster management. For example, personal protective equipment such as masks and gloves will be required in a pandemic. These are
things used in everyday practice, and the initial response will utilise those immediately
available. It is critical to identify where those existing supplies are, and their manufac-
ture, supply and distribution systems, so that ongoing supplies will be available in the
event of a major incident. It will also be important as part of an initial response to secure
the embedded stockpile, as this is the first tier of resources critical to effective
management.

Response and relief

The response and relief phase of disaster management concerns the period immediately
following the event. This phase is the focus of much of disaster management, often led
by key response agencies such as police, ambulance, fire or the state emergency management services. Health is not often the lead agency (sometimes referred to as 'combat
agency') except in the management of major disease outbreaks. However, health is
almost always involved as a partner agency in any event that is associated with significant injury to people.

The declaration of an event as a disaster is a critical point in the disaster response
sequence. However, a response should never await such a declaration. Disaster declaration initiates additional assistance and permits special authority for response
agencies.

The management of the response and relief phase is complex, but may be considered
according to the *eight Cs of response management*:

- *COMMAND* refers to the direction of members of an organisation in the
  performance of roles and tasks. Command arrangements operate vertically
  within an organisation, and ensure that the organisation's resources can be
  directed to the delivery of its roles and responsibilities.

- *CONTROL* refers to the overall direction of emergency management activities in an emergency situation. Control arrangements operate horizontally across organisations, and seek to ensure that various organisations act in a coordinated and collaborative fashion. Establishment of command and control arrangements is a critical first step. If you could only do one thing to improve disaster management it would be to put someone in charge, and then allow that person to take charge.
- *COORDINATION* describes the bringing together of organisations and elements to ensure an effective response. Coordination is mainly concerned with the systematic acquisition and application of resources from various agencies and locations. Coordination operates both vertically and horizontally as an adjunct to the authority to command and control.
- *COMMUNICATION* refers to the provision of information, which facilitates an efficient and effective response. Communication refers to the design and development of the message, including its clarity, as well as the means of communication. Most response personnel complain about breakdowns in communication, and, in reality, communication is most difficult to maintain. It is worth considering the vulnerability of normal means of communication. Recent disasters in Queensland, for example, demonstrated the vulnerability of modern communications, with power failures affecting transmission towers, etc. Often non-technological means, such as runners, may prove more reliable and resilient.
- *CLINICAL*—Disasters may directly affect the health and wellbeing of individuals, who will require clinical care. Disasters may also disrupt the health infrastructure, resulting in a lack of a capacity to manage health needs.

   Ongoing care of people in the vicinity of the event is critical. A major event may impact on the capacity to provide clinical care. For example, patients may lose access to dialysis or their regular medications, and not be able to obtain ongoing supply and prescriptions, if the health services have been damaged.

   The key issues to be addressed include the following:
   - *Triage* is a necessary component of disaster health management. Triage is the sorting of patients, according to their urgency and severity, into groups that determine their healthcare. Triage is a continuous process which needs to be reinforced at key points, such as extrication from the scene, arrival at hospital, presentation to theatre, etc.
   - Rapid development of *clinical standards* for the particular challenge is essential. Clinical care in a disaster should be based on the principles of maximum benefit, so immediate interventions should be restricted to life and limb preservation with deferred definitive care.
   - *Clinical documentation* is essential. Triage tags are the subject of considerable debate, but some form of initial documentation is essential to ensure the safety of ongoing care, as well as to inform the incident management.
   - *Definitive diagnosis* of the nature and extent of injuries or illness is essential to defining the healthcare requirements. Particularly during pandemics, accurate diagnosis is essential to inform the development of clinical standards and disease control strategies.

There is a need to determine the requirements for *decontamination and isolation.*

○ There is a need to ensure care for the *family and contacts* of those suffering directly from the event.

- *CAPABILITY*—Planning and response management must address the need for the maintenance of the health services' capability. *Health is a critical service* in disasters, and the maintenance of critical services is a key aspect of effective management.

  In order to maintain health services, attention must be given to a number of significant issues, including:

  ○ *Critical infrastructure protection*, including workforce protection with enhanced infection control, personal protective equipment (PPE), isolation of patients, and administration of antiviral agents.

  ○ *Maintaining access to services* and health business continuity throughout an event that may have impaired not only the stability of the infrastructure and the availability of key personnel, but also power, fuel and supplies.

  ○ There may be a need to create *additional capability*. There is value in taking a hierarchical approach to the mismatch of demand for healthcare and the capability available. The following approach to infrastructure creation or capability development may serve as a guide:

    – *Level 1* events require concentration of expertise utilising existing infrastructure.

    – *Level 2* events require the preservation of infrastructure for the event by early discharge of patients and limiting non-urgent activity.

    – *Level 3* requires expansion of health infrastructure through system-wide management, growing capacity and importing capacity (e.g. field hospitals).

    – *Level 4* requires rationing of access to health infrastructure through triage of patients.

- *CONTAINMENT* refers to the strategies required to limit the scope and spread of an event. The concept has most relevance for pandemic preparedness, whereby strategies seek to limit the spread of an infectious disease through quarantine, isolation and containment strategies, or through *ring immunisation* of family, contacts and neighbours. However, the concept is also relevant to other events where we seek to limit the extent and impact of the incident. Patients injured or exposed to a major toxin may independently seek medical aid and thus continue to spread the exposure. Likewise, people involved in a major traumatic incident often depart independently from the scene, thus making it difficult to determine the extent of the problem and to ensure appropriate care. Often the walking wounded will crowd the nearest hospital, limiting its capacity to deal with the critically ill or injured.

  Containment in pandemic responses is achieved though isolation and quarantine. Immunisation of family, contacts and neighbours, if available, or through the prophylactic use of antiviral or antibacterial agents, may also limit the spread of the disease. Social distancing measures, such as school closure or the banning of mass gatherings, may reduce disease transmission opportunities.

Containment is an important aspect of response management, as we attempt to focus the available resources on the incident and to achieve maximum benefit. It enables the responders to manage the site more effectively, and to ensure maximum utilisation of available resources.

At the macro level, containment is about stopping the spread of hazards between countries. Border control is a first strategy in pandemic management, although unlikely to be successful, even in Australia where our large 'moat' is no protection against diseases brought into the country by airline passengers during the disease's incubation period.

- *CONTINUITY* describes the strategies needed to maintain functionality. When events are long-term, it is neither possible nor safe to maintain key personnel on duty. They need to be relieved from duty, particularly if their own families are under threat, or if they have suffered personally from the incident. Sometimes, effort put into securing the safety of the families of key personnel will free them to maintain activity.

  o It is necessary to maintain *supplies* through a prolonged event, and supply and distribution systems are necessary. There is a need to secure supplies, as the imbedded stockpile will be consumed first in an uncoordinated manner.

  o *Data and information systems* need to be maintained. Often staff lists are stored on computer and we need to ensure that through sensible preparedness we have access to such material when power may not be available.

  o *Volunteer management* is a critical aspect of this maintenance of functions. Volunteers can be used to support staff and allow them time for relief, but be aware that the use of volunteers may conflict with the principle of familiarity.

  o Appropriate *education* will expand capability. Smart use of resources is needed to concentrate expertise while maximising support from volunteers and less-trained personnel. For example, general practitioners may be useful as surgical assistants, to care for families, or provide vaccinations and counselling.

Look at the example of the eight Cs of response management in practice in Table 13.1, then consider Activity 13.3 and Reflection 13.3.

Recovery, rehabilitation and redevelopment

The aim of disaster management is to restore functionality as soon as possible. Indeed, in the best circumstances, the aim of the recovery phase is to utilise the opportunity posed by reconstruction to develop and improve. For example, after the destruction caused by cyclones it is often a time to rebuild to more modern and resilient standards.

There are both human and economic costs of disasters. The human costs are those of the injured, people deprived of healthcare, and the deceased. Often, public analysis focuses on the deceased when, for each person who dies, numerous people suffer injuries, even if the injury is the mental anguish of loss.

However, the economic impact also has significant health consequences, particularly in developing countries. Loss of production means that industries fail and

TABLE 13.1 Example of the eight Cs of response management in practice

The Queensland floods of 2010/2011	
Response principle	Example
Command	The Premier took charge of the operation
Control	The Disaster Management Group was established
Coordination	The new Disaster Coordination Centre was activated
Communication	Press conferences were conducted several times each day by the Premier
Clinical	Aerial retrieval of patients from vulnerable health facilities occurred
Capability	Additional resources were sourced from unaffected areas and interstate
Containment	Evacuations occurred in vulnerable areas
Continuity	Food and other supplies were flown into affected areas.

ACTIVITY 13.3 Managing Fukushima

- Imagine you were a public health official in the vicinity of the Fukushima nuclear power plant in northern Japan, which was disabled by an earthquake and subsequent tsunami, resulting in a loss of cooling to the reactor and the leakage of radioactive material into the seawater and atmosphere.
- What actions would you take to protect the health of the people in the surrounding community?

REFLECTION 13.3

Imagine the difficulty in responding to a tsunami warning at a five-storey hospital on the seafront in northern Japan. You have 20 minutes to respond. What would you do with the patients? You can't move them outside as that would place them at added risk, and you have no idea how high the water might be or whether the building will withstand the waves.

employment is lost, at a time when individuals and families are seeking to restore their livelihood and their normality. There is an association between disaster and the overall economy (Asian Disaster Reduction Center 2005). Major disasters have been shown to reduce economic development and recovery, and rehabilitation strategies are aimed at reducing the long-term economic and health impacts.

The recovery phase is a critical aspect of disaster health management which is often relatively neglected or devalued by those interested in the emergency response aspects. Poorly managed recovery can lead to the 'secondary disaster', whereby the consequences of poor management create additional distress. Psychological effects may last a lifetime, and the cost of recovery leads to lost opportunities for development. Most commonly, the need for financial and material assistance is in the months and years after a disaster, but often the media scrutiny is gone and the world's compassion has shifted to the next issue.

The aim of recovery management is to restore functionality; not only economic but also social functioning. The key elements of the recovery phase include the following:

- *Restore essential services* to ensure that the basics of population health, water, food and security are restored as soon as possible.

- *Rehabilitate the community* and its structures, including the functioning of community systems of government and the societal structures, including community organisations.
- *Provide for immediate needs*, including safe housing and financial support.
- *Provide information*, including health and safety and public health information.
- *Identify ongoing healthcare needs*, particular mental health needs.
- *Restore and develop the community infrastructure.*
- *Develop the economy and restore economic activity.*

Reporting is a critical aspect of disaster management throughout the full cycle of disaster preparedness, response and recovery; it is important not only to contribute to the lessons learned, but also as a means of reassuring the community and validating the experiences of people impacted by the disaster. Reporting is also important in terms of informing and improving the quality of response to future events, and is designed to inform and not to serve as a medium for criticism. Linked to reporting is the need for evaluation, which is important, as it not only informs the community about what worked well and what did not, but it is also a means by which the community reaches some degree of closure, enabling it to move on to the new, and probably different, reality. We cannot reconstruct lost lives or families, nor can we readily reconstruct the damaged natural environment.

These are opportunities for research and analysis to inform future planning, preparedness, response and recovery, and to complete the disaster management cycle. However, there is a real risk that the reporting and evaluation may be as destructive as the original event. In Australia we have seen highly destructive post-event enquiries, which have victimised and blamed individuals rather than focus on system and structural issues. These may create a third wave of injuries among the very people who sought to render aid.

There is a need to ensure that aid and assistance are designed in such a way as to contribute to the restoration of economic and social functioning. For example, donations of food may be necessary in the short term, but if the donated food removes the ability of local business to sell their goods, or farmers to restore their livelihoods, then the result may be negative in terms of adding to the economic and social distress. The principal focus of recovery should be to develop local industry and restore normality. Accordingly, ongoing donations of food or other essential supplies may be counterproductive if they impair any local markets and prevent reconstruction of local businesses.

Redevelopment, or enhanced development, is an important aspect of the recovery phase. Cyclone Yasi, which struck North Queensland in 2011, did less damage to Innisfail compared with other areas, as Innisfail had been rebuilt to more modern standards after the destruction of Cyclone Larry in March 2006. In developing countries, disasters may be an opportunity to build anew to better standards, and to develop new industries. Often, infrastructure destruction offers the opportunity to rebuild better infrastructure. The economics of building stronger is appropriate in developed countries where there is capacity to make the necessary investments. Conversely, in developing countries, the capacity may not be there. People know their mud huts will wash away in the next flood, but that is all they can afford.

An important aspect of community resilience is to rebuild community infrastructure, not only the buildings and business, but also the social structures and networks that characterise 'community'. For example, re-establishing sports groups, clubs and societies may not be seen as an immediate priority, but it is an important part of the healing process. It is these organisations that define the community and provide the mutual aid and support necessary for full recovery. Similarly, it is important to reopen schools as soon as possible. Not only does this restore a sense of normality, but it also frees up parents for reconstruction and employment.

Systems and structures

The Australian disaster management system is based on local authorities being the first responders, and the prime responsibility of district, state and national agencies is to assist the local authorities. Restoration of community functionality is local and dependent on restoration of the normal functions of the community.

Figure 13.4, from the Queensland Government Disaster Management website, outlines the coordination groups at each level.

The Australian Government maintains Emergency Management Australia (EMA), whose role is to set national standards and conduct education, and to provide operational support to the Australian Government in the event of an incident that requires their involvement.

Each of the states and territories in Australia has a similar body with responsibility for facilitating planning, providing support to state agencies, and coordinating response and recovery arrangements. All states and territories also maintain a volunteer-based organisation which provides initial support. The State Emergency Service (SES) comprises volunteer units in each local authority, supported by the local authority as well as by the state, particularly through educational, equipment and standards support.

Each of the states has disaster management legislation that prescribes planning and response arrangements, and provides the authority to create the relevant systems and structures. Many other items of legislation have significance for disaster management.

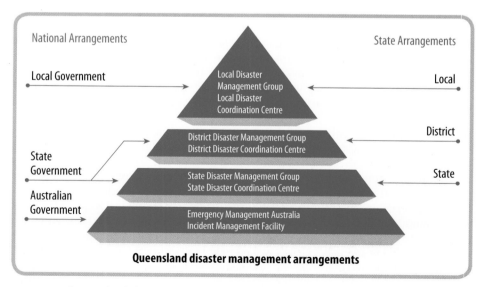

FIG. 13.4 Queensland disaster management arrangements.
(Source: Queensland Government Disaster Management website 2014)

These laws could be divided into those specific to disaster management (e.g. the Disaster Management Act), those that have direct relevance or include specific provisions for disaster response (e.g. the Public Health Act), and those that have general application but contribute to risk reduction (e.g. the Traffic Act).

Many agencies provide aid and assistance during disasters. These include: government agencies, such as health, fire and police; non-government agencies, such as St John Ambulance and the Red Cross; and charitable and community organisations, such as Lions and Rotary. The Salvation Army, in particular, has a long tradition of providing immediate aid and support to emergency responders.

In Australia, the military has traditionally played a significant role in disaster response, more so than in many other countries. The military generally has access to significant assets, such as aircraft and ships, which can facilitate responses, particularly for overseas disasters. In addition, the military has personnel who are rapidly deployable and are supported by appropriate resources to ensure that they are self-sustaining.

An essential component of disaster response is the establishment of central coordination and control centres (see Activity 13.4). Highly sophisticated centres are available in most states, and the Commonwealth has similar centres available as lead agencies.

> **ACTIVITY 13.4 Local disaster health committees**
>
> - Consider the structure of a local government disaster health committee. Who should be involved in the committee and what should their roles be?

Special considerations

There is insufficient space to consider the full range of special issues that must be considered in disaster health management. The following comprise some of the more common observations. This commentary does not attempt to explain these in detail, but rather to provide an introduction.

Floods

Flooding is the most common natural hazard, and causes almost half of all events, deaths and injuries. It has an extensive impact on health, ranging from drowning through to the health consequences of poverty from destroyed livelihoods.

Floods are caused by precipitation of rain or snow, or by displacement of stored water supplies. Floods may be categorised into flash floods, which occur as a result of a sudden downpour or dam failure, or slower riverine flooding caused by raised water levels. Other causes of flooding include tsunami, storm surge, and rising sea levels from global warming.

The most dangerous form of flooding is the sudden flooding associated with flash flooding or tsunami. These events may be complicated further when accompanied by debris that smash into infrastructure, such as bridges and houses, or directly injure people.

The key elements of flood management are mitigation strategies to divert or store water, construction standards to withstand the floods, and evacuation strategies to remove people from the danger. In developed countries, most deaths occur due to the decision by individuals to enter floods, either in vehicles or on foot. In Australia, 90% of flood-related deaths occur in this way (FitzGerald et al. 2010). The 2011 floods at Toowoomba and Grantham in Queensland were a notable exception; in these cases, debris-laden flash flooding isolated and swept away people who were essentially unaware of the danger confronting them.

Pandemics

Pandemics are common, characterised by a slower onset of development and the wide-spread nature of the outbreak. Pandemics may be relatively sudden, as exemplified by the outbreak of SARS (severe acute respiratory syndrome), or may be slower in onset and relatively silent, such as the HIV/AIDS pandemic. The key aspects of pandemic management include:

- early isolation and containment
- enhanced infection control procedures
- rapid development of immunisation.

Mass gatherings

Mass gatherings may be either spontaneous or planned. Mass gatherings are difficult to define, but the common theme is the accumulation of people in a relatively restricted area to a level that exceeds the reasonable capacity of the area.

The risks associated with mass gatherings are a combination of the risks of the event, determined by the nature and locality of the event, and the normal risks of so many people gathered together, aggravated by the often-confined nature of the location and the lack of normal infrastructure. The impact of mass gatherings is determined by the nature of the event, the nature of the location, and the size and demographics of the population.

Mental health

Mental health is a relatively silent, but exceedingly important aspect of disaster health. Exposure to terrifying images or events, injury and permanent disability, loss and grief, and the ongoing distress caused by the direct and indirect effects of disaster, can have a long-lasting effect on individuals and therefore on the community. Effects can range from immediate distress and adjustment, through to chronic depression associated with post-traumatic stress disorder (PTSD).

Effective management of the mental health consequences of disaster can reduce their potential impacts. Effective psychological first aid will help individuals to adjust to often understandable reactions to traumatic events. Monitoring of affected individuals will provide an opportunity for early recognition and intervention for those most at risk.

The incidence of chronic issues is often associated with repeated exposure, which can be related to ineffective management of often relatively basic recovery issues, such as food, accommodation and protection.

Public health considerations

Much of disaster health management is associated with the maintenance of public health systems. The key aspects include:

- maintenance of clean water
- food supplies
- shelter and protection
- waste disposal
- immunisation status for known risks
- preventing the spread of vectors (e.g. mosquitoes breeding in flood waters).

There are some myths associated with public health. The real risks are those associated with a breakdown in public health protection, or those associated with the collection of large numbers of people, which may facilitate person-to-person spread of illnesses. There is no evidence of risks that would not normally be present in a community. For example, we would not anticipate an outbreak of cholera in an Australian disaster, as the organism is not normally present.

Displaced persons

Individuals displaced during a disaster have an increased risk of harm. The process of evacuation may endanger individuals in circumstances where their escape routes may be blocked or endangered. For example, during cyclones or bush fires it is important to leave early, or 'stay and defend'—where residents remain at their homes to protect them from fire—as the roads may be more dangerous during the height of the event. Facilities are required for the displaced; these include providing for their basic human and health needs, such as healthcare, accommodation, food and water, and safety and security.

International aid

One of the most significant contributors to improved health outcomes following disaster has been the capacity and willingness of countries to provide assistance to each other in times of need. This assistance may be specific in terms of finance or particular needs, or it may take the form of aid teams, including health teams. The nature of international health teams (often referred to as 'disaster medical assistance teams') is determined by the event, but such teams should comprise individuals who are trained and aware of disaster health, are self-sufficient as to their own needs, and operate with flexible management structures in place to enable the teams to adapt to the communities' needs.

Volunteers and donations

Major incidents typically induce a significant outbreak of compassion and support. The 2011 floods in Brisbane were marked by an enormous outpouring of support for the clean-up, with tens of thousands of people volunteering to help clear the mud. However, the use of untrained volunteers has some risks. The volunteer teams may lack coordination and control, and at worst present an additional burden, such as when they require accommodation, food, water and sanitation.

Similarly, inappropriate donations can add to distress. Often, donors are generous in terms of things they do not need, but usually the recipients do not need them either. Culturally inappropriate donations (particularly food), or drugs that are past their use-by date, add to the confusion. Donations also have the potential, as mentioned earlier, to destroy the fragile attempts of local industry to return to full function.

Vulnerable populations

There are a number of people who are particularly vulnerable in disasters. These include people who are unable to evacuate the area because they are isolated and unaware, physically incapable (disabled or ill), or contained (e.g. prisoners).

The elderly are particularly vulnerable. Not only does their fragility make them vulnerable to injury, but they also often suffer from chronic illnesses and are dependent on medical care, which may become inaccessible. The evacuation of nursing homes is particularly troublesome, because of the combination of ill health and disability. There is evidence of a significant increase in mortality rates associated with the evacuation of nursing homes, not only because of the circumstances of the event, but also because of the normal mortality risk of this population group.

Management of exercises

Exercises are an essential element of disaster preparedness, providing an opportunity not only to test plans and preparedness arrangements, but also to familiarise people with the concepts and practice of disaster health management, and with each other.

The organisation of exercises requires reasonable experience and skills. Special tools are available—for example, the Emergo Train System® (Emergo Train System® website 2007)—to provide a structured approach to the management of exercises. Tabletop exercises allow key executives to test their thinking and awareness in an environment that does not risk further injury or unnecessarily impede the normal operations of the organisation.

Field exercises are more difficult to arrange and can be extremely complex, and include high-fidelity simulations. There are often dangers associated with field exercises, so they should not be undertaken lightly. There are also significant risks associated with allowing field exercises to impede the normal operations of health facilities. We cannot stop treating the sick to practise for a disaster.

ACTIVITY 13.5 Disaster health management

- Draw up a table that outlines the principal issues that public health practitioners may face in the prevention, preparedness, response and recovery phases of disaster health management.

REFLECTION 13.5

Community resilience describes the ability of a community to withstand and recover from major incidents. The concept implies that the whole community has a role in minimising the impact of disasters. Community resilience includes strategies to design infrastructure to withstand the event (e.g. cyclone-resistant buildings), effective community-wide planning and preparedness, and whole-of-community commitment to response and recovery. Identify other strategies that you consider would build resilience in your community.

The role of the public health practitioner

Public health practitioners have a critical role to play in disaster health management. Not only do they have a responsibility to be informed and aware of disaster health requirements and principles, but they also need to be mindful that the restoration and maintenance of public health systems are critical to avoid the second wave of disaster health impacts.

Public health practitioners are responsible for planning and preparing for disasters, and for surveillance and early intervention. They are also responsible for monitoring the public health consequences of disasters, such as disease outbreaks, and for the provision of clean water, food and waste disposal (see Activity 13.5 and Reflection 13.5).

A final word

Disaster health management is an important part of public health. Disasters are becoming more frequent, and their impact potentially more significant, as large populations are exposed to natural and man-made risks. However, effective management of disasters through preparation and response management can reduce the health consequences to the community. This chapter has provided you with an overview of the principles of disaster management to inform your understanding.

REVIEW QUESTIONS

1 What do the letters 'PPRR' stand for?

2 What are the eight Cs of response management?

3 What are some of the key issues to be addressed in 'clinical' response management?

4 If you could do only one thing to improve disaster management, what would it be?

5 What are the seven key elements of the recovery phase?

6 What is the role of the public health practitioner in disaster health management?

7 Why are exercises essential elements of disaster preparedness?

8 What are some of the impacts of disasters on mental health, and how can these impacts be managed?

9 How can the process of planning for disaster preparedness be more significant than the plan itself?

10 What do you understand by the principle of familiarity with respect to disaster management?

References

Asian Disaster Reduction Center, 2005. Total disaster risk management—good practices. Online. Available: <http://www.preventionweb.net/files/9055_TDRM05.pdf> (15 Apr 2014).

Du, W., FitzGerald, G., Clark, M., et al., 2010. Health impacts of floods: a comprehensive review. Prehospital and Disaster Medicine 25 (3), 265–272.

Emergency Management Australia, 1998. Australian emergency management 3: glossary. Australian Emergency Manuals Series Part I: the fundamentals. Online. Available: <http://www.em.gov.au/Documents/Manual03-AEMGlossary.PDF> (15 Apr 2014).

Emergo Train System® website, 2007. Available: <http://www.emergotrain.com/> (15 Apr 2014).

FitzGerald, G., Du, W., Clark, M., et al., 2010. Flood fatalities in contemporary Australia (1997–2008). Emergency Medicine Australasia 22, 183–189.

Guha-Sapir, D., Below, R., Hoyois, Ph. EM-DAT: Interantional Disaster Database (www.emdat. be), Université Catholique de Louvain, Brussels, Belgium.

Hodgetts, T., Porter, C., 2002. Major Incident Management System. BMJ Books, London.

Intergovernmental Panel on Climate Change, 2007. Climate change: synthesis report 2007. Online. Available: <http://www.ipcc.ch/publications_and_data/ar4/syr/en/contents.html> (15 Apr 2014).

Queensland Government Disaster Management website, 2014. Queensland disaster management arrangements. Online. Available: <http://www.disaster.qld.gov.au/About_Disaster_Management/DM_arrangments.html> (3 Sep 2014).

Steering Committee for the Review of Government Service Provision (SCRGSP), 2011. Report on Government Services 2011. Productivity Commission, Canberra. Online. Available: <http://www.pc.gov.au/research/recurring/report-on-government-services/2011/2011> (15 Apr 2014).

Sundnes, K.O., Birnbaum, M.L., 2003. Health disaster management: guidelines for evaluation and research in the Utstein style. (Chapter 1: Introduction.). Prehospital and Disaster Medicine 17 (Suppl. 3), 1–24.

World Health Organization Collaborating Centre for Research on the Epidemiology of Disasters (CRED), 2009. Emergency events database EM-DAT. Online. Available: <http://www.emdat.be/disaster-trends> (3 Sep 2014).

CHAPTER 14

Health promotion

Elizabeth Parker

Learning objectives

After reading this chapter, you should be able to:

- define 'health education' and 'health promotion', and understand their histories and place in public health

- discuss health promotion actions and strategies, and their applications in various settings and populations

- identify levels of prevention, and how health promotion works across these levels

- discuss different practices in health promotion for health professionals

- discuss the use of internet social networking, smart phones and self-tracking technologies in health promotion.

Introduction

The promotion of health has become everybody's business, including: the marketers of 'healthy' products and lifestyles, and gym memberships; government media campaigns such as Go for 2&5© (fruit and vegetables); special 'extra' benefits for joining a private health insurance fund; workplace wellness programs; and the technological explosion of internet and smart phone devices. Health professionals need to understand the background to this growth in promoting 'health', and its role in public health. We begin with health education, continue with the development of health promotion strategies and settings, and conclude with challenges for health promotion.

History of health education

Education concerning prevailing health problems, and the methods of preventing and controlling them, is the first of the eight basic elements of primary healthcare (World

Health Organization (WHO) 1978). Health education is about educating individuals about specific illnesses so that they can make informed decisions about preventing the onset of these conditions, or maintaining and restoring health, usually by changing their behaviour.

Ritchie (1991) described four stages of health education activity in Australia. The first was education through the provision of health information. Health professionals were considered to have the relevant knowledge and were 'the prime source responsible for the health of individuals' (Ritchie 1991 p 157). Although great efforts were made in providing information to patients, information alone was not producing the desired effects. In stage 2 (the early 1970s), health information and education programs were delivered through audiovisual channels, such as films, leaflets, posters and teaching kits. Even with all these additions health professionals were still disregarded, and some of the brochures were inaccessible as they were written in obscure scientific language (Ritchie 1991). In stage 3, health educators used adult education principles of empathy, experiential learning, participation and authenticity (Boshier 1998). Adults learned by building on their own experiences, particularly in groups with other adults. Group work that used these principles was pursued, with the assumption that being informed would automatically lead to behaviour change. When people did not change, they tended to be 'blamed' (Ritchie 1991). Stage 4 was the combination of improving individuals' knowledge, skills and understanding, but within the context of their social and environmental milieu.

Mass health education campaigns in the 1970s and 1980s broadened from a focus on individuals, to health education campaigns aimed at changing the behaviour of populations. One of the earliest of these large programs was the *North Karelia Project* in Finland. The study in North Karelia (population of 180,000) showed that Finnish men had the world's highest mortality rate from ischaemic heart disease in 1972. A health education program was started to see whether the main risk factors of high blood pressure, high cholesterol and smoking could be reduced in the population, and whether this would in turn reduce mortality from cardiovascular diseases (Vartianen et al. 2000).

Knowledge of effective health education strategies, particularly the application of theories of individual behaviour change, is essential for health professionals who work with individuals. Behaviour change is complex because, while knowledge about a health problem is easily found, modifying behavioural risk factors related to the problem is not necessarily easy. Tested theories of behaviour change, such as the theory of reasoned action and planned change, and the transtheoretical (stages of change) model, are two theories which have been effective in underpinning programs focused on individual change. You will learn more about these in your future studies in health promotion; see Nutbeam et al. (2010). Understanding of this takes on a special significance as the health profile of the population changes, with the consequent rise in chronic diseases. Health education definitely has a place for nurses and allied health professionals to counsel patients about self-management. Patients have the right to know about their care, but, as a whole-of-population approach, health education alone is limited.

The concept of wellness

Unsatisfied with the term 'health' and its origins in the 'absence of disease', some American health professionals thought that health education should be about improving 'wellness'—that is, people's sense of wellbeing. Wellness programs have sprung up in many organisations. These focus not only on keeping employees physically active and healthy, but also on the spiritual, emotional and social aspects of health.

Evolution and evidence for health promotion

The concept of health promotion emerged with the *Declaration of Alma-Ata* in 1978 (WHO 1978), and its *Health for All* strategy. Catford (2004) argued that 'health promotion' was becoming increasingly used by a new wave of public health activists who were dissatisfied with the traditional top-down approaches of 'health education' and 'disease prevention'. Health promotion was a more radical approach, because it assumed that people's health was determined not only by their own behaviour but also by the contexts in which they lived and worked. We discussed contexts and the importance of socio-economic influences on health in Chapter 7. To improve health within a population, a 'new public health' was needed to tackle these determinants, as research revealed that multiple strategies across many sectors—government, non-government and industry— were needed to ensure health opportunities for all.

Catford (2004) identified three stages in the development of health promotion. The *first stage* was 'tackling preventable diseases and risk behaviours' (e.g. heart disease, cancer, tobacco and poor nutrition) through education (Catford 2004 p 3), commonly termed 'health education'—for example, the North Karelia program. The *second stage* of health promotion was the 'complementary intervention approaches' (Catford 2004 p 3), with a range of action areas such as the development of healthy public policy, personal skills, supportive environments, community action and health services. The *third stage* was 'the value of reaching people through the settings and sectors in which they live and meet' (Catford 2004 p 3). This became known as the 'settings' approach for health promotion. There is a fourth dimension for the twenty-first century, and that is the social determinants of health in an increasingly globalised world. The issues include: the migration and movement of people in Europe; the pressure on the world's cities as increasing numbers of people move from agrarian-based economies to market-based economies—for example, the mass migration to cities in South East Asia to work in sewing and technology-based industries; increasing disparities in the standards of living between developed countries and developing countries; changing weather patterns that impact on agriculture; and war and the consequent displacement of millions of people. All of these factors create challenges for public health. Therefore, health promoters need the skills to analyse the impact of these factors on health and to advocate for healthy public health policies.

There is mounting evidence for the cost–benefit of health promotion, and thus the need to devote resources to the prevention agenda to improve the health of the population (Catford 2009, Trust for America's Health 2008).

In Australia, Vos et al. (2010) analysed the cost–benefit of over 150 preventive health interventions,

---

ACTIVITY 14.1 Health education and promotion

Discuss the following questions with other students.

- Why were the early community health education programs—which tried to produce behaviour change by educating the public about multiple risk factors for cardiovascular disease—not as successful as expected?
- Are there lessons to be learned from Ritchie's (1991) analysis of health education?
- Define 'wellness', and comment on whether you believe there is a lot of attention in the community to 'wellness', and does this include complementary medicine?
- Identify two other changes in the increasingly globalised world that will prove a challenge for health promotion.
- Write a short summary on the case for financial investment in preventing premature mortality in Australia.

and their actual impact on people's health. Some of the proven interventions included a 30% increase in tax on tobacco. In the May 2010 budget, the federal government increased the tax on tobacco by 25% and on alcohol by 10%. In December 2013, a further 12.5% tax on tobacco—a rise on a packet of 20 cigarettes of $2.50—was implemented. On 1 July 2014, there was an increase in the tax on beer and spirits—29 cents per 'slab' (24 cans) of full-strength beer, and 11 cents per slab of light beer (Australian Government Department of Health 2014b).

Principles of health promotion

> **REFLECTION 14.1**
>
> Did you consider that it is difficult for people to change their behaviour and that education alone may not be enough motivation? Health education is only one aspect of health promotion, and community change requires numerous strategies in a variety of settings. If your group thought that more people were interested in alternative paths to wellness, what does this mean for the education of health professionals or health science students?

In 1986, the WHO declared a set of principles that underpinned health promotion: '... "health" as the extent to which an individual or group is able ... to realise aspirations and satisfy needs; and ... to change or cope with the environment' (Health Promotion International 1986 p 73). The principles underpinning health promotion are:

- Health promotion involves the population as a whole in the context of their everyday life, rather than focusing on people at risk for specific diseases.
- Health promotion is directed towards action on the determinants or causes of health.
- Health promotion combines diverse, but complementary, methods or approaches, including communication, education, legislation, fiscal measures, organisational change, community development, and spontaneous local activities against health hazards.
- Health promotion aims particularly at effective and concrete public participation.

Health professionals, particularly in primary healthcare, have an important role in nurturing and enabling health promotion (WHO 1984 p 20).

The *Ottawa Charter for Health Promotion* (WHO 1986) used the WHO (1984) health promotion principles as a foundation for five action areas. The specific prerequisites for health were 'peace, shelter, education, food, income, a stable ecosystem, sustainable resources, social justice and equity' (WHO 1986 p 1). These prerequisites are still the cornerstone for health actions. Health was seen as a 'resource for everyday life, not the object of living' (WHO 1986 p 1). This represents a positive concept of health instead of it merely being the absence of disease. The definition of health promotion was to 'enable people to take control over their health'. The concept of empowerment was implicit in health promotion, and was described as 'a process through which people gain greater control over decisions and actions affecting their health' (WHO 1998). The role of health professionals in health promotion is to practise *with* people not *on* them.

The Ottawa Charter (WHO 1986) was based on the social democratic principles of justice, equity and access. This translates to a public health practice that addresses the determinants of ill health in societies. There are five essential actions (see Figure 14.1):

1 *Build public policies that support health*—Health promotion goes beyond healthcare (e.g. hospitals that treat the sick) and makes health an agenda item for policymakers in all areas of governmental and organisational action. The aim must be to make healthier choices easier.

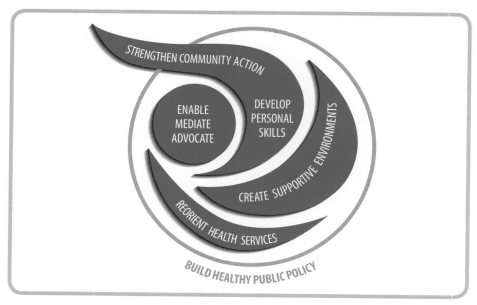

FIG. 14.1   The Ottawa Charter emblem for health promotion.
(Source: WHO 1986)

2 *Create supportive environments*—Health promotion recognises that, at both the global and the local levels, human health is tied to nature and the environment. Societies that exploit their environments without attention to ecology reap the effects of that exploitation in ill health and social problems. Health promotion must create living and working conditions that are safe, stimulating, satisfying and enjoyable.

3 *Strengthen community action*—Health promotion works through effective community action. Communities need to have control of their own initiatives and activities. Health professionals must learn new ways of working with individuals and communities—working *for* and *with*, rather than *on*, them.

4 *Develop personal skills*—Health promotion supports personal and social development through providing information and education for health, and by helping people to develop the skills they need to make healthy choices.

5 *Reorient health services*—The responsibility for health promotion in health services is shared among individuals, community groups, health professionals, medical care workers, bureaucracies and governments (WHO 1986).

Here are some examples of the application of these action areas to contemporary health problems:

- *Building public policies that support health*—Government policies developed to prevent smoking through banning smoking in workplaces, public transport, hospitals and schools.
- *Create supportive environments*—Actions to ensure sustainable physical environments; for example, not building housing on toxic landfills, or ensuring a safe working environment through workplace health programs.

	TABLE 14.1 WHO Global health promotion conferences	
Year	Place	Theme/scope
1986	Ottawa, Canada	Action to achieve Health for All by the year 2000 and beyond (WHO 1986)
1988	Adelaide, Australia	Healthy public policy (WHO 1988)
1991	Sundsvall, Sweden	Creating supportive environments for health (WHO 1991)
1997	Jakarta, Indonesia	Partnerships and settings (WHO 1997)
2000	Mexico City, Mexico	Bridging the equity gap, with a focus on the determinants of health (WHO 2000)
2005	Bangkok, Thailand	'… identifies actions, commitments and pledges required to address the determinants of health in a globalized world through health promotion' (WHO 2005)
2009	Nairobi, Kenya	'Promoting health and development: closing the implementation gap' (WHO 2009)
2013	Helsinki, Finland	'Health in All Policies' (HiAP) and how to implement them (WHO 2013)

- *Strengthen community action*—Health professionals who work with and advocate for newly arrived refugee communities to ensure that health services are accessible and that interpreters are available.
- *Develop personal skills*—Health professionals who educate diabetic patients about managing their diabetes.
- *Reorienting health services*—Integrating a health promotion orientation within health services. This could require staff development and organisational support for such change. In some hospitals, individual lifestyle assessments are conducted during the patient intake process, and when follow-up post-hospital discharge is undertaken.

Since 1986, the WHO global conferences focusing on health promotion have been held regularly, each exploring specific aspects of health promotion (see Table 14.1).

These conferences and actions provide frameworks for propelling continued action for advancing health. They continue to embed the principles of health promotion as an integral part of public health.

Aboriginal and Torres Strait Islander peoples' concepts of health promotion

For Aboriginal and Torres Strait Islander people, 'health' is interlinked with families, communities and land, and so health promotion needs to consider the individual, family and community. Health professionals need to understand the dynamics of the cultures of Aboriginal and Torres Strait Islander peoples and be culturally competent.

Health promotion uses a primary healthcare and a 'strength-based' approach to improve health in communities. A primary healthcare approach integrates 'both an individual and the population' (Couzos & Murray 2003 p xxxi). 'Primary healthcare', according to the National Aboriginal Community Controlled Health Organisation (NACCHO), is designed as 'essential, integrated care based upon scientifically sound and socially acceptable procedures and technology made accessible to communities (as close as possible to where they live) through their full participation, in the spirit of self-reliance and self-determination' (Couzos & Murray 2003 p xxxii). There are more than 150 (NACCHO website) Aboriginal community-controlled health services (ACCHSs) that are managed by boards of elected Aboriginal members. These ACCHSs offer integrated care for the community through individual treatment and promotion programs, as well as extensive community health screening and health promotion programs. The ACCHS organisations exemplify how health services mix successfully the incorporation of medical services and health promotion, and thus enact the 'reorienting health services' action step from the Ottawa Charter. Case Study 14.1 illustrates the application of reorienting health services in the Townsville Mums and Bubs Program.

CASE STUDY 14.1

Aboriginal and Torres Strait Islander peoples' health promotion

The Townsville Aboriginal and Islander Health Services' *Mums and Babies Program* illustrates 'developing personal skills', 'reorienting health services' and 'creating supportive environments' towards their goal of improving the health of young mothers and children in Townsville.

The program was established in 2000—a morning clinic for pregnant women and young mothers—with limited staff (two doctors, two health workers, a childcare worker and a driver). The service responded to 'long waiting times and a historically unwelcoming hospital environment that had kept many Indigenous women from using mainstream health services' (Panaretto 2007 p 8). In the first month, the service saw 40 clients; in 2001, there were 500 clients a month, and now there is a purpose-built family-friendly centre with a growing number of clients from outside Townsville. There has been a reduction in low-birth-weight babies (<2500 g, Panaretto et al. 2007) from 16% to 11.7%; and mean birth weights have increased by 170 g; perinatal deaths have fallen from 58 per thousand to 22 per thousand. 'We wanted to create an environment where women felt comfortable, treated as people and where they could bring children along' (Panaretto 2007 p 8). Additional programs were added: encouraging breastfeeding, nutrition support, increasing immunisation rates, and monitoring healthy child development. In 2014, a new building was opened to accommodate the staff needed for this growing program. This program demonstrates health promotion in action, in a supportive health service where the majority of the staff are Indigenous. Shanahan (2010) highlighted the strong concept of self-determination and empowerment that underpins this community-controlled initiative. Additionally, immunisation services are provided through collaboration with child health nurses from Queensland Health's Townsville Hospital and Health Service.

Brough et al. (2004) argue that health promotion with Aboriginal and Torres Strait Islander peoples should begin with the 'strengths' that exist within communities, rather than a more traditional approach that focuses on 'deficits', such as people's unhealthy behaviours. The authors asked over 100 Aboriginal and Torres Strait Islander people in urban Brisbane to identify the strengths in their community. Five key strengths were identified: extended family, commitment to community, neighbourhood networks, community organisations, and community events. These community 'assets' laid the foundation on which to strengthen existing initiatives, such as 'the provision of a youth nutrition program in an Indigenous youth organisation' (Brough et al. 2004 p 219). This approach clearly links with the Ottawa Charter's action step 'strengthen community action'. For a comprehensive discussion on Aboriginal and Torres Strait Islander peoples' health, see Chapter 16.

One principle of health promotion is that the strategies need to be intersectoral and engage participants, as the focus of health promotion is to 'enable all people to achieve their fullest potential' (WHO 1986). The WHO articulated a broad range of approaches to health promotion:

- Changing public and corporate policies to make them conducive to health, and reorienting health services towards the maintenance and development of health in the population, regardless of current health status.
- Developing an environment conducive to health, especially in conditions at work, at home and in the community. Since this environment is dynamic, health promotion involves the monitoring and assessment of technological, cultural and economic influences on health.
- Health promotion should strengthen social networks and social support. This recognises the importance of social forces and relationships as determinants of values and behaviour relevant to health, and as significant resources for coping with stress and maintaining health.
- Promoting healthy lifestyles gives consideration to personal coping strategies and dispositions, as well as to beliefs and values relevant to health, all shaped by lifelong experiences and living conditions.
- Providing information and education assists people to make informed decisions about their health choices (Health Promotion International 1986).

ACTIVITY 14.2 Reducing alcohol- or drug-related violence

- With a group of students, apply the five action steps of the Ottawa Charter (WHO 1986) for reducing alcohol- or drug-related violence in or outside night club precincts in your capital city. (See the bullet points to the left of this Activity for tips.) Begin by researching whether there have been national recommendations on the issue, explore your state or territory's approach, and identify evidence that particular strategies are effective. Can you assess which combination of the five action steps of the Ottawa Charter (WHO 1986) are the most effective?
- Explain how the concepts of health and health promotion in Aboriginal and Torres Strait Islander peoples' communities may differ from those of non-Indigenous people.
- If you are a non-Indigenous health professional working in an Aboriginal and Torres Strait Islander community, what influence would a strength-based approach have on your professional practice?
- How would you use the definition of health as a 'resource for every life' (WHO 1986 p 1) in a nutrition program when working with a group of homeless young people?

REFLECTION 14.2

In alcohol-related violence at night club precincts, you can see how extensive the application of the five action steps can be. There are differences in Aboriginal and Torres Strait Islander peoples' and non-Indigenous concepts of health promotion because of the significance of ties to the land and community for Aboriginal and Torres Strait Islander peoples, and therefore a particular focus on local community-based services and building on cultural assets within communities.

Nutbeam (2008a) provides some commentary on how the Ottawa Charter (WHO 1986) would appear if written now. Health promotion 'will almost certainly involve partnership with the private sector in ways that were inconceivable in 1986' (Nutbeam 2008a p 437). For example, a range of businesses promote fund-raising for breast cancer research through selling pink ribbons and sponsoring fun-runs. Several years ago, such promotions would have received scant attention in the media.

If we use 'supportive environments for health' to focus on the physical environment, climate change and environmental damage were primarily the domain of environmentalists. Now, these professionals collaborate, because degradation of rainforests increases mosquito-borne disease, and climate change alters ocean flows, with the consequential depletion of fish stocks and therefore food resources. (See Chapter 12 for more on environmental health.) But it is the area of the globalisation of trade, and its influence on health in many countries, that challenges the building of a national healthy public policy, which demonstrates the impact on population health of 'national public policies' (Nutbeam 2008a p 436).

Jackson et al. (2006) analysed eight reviews of the efficacy and cost-effectiveness of health action areas of the Ottawa Charter. Significant lessons are:

- *Investment in building healthy public policy is a key strategy*—'investment in government and social policy, creation of legislation and regulations and intersectoral and inter-organisational partnerships and collaboration' (Jackson et al. 2006 p 76). Multiple strategies and actions are needed. Road safety legislation is an example.
- *Supportive environments need to be created at all levels*—For example, in a youth health promotion program, multiple strategies to ensure counselling and outreach, and the involvement of parents and other professionals, are necessary (Jackson et al 2006).

Successful health promotion actions featured the following elements:

- *Intersectoral collaboration and inter-organisational partnerships at all levels*—Develop strategic partnerships with like-minded organisations to solve health issues.
- *Community participation and engagement in planning and decision-making*—Engage clients in design, implementation and evaluation. For example, survey users of a multicultural health service to ensure that the hours of opening are suitable for their needs and that interpreters are available if necessary.

Strategies for health promotion

Multiple strategies are used in health promotion: individual counselling and group work; development of print and web-based interactive sites; individual tracking on smart phones; social marketing television campaigns; patient, health professional and community special-interest advocacy, political lobbying, policy and legislative changes; and the development of networks.

Social marketing in Australia has been used successfully in a number of campaigns. Social marketing is 'the application of commercial marketing techniques to the achievement of socially desirable goals' (Egger et al. 2005 p 96); these are used in Australia to raise awareness of specific health issues. 'Slip, Slop, Slap, Seek, Slide' is one of Australia's best-known health slogans, and has played a key role in producing a dramatic shift in sun protection attitudes and behaviour (Cancer Council Australia website 2013). Donovan and Henley (2003, in Egger et al. 2005) propose that while campaigns target families as 'consumers' of junk food, these campaigns should simultaneously target food manufacturers to reduce the fat and sugar content in their products, and to stop advertising such products during children's television programs. To demonstrate the impact of social marketing and other strategies, we examine tobacco control.

The most successful nations at reducing smoking prevalence (indicated by total population smoking rates) are Sweden, Canada, Australia and the United States, with rates of between 16% and 20% (Chapman 2007). Tobacco control is one of the most successful public health efforts in Australia, through the use of integrated, broad-based and consistent approaches (WHO Tobacco Free Initiative website 2011) (see Case Study 14.2 and Figure 14.2). These achievements in tobacco control are the result of a variety of strategies (see Box 14.1).

Tobacco smoking still presents challenges for public health. In the past, tobacco companies lured young people through messages that made tobacco smoking 'cool'. Professor Ian Olver of the Cancer Council Australia raised concerns about the sale of

---

CASE STUDY 14.2

Tobacco control

In Australia, smoking rates have been declining for several decades. A report by the Australian Institute of Health and Welfare (Australian Institute of Health and Welfare (AIHW) 2014) demonstrates this steady decline by referring to the latest National Drug Strategy Household Survey, conducted in 2013, which showed that in 2013 approximately 2.5 million Australians (aged 14 years and over) smoked daily; however, there was a reduction in the amount of tobacco smoked by more than one in three smokers, and more than 'a month before the survey' 20% had successfully stopped smoking (AIHW 2014 p 27). More men smoke daily than women (18% and 15.2%, respectively), and, significantly, more than half of the population had never smoked (55.4%). 'Different groups in the population were more likely than others to smoke—those unemployed (32%), unable to work (33.7%), living in areas with the least socioeconomic resources (25.9) and Indigenous Australians (34%)' (AIHW 2010 p 84).

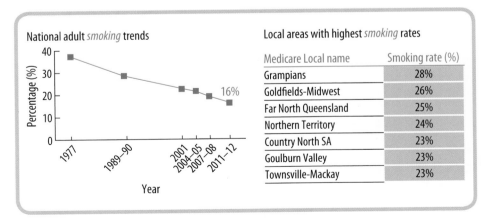

FIG. 14.2   Tobacco smoking rates across Australia, 2011–12.
(Source: National Health Performance Authority, 2013)

BOX 14.1

AUSTRALIAN TOBACCO CONTROL STRATEGIES

- *Harm reduction*—'Australian advocates were among the first to arrange for the tar and nicotine content of cigarettes to be tested' (Chapman & Wakefield 2001 p 275).
- *Advertising bans*—'Australia was one of the first democracies to ban all tobacco advertising and sponsorship' (Chapman & Wakefield 2001 p 275).
- *Pack warnings & plain packaging*—Since 1 December 2012, cigarettes and tobacco 'must be in plain packaging and be labelled with the new and expanded health warnings' (Australian Government Department of Health 2014a).
- *Mass-reach campaigns*—Mass community antismoking campaigns were one of the first, and were countered forcefully by the tobacco industry (Chapman & Wakefield 2001).
- *Civil disobedience*—'Health and community activists "graffitied" tobacco billboards' (Chapman & Wakefield 2001 p 276), focusing on the harm the tobacco industry was causing.
- *Smokeless tobacco*—South Australia banned smokeless tobacco in 1986. This was a world-first. All states followed. Similarly, South Australia banned small 'kiddie' packs (fewer than 20 cigarettes) (Chapman & Wakefield 2001).
- *Tax*—'Australia has a relatively high tobacco tax', with intense lobbying against this by the tobacco industry (Chapman & Wakefield 2001 p 276). Worldwide, Australians pay the second-highest price for a pack of cigarettes (behind Norway); however, relative to income, cigarette prices in Australia are among the cheapest (World Lung Foundation).
- *Replacement of tobacco sponsorship*—Victoria paved the way by establishing the Victorian Health Promotion Foundation (VicHealth), which was funded by an extra tax on tobacco. This enabled 'the buyout of tobacco sponsorships'—that is, tobacco advertisements were replaced by messages about skin cancer prevention and quitting smoking (Chapman & Wakefield 2001 p 285).
- *Clean indoor air*—'Australia has one of the highest rates of smoke-free workplaces' and environments, such as restaurants, bars and clubs, and all public transport (Chapman & Wakefield 2001 p 276).
- *Subsidised nicotine replacement therapy (NRT) for all*—1 x 12-week supply each year, on the Pharmaceutical Benefit Scheme, even cheaper for concession card holders (Australian Government Department of Health website).

---

non-nicotine electronic cigarettes (e-cigs) to young people; he stated that there are risks to 're-normalising' cigarette use in young people with various vapour flavours, such as fruit juice, energy drinks and the flavour of tobacco (Olver 2014). The e-cigarette is a device that converts liquid into a vapour, and is inhaled in the same way that a cigarette is smoked ('vaping'). E-cigarettes (non-nicotine) are not tested, and can be purchased over the counter at service stations and some clubs. 'Unlike Nicotine Replacement

Therapy (NRT) that has been rigorously assessed for efficacy and safety, and … approved by the Therapeutic Goods Administration (TGA) for use as an aid in withdrawal from smoking, no assessment of electronic cigarettes has been undertaken' (Therapeutic Goods Administration 2014). However, such products containing nicotine have been promoted to assist with quitting tobacco smoking, and are available online and so therefore difficult to control. Moreover, the Victorian Poisons Information Centre stated that the service had nine calls in 2013 about nicotine poisoning related to e-cigarettes, including five cases involving children aged one to four years (Hagan 2014).

In light of this, the federal Department of Health (2014c) is now examining a regulatory framework governing e-cigarettes. It will use the World Health Organization's Framework Convention on Tobacco Control Treaty as a guide. This treaty aims to protect present and future citizens from the health, social and economic consequences of tobacco smoking and its exposure.

Public health officials in the United States are also concerned about the impact of e-cigarettes on youth. In the United States, e-cigarettes with and/or without nicotine are easily available and are advertised on television and through other media channels. The United States Food and Drug Administration's Center for Tobacco Products (Food and Drug Administration (FDA) 2014) is proposing an extension of its jurisdiction over nicotine-related devices, including e-cigarettes. The director has stated that 'any use of a tobacco or a nicotine-containing product by young people is detrimental to public health' (FDA 2014). Vapour device sales (including non-nicotine devices) in the United States were estimated to have reached $2.5 billion in 2014 (PACT website).

The next section extends our discussions on health promotion by seeing how it is linked across various levels of prevention.

> ### REFLECTION 14.3 E-cigarettes
>
> What views do you have about increasing sales of vapour devices that do not contain nicotine? Do you agree with Professor Olver that these devices create risks of re-normalising tobacco smoking? What are the challenges for the federal Department of Health in developing a framework for e-cigarettes?

> ### ACTIVITY 14.4 Strategies for healthy change
>
> - Would the decline in tobacco smoking in Australia have been achieved without the identified actions? How could some of these strategies be applied more intensively to groups that are socioeconomically disadvantaged? For guidance, see Chapter 7. What strategies worked in the Mums and Babies Program in Townsville?

> ### REFLECTION 14.4
>
> Did you note that the decline in tobacco smoking has taken many years and concerted efforts? Often in health promotion, there are expectations that population health change is simple and can be done quickly. Did you find that the strategies that worked in Townsville utilised a unified approach across services?

Levels of prevention in public health and health promotion

The health promotion paradigm is one of prevention at three levels: primary, secondary and tertiary (see Figure 14.3). *Primary prevention* 'refers to strategies to reduce incidence and prevent occurrence of poor health' (Oldenburg et al. 2004 p 218). These include tobacco control measures, such as banning cigarette advertising in all media, and implementing legislation or public policies that will assist people to make 'healthy choices'. Strategies such as these are sometimes called *upstream strategies*, as they work on creating healthy public policy. *Secondary prevention* aims at detecting and curing the disease before it causes symptoms—for example, cervical cancer screening. *Tertiary prevention* aims at minimising the consequences for a patient who already has a disease,

	Primary prevention	**Secondary prevention**	**Tertiary prevention**
Target group	Healthy individuals Whole populations	Individuals at risk The early stages of a condition	Individuals with the condition Conditions that have already occurred
Aim	Prevent occurrence Reduce incidence	Prevent progression Slow progression Minimise duration Risk reduction	Minimise complications Optimise functioning Limit recurrence
Strategies	Promote health-enhancing and preventive practices Create supportive environments Develop healthy public policy	Screening Early detection Early intervention Risk assessment and reduction	Treatment or rehabilitation Reduce psychological, social, physical distress Enhance support networks Enhance self-management

FIG. 14.3   The relationship between primary, secondary and tertiary levels of prevention. (Reproduced by permission of Oxford University Press Australia from Cromar, N., Cameron, S., & Fallowfield, H., Environmental health in Australia and New Zealand © 2004 Oxford University Press)

such as cardiac rehabilitation programs for heart disease (Couzos & Murray 2003 p xxxv).

Health promotion in practice

Settings for health promotion

'A setting refers to a socially and culturally defined geographical and physical area of factual social interaction, and a socially and culturally defined set of patterns of interaction to be performed while in the setting' (Wenzel 1997). Thus, a health service could be the focal point for health education television programs in waiting rooms; schools can promote healthy messages for children; workplaces could offer healthy options in canteens. Additionally, in shopping centres, it is not uncommon to see blood glucose testing booths promoting diabetes prevention, healthy heart information programs, and walking programs.

WHY A SETTINGS APPROACH?

Health is promoted where people live, work and play. A settings approach also aligns with a population health approach, rather than merely a focus on individuals. Some of the initial thinking about a settings approach stemmed from the work of Hancock and Duhl (1988) who began working on the concept of the 'healthy city'—a setting where health opportunities or lack of them occurred. This work was extended to include settings outside the health system or health services, such as sport and recreation facilities, service clubs, prisons, shopping malls, and hair salons.

Schools

Kolbe (2005) claimed that schools have the potential to do more than any other single agency in society to help young people live healthier, longer and more satisfying and productive lives. An emphasis on healthy food has seen tuckshops change their food selections, fruit and vegetables grown in schoolyards, and sun protection programs enacted. Visiting dental staff promote tooth-brushing and provide regular check-ups. Positive emotional health programs are integrated into teacher training, and anti-bullying policies are common. Sustainable environments are encouraged through planting trees, learning to be 'water wise' and recycling.

The *Health Promoting Schools* (HPS) framework has guidelines for development (International Union for Health Promotion and Education 2008): integrate the school health curriculum, the school ethos, school health policies and practices, the community in which the school resides, and the school environment (physical, social and emotional); promote the development of students' skills and understanding of taking care of their own health; and emphasise that local health services should be a partner in developing a health promoting school. An HPS focuses on:

- 'caring for oneself and others
- making healthy decisions and taking control over life's circumstances
- creating conditions that are conducive to health (through policies, services, physical/social conditions)
- building capacities for peace, shelter, education, food, income, a stable ecosystem, equity, social justice, sustainable development
- preventing leading causes of death, disease and disability: helminths, tobacco use, HIV/AIDS/STDs, sedentary lifestyle, drugs and alcohol, violence and injuries, unhealthy nutrition
- influencing health-related behaviours: knowledge, beliefs, skills, attitudes, values, support' (WHO School and youth health website).

Lister-Sharp et al. (1999) conducted a systematic review of studies to evaluate the effectiveness of HPS programs. Their analysis showed 'that school health promotion initiatives can have a positive impact on children's health and behaviour through changes in the social and physical environment, staff development, school lunch provision and exercise programmes but do not do so consistently' (Lister-Sharp et al. 1999 p 5). Thus, clear guidelines are needed to ensure quality and consistent implementation (Samdal & Rowling 2013).

Despite the complexities of evaluating such a multifaceted approach to school health, schools do have the potential to be a vital resource in the community where children's attitudes and values about health can be formed.

Communities

'Community' in health promotion is interpreted in a number of ways. First, community can be a geographical place; secondly, groups of people who share common bonds (such as age and cultural identity) or are linked through a common cause (such as protecting the environment) can be a community. Thirdly, communities of people who are coping with the same health condition (such as cancer 'survivors') represent another type of community where health promotion is practised (Fleming & Parker 2007).

Health promotion practice varies in different communities. Community health nurses provide patient self-management in the home, and young mothers and babies' health education programs. Community nutritionists, physicians and exercise physiologists collaborate to plan healthy walking and weight control programs in health and

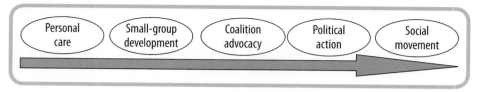

FIG. 14.4   The empowerment continuum.
(Source: Adapted from Labonte 1992, Figure 2. Labonte, R., 1992. Heart health inequalities in Canada: modules theory and planning. Health Promotion International 7 (2), 119–128.)

fitness centres. Service clubs can provide a venue for promoting cancer-screening programs, and hair salons can promote cervical and breast screening services.

Communities also need to identify their own health problems and possible solutions, thereby gaining control over the initiatives and solutions. The health professional is a facilitator of actions and solutions, and thus works as an advocate for communities. This adheres to the 'enabling' and 'advocating' approaches to health promotion, as indicated in the Ottawa Charter for Health Promotion (WHO 1986).

Strengthening community action broadens the role of the community health promotion worker, from solely providing health education and information to encouraging collaborative partnerships with communities in the development, implementation and evaluation of programs.

Community development is central to community health promotion—that is, 'working in ways that facilitate people and communities developing their strength and confidence while at the same time, addressing immediate problems' (Butler & Cass 1993 p 8). Recalling that health promotion has, at its roots, the fundamental concept of empowerment, and that practice is 'with' people not 'on' them, then the empowerment continuum is helpful in thinking about the strategies to implement to make a difference (see Figure 14.4).

In practice, it can be difficult to achieve community participation for a number of reasons. This can stem from the lack of clarity that health professionals have about the specific purpose of participation. Why are you engaging with a community? To provide feedback on your own agenda? To really listen to the community, and subsequently to be sufficiently flexible to adapt your agenda? Or to really adopt a community's agenda for health action? You should always be very clear about your purpose when you invite a community to participate in a consultative process; otherwise you are potentially raising unrealistic community expectations.

Personal care is individual care or an education/information program with individuals, such as patients. *Small-group development* can be discussion on issues of concern and needed action, or an education program could be a catalyst for broader actions. For example, a group of women in a smoking cessation program may discuss the lack of daycare facilities in their neighbourhood. Through mutual support, the group is strengthened, and friendships extended through other networks. *Coalition advocacy* is about issue identification, and joining together with other networks to build strong coalitions to bring about change. *Political action* is about working 'upstream' and engaging political support for policy change, resource allocation, research funding, networking and advocacy. For example, without the grass-roots activism, sound research, advocacy and lobbying, the policy changes on smoking, and the subsequent reduction in tobacco-smoking rates, would not have occurred. *Social movement* refers to the swell in activity and the changing community consciousness of issues. Environmental issues and the concept of sustainability were quite alien terms for the majority of Australians 50 years ago—the domain of radicals! Fast-forward, and climate change, destruction of forests and the shortage of water are now on the political agenda.

Workplaces

Promoting health in the workplace is good for business, because healthy workers are productive workers. Many workplace health promotion programs complement, and are integrated with, the occupational health and safety programs. Since legislative change in Australia in the 1980s, there has been a *duty of care* imposed on employers to provide a safe and healthy working environment for their employees, and to train some employees as occupational health and safety representatives (National Health Strategy Unit 1993); this has led to an increase in workplace health promotion programs.

Workplace health promotion programs can include the provision of daycare centres, healthy food options in the canteen, employee health checks, gymnasiums, and employee assistance programs. Hess et al. (2011) implemented a workplace nutrition and physical activity promotion program, using pedometers, for workers at Liverpool Hospital. Overall, the program improved participants' physical activity levels and diets (Hess et al. 2011).

Australians spend approximately one-third of their life at work. A comprehensive workplace strategy has clearly defined policies, builds organisational and individual efficacy (empowerment), eliminates unnecessary organisational stress, and commits to and works towards a healthier organisational culture (Dooner 1990–91).

The internet and interactive technologies

The internet is a setting for health promotion. The explosion in the growth of social media tools, such as Facebook, Twitter, blogs, wikis, YouTube, chat rooms, SMS messaging, telephone-assisted devices (TADs), smart phones, and self-tracking devices, expand the repertoire for all health professionals. The worldwide upsurge of social media through Twitter, special Facebook pages and phone texting was evident during the 2011 natural disasters in Australia and unfolding political crises worldwide. Mobile phones and smart phones have transformed communication. Access to the internet at home has risen. For the period 2012–13, 7.3 million Australian households had 'access to the internet at home', which is 83% of all Australian households, an increase from 79% in 2010–11 (Australian Bureau of Statistics 2014).

Consumers can converse with each other and with health professionals, and search for information through these media. These health information pages, some of dubious quality, 'represent passive, non-intrusive attempts at promoting health online' (McFarlane et al. 2005 S60). Health consumers are becoming educated about their own illnesses; this can present a challenge to health professionals, whose traditional role was to know more than their patients. There are interactive online outreach programs—for example, in Houston, Texas, the Montrose Clinic staff conduct online outreach through an instant messaging chat room for question and answers, information and referrals as part of *Project CORE* (Cyber OutReach Education) in a sexually transmitted disease program (McFarlane et al. 2005 p S60), and Ybarra and Bull (2007) claimed the internet and cell phones as plausible communication technologies in HIV programs. In a review of 21 international studies on the use of smart phones by professionals and patients, the majority of apps were for nutrition (calorie counting and food diaries) and physical exercise (Bert et al. 2014). Possible risks related to the use of these apps include inadequate monitoring of content and data confidentiality

TLC Diabetes Project

The *Telelphone-Linked Care (TLC) Diabetes Project* is a computer-based, interactive telephone system that acts as an educator, monitor and counsellor for patients between ages 18 and70 years diagnosed with type 2 diabetes. Patients will be randomised to either routine care or the TLC intervention for six months. Using sophisticated speech recognition software, the interactive telephone system receives calls from diabetic patients using a regular phone, and provides information and feedback to these patients. This telehealth system is designed to educate, monitor and coach patients to improve self-care behaviours essential to diabetes management. These behaviours include nutrition, physical activity, blood glucose testing, and using medication as prescribed. The system is being trialled in Brisbane (Bird et al. 2010).

systems (Bert et al. 2014). Ding et al. (2013) designed an app called ManUp, targeting physical activity lifestyle modifications for middle-aged men because of the prevalence of chronic diseases. Motivational feedback via SMS messages is provided. ManUp is being trialled currently in Queensland. There is a surge in wearable self-improvement tracking devices, such as Fitbit. These tools can keep track of a person's sleep patterns, heart rate and numbers of daily walking/running steps. Could this 'quantified self' movement be a way of the future in health promotion? Bottles (2012 p 74) believes that members of this group share 'a belief that gathering and analysing data about their everyday activities can help them improve their lives'. He suggests that users are an eclectic mix of 'early adopters, fitness freaks, technology evangelists … and patients with a wide variety of health problems' (Bottles 2012 p 74).

Case Study 14.3 provides an example of one of these communication technologies.

Bennett and Glasgow (2009) conducted a major assessment of the potential of the internet for public health interventions, with some evidence that online 'quit smoking' support programs are an effective mechanism to recruit and support individuals who wish to quit smoking.

Interactive technologies can be used for advocacy purposes. For example, GetUp! is a community-based advocacy organisation that gives Australians opportunities to get involved in the political process by sending emails to politicians on topics of community concern, or raising issues in the media (see Case Study 14.4). Social media is an innovative platform for individual and community engagement. Neiger et al. (2012) outline potential key performance indicators and evaluation metrics for social media in health promotion. These will assist you in designing robust programs.

ACTIVITY 14.5 Technology and health promotion

- What other settings and interactive technologies can you identify that might be useful for health promotion actions? At what level of the empowerment continuum would your health promotion practice be situated? Write a sentence describing the three levels of prevention.

- What health apps do you have on your smart phone or tablet? Which, if any, do you use? How would you integrate and monitor an app in a health promotion program related to your profession?

- What are the strengths and limitations of individually-focused self-tracking apps? To guide your answer, recall that health promotion is a holistic practice that embraces multiple strategies to be effective.

Blogging

The skilful use of online communication in health promotion was used in the study by Carroll et al. (2008) to assess whether there was an association between living environments and the physical activity of residents from low socioeconomic backgrounds who had recently moved into a mixed urban environment that featured amenities such as walking paths, parks and a pool.

A blog was used to gather information from 16 newly settled female adult residents who had little, if any, familiarity with the internet. However, after a short training period they became adept not only with technology, but with the freedom that a blog as a communication tool provides to speak openly about the barriers, and as enablers to physical activity in their lives. The blog provided a venue for anonymous postings of responses to research questions, and the opportunity to view others' comments, and, for the researchers, an opportunity to analyse the collective responses.

Interactive technologies are transforming the way health professionals deliver health education and promotion programs. They provide an exciting repertoire of communication and engagement tools for education and promotion, and they steer health promotion research and data gathering in new directions. See the blog for more information: http://theeffectsofanewurbancontextonhealth.blogspot.com/.

(Source: Carroll et al. 2008)

Emerging challenges for health promotion

In this final section, we present some future challenges for health promotion and health education. Despite the plethora of information about being and maintaining health or wellness, disparities in health status within the Australian population persist. For example, there are still cases of trachoma (eye disease) in remote Aboriginal and Torres Strait Islander communities. This health issue is virtually unheard of in other developed countries, so one of the challenges of health promotion within public health is to maintain a steady focus on addressing the social determinants of health (Marmot 2003, WHO 2007).

> **REFLECTION 14.5**
>
> You can think about settings as the place people live, work or play, and can be creative in planning your approach. Night clubs, sporting clubs, the streets, parks, and beaches are possible settings. Remember to match the technology to the skill level of the population you are targeting. The empowerment continuum will help you think about where your program starting point is, and how it expands opportunities for strategic community engagement.

Another current health promotion challenge is diabetes. McKinlay and Marceau (2000) present a succinct overview of diabetes mellitus in the United States as a focal point within the 'new public health'. They claim that there are three levels of public health intervention used to address the challenge of diabetes. *Downstream or curative efforts* consume most of the available resources; *midstream or primary and secondary prevention* is about community-based primary prevention programs such as diet and exercise. However, *upstream or healthy public policies* are required if there is to be a change in the patterns of diabetes-related mortality and morbidity. Figure 14.5 illustrates points of intervention for a new public health approach to diabetes. As a future

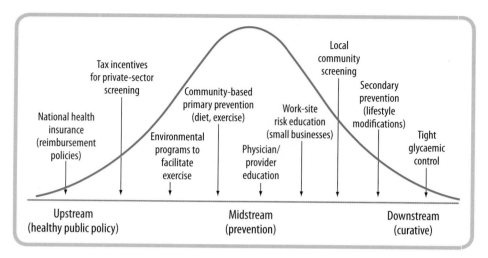

FIG. 14.5   Some possible points of intervention for a new public health approach to diabetes, given the distribution of risk.

(Source: Reprinted from McKinlay, L., Marceau, L., 2000. US public health and the 21st century: diabetes mellitus. Lancet 356 (9231), 757–761, with permission from Elsevier.)

health professional, do you see yourself working in the upstream (healthy public policy), midstream (prevention) or downstream (curative) area?

Health education faces challenges. Nutbeam (2008b) argues that health education has evolved into a new form. We have termed this the 'new health education'. Literacy is obviously a common term in education—the ability to read, write and comprehend. There are three forms of health literacy. The first is *functional literacy*, which is 'sufficient basic skills in reading and writing to be able to function effectively in everyday situations' (Nutbeam 2000 p 263). The roots of health literacy stem from clinical care and public health (Nutbeam 2008b). Patients need to be able to read prescriptions and labels, and directions for home healthcare. With over 100 languages spoken in Australia, English is not the first language of many. Thus, functional literacy enables better access to health services and health information. The second is *communicative/interactive literacy*—the ability to engage in everyday activities, and to apply new information and skills to exert greater control over their changing circumstances (Nutbeam 2008b). The third, *critical literacy*, presupposes advanced cognitive and social skills, and the ability to analyse information to be able to exert control over life events. It is the bedrock for personal and community empowerment, as people then have the skills, abilities and confidence to make changes to their lives and circumstances. Education and health can work together to further health literacies within the community. Internet-based technologies can aid in skills development, not only in functional literacies—reading and writing and understanding—but also in communicative and critical literacies.

Self-management

An ageing population, an increase in chronic diseases—such as diabetes, mental health problems, cancer, arthritis and chronic heart disease—and the increasingly complex care needs in communities have an impact on current and future health promotion practice. Health professionals need to be conversant with self-management theories and practices in their work with patients. Skills in motivational interviewing will be needed (Rollnick et al. 1999). Expanded scopes of practice may be required through mixed general practices, community health centres, hospitals and the non-government sector, in designing programs to keep people in their homes as long as possible, and for educating patients/clients about managing their conditions. This self-management practice can include those technologies discussed in this chapter. The context for health promotion practice is, therefore, a dynamic one.

A final word

Health promotion, as part of the 'new public health', focuses on *enabling* people to take control of their health. Its main focus is on addressing the determinants of health through upstream policy advocacy and downstream personal skills development, community empowerment and action; and it works through developing strategic partnerships across sectors to create health opportunities for all.

From its earliest roots in health education to the contemporary comprehensive approach across the prevention continuum, health professionals embrace health promotion knowledge and skills to make a difference to the health of individuals, communities and populations.

ACTIVITY 14.6 Health promotion strategies

- Define 'upstream' and 'downstream' strategies, by examining Figure 14.5. Why is health literacy important for a changing demographic in Australia? With a group of students, write your own definitions of 'self-management'.
- Name three other settings for health promotion practice that have not been presented.

REFLECTION 14.6

The upstream and downstream strategies illustrated through the diabetes example (Figure 14.5) can be applied to other health issues, such as mental health. Such schemata provide a framework for thinking about how you can plan a number of strategies.

Did you think about the changing multicultural profile of Australians, and how we make assumptions about people's ability to comprehend the health information available? With the increasing emphasis being placed on patients to understand and manage their own chronic diseases, it is important to understand self-management.

REVIEW QUESTIONS

1 What, if any, are the differences between 'health education', 'wellness' and 'health promotion'?

2 What are the strengths of using a 'settings' approach for health promotion?

3 Is there a role for health promotion for most health professionals?

4 What is meant by the 'new health education'?

5 How do the levels of prevention influence the choice of health promotion strategies in developing a health promotion program?

6 Define 'health literacy'. Name three assumptions we make about people's literacy levels.

7 What are the strengths and limitations of digital technologies in promoting health literacy?

8   What does it mean to focus on strengths rather than deficits in Aboriginal and Torres Strait Islander health promotion, and how could this approach be used more widely?

9   Discuss with a group of students your role in health promotion in the future.

10 How can the Ottawa Charter for Health Promotion framework be utilised to address adult obesity in Australia?

Useful websites

- Australian Health Promotion Association: http://www.healthpromotion.org.au
- Victoria Health Promotion Foundation: http://www.vichealth.vic.gov.au

References

Australian Bureau of Statistics, 2014. 8146.0—Household use of information technology, Australia, 2012–2013. Online. Available: <http://www.abs.gov.au/ausstats/abs@.nsf/Lookup/8146.0Chapter12012-13> (25 Mar 2014).

Australian Government Department of Health website. The extension of the listing of nicotine patches on the Pharmaceutical Benefits Scheme from 1 February 2011. Online. Available: <http://www.pbs.gov.au/info/publication/factsheets/shared/Extension_of_the_listing_of_nicotine_patches> (30 Oct 2014).

Australian Government Department of Health, 2014a. Plain packaging of tobacco products. Online. Available: <http://www.health.gov.au/internet/main/publishing.nsf/Content/ictstpa> (4 Sep 2014).

Australian Government Department of Health, 2014b. Taxation—the history of tobacco excise arrangements in Australia since 1901. Online. Available: <http://www.health.gov.au/internet/main/publishing.nsf/Content/tobacco-tax> (4 Sep 2014).

Australian Government Department of Health, 2014c. Tobacco product regulation and disclosure: overview of tobacco product regulation and disclosure in Australia. Online. Available: <http://www.health.gov.au/internet/main/publishing.nsf/content/tobacco-prod-reg> (17 Nov 2014).

Australian Institute of Health and Welfare, 2008. 2007 National Drug Strategy Household Survey: first results. CAT. No. PHE98. AIHW, Canberra.

Australian Institute of Health and Welfare 2010. Australia's Health 2010. Cat. No. AUS 122. AIHW, Canberra.

Australian Institute of Health and Welfare, 2014. National Drug Strategy Household Survey detailed report 2013. Drug statistics series No. 28. Cat. No. PHE 183. AIHW, Canberra.

Bennett, G., Glasgow, R., 2009. The delivery of public health interventions via the internet: actualizing their potential. Annual Review of Public Health 30, 273–292.

Bert, F., Giacometti, M., Gualano, M., et al., 2014. Smartphones and health promotion: a review of the evidence. Journal of Medical Systems 38 (1), 9995–9997.

Bird, D., Oldenburg, B., Cassimatis, M., et al., 2010. Randomised controlled trial of an automated, interactive telephone intervention to improve type 2 diabetes self-management (Telephone-Linked Care Diabetes Project): study protocol. BMC Public Health 10, 599.

Boshier, R., 1998. Malcolm Knowles, archbishop of andragogy. Adult Education Quarterly 48 (2), 64.

Bottles, K., 2012. Will the quantified self movement take off in health care? Physician Executive 38 (5), 74.

Brough, M.K., Bond, C., Hunt, J., 2004. Strong in the city: toward a strength based approach in Indigenous health promotion. Health Promotion Journal of Australia 15 (3), 215–220.

Butler, P., Cass, S. (Eds.), 1993. Case Studies of Community Development in Health. Centre for Development and Innovation in Health, Melbourne.

Cancer Council Australia website, 2013. Slip Slop Slap Seek Slide. Online. Available: <http://www.cancer.org.au/preventing-cancer/sun-protection/campaigns-and-events/slip-slop-slap-seek-slide.html> (20 Feb 2014).

Carroll, J.A., Adkins, B., Parker, E., et al., 2008. My place through my eyes: a social constructionist approach to researching the relationships between socioeconomic living contexts and physical activity. International Journal of Qualitative Studies on Health and Well-being 3 (4), 204–218.

Catford, J., 2004. Health promotion's record card: how principled are we 20 years on? Health Promotion International 19 (1), 1–4.

Catford, J., 2009. Advancing the 'science of delivery' of health promotion: not just the 'science of discovery'. Health Promotion International 24 (1), 1–5. doi:10.1093/heapro/dap003.

Chapman, S., 2007. Falling prevalence of smoking: how low can we go? Editorial. Tobacco Control 16, 145–147.

Chapman, S., Wakefield, M., 2001. Tobacco control advocacy in Australia: reflections on 30 years of progress. Health Education and Behavior 28 (3), 274–289.

Couzos, S., Murray, R., 2003. Aboriginal Primary Health Care: An Evidence-Based Approach, second ed. Oxford University Press, Melbourne.

Cromar, N., Cameron, S., Fallowfield, H. (Eds.), 2004. Environmental Health in Australia and New Zealand. Oxford University Press, Melbourne.

Ding, H., Karunanithi, M., Duncan, M., et al., 2013. A mobile phone enabled health promotion program for middle-aged males. Conference Proceedings of the IEEE Engineering in Medicine and Biology Society, 1173–1176.

Donovan, R.J., Henley, N., 2003. Social marketing: principles and practice. IP Communications, Melbourne. Cited. In: Egger, G., Spark, R., Donovan, R. (Eds.), Health Promotion Strategies and Methods, second ed. McGraw-Hill, North Ryde. 2005.

Dooner, B., 1990–91. Achieving a healthier workplace. Health Promotion Canada 29 (3), 2–6.

Egger, G., Spark, R., Donovan, R., 2005. Health Promotion Strategies and Methods, second ed. McGraw-Hill, North Ryde.

Fleming, M.L., Parker, E., 2007. Health Promotion: Principles and Practice in the Australian Context, third ed. Allen & Unwin, Crows Nest.

Food and Drug Administration, 2014. Deeming—extending authorities to additional tobacco products. Online. Available: <http://www.fda.gov/TobaccoProducts/Labeling/ucm388395.htm> (14 Nov 2014).

GetUp! Action for Australia. Online. Available: <http://www.getup.org.au/> (25 Feb 2014).

Go for 2&5® campaign: an Australian Government, state and territory health initiative. Online. Available: <http://www.gofor2and5.com.au/> (24 Feb 2014).

Hagan, K., 2014. E-cigarettes poisoning Victorian toddlers. The Age, 7 Jun 2014. Online. Available: <http://www.theage.com.au/national/ecigarettes-poisoning-victorian-toddlers-20140606-39ohu.html?skin=text-only> (17 Nov 2014).

Hancock, T., Duhl, L., 1988. Promoting Health in the Urban Context. FADL, Copenhagen.

Health Promotion International, 1986. A discussion document on the concept and principles of health promotion. Health Promotion International 1 (1), 73–76.

Hess, I., Borg, J., Riseel, C., 2011. Workplace nutrition and physical activity promotion at Liverpool Hospital. Health Promotion Journal of Australia 22 (1), 44–50.

International Union for Health Promotion and Education (IUHPE), 2008. Achieving health promoting schools: guidelines for promoting health in schools. Online. Available: <http://hps.tki.org.nz/Media/Files/Achieving-Health-Promoting-Schools-Guidelines-International-Union-for-Health-Promotion-and-Education> (19 Mar 2014).

Jackson, S., Perkin, F., Khandor, E., et al., 2006. Integrated health promotion strategies: a contribution to tackling current and future health challenges. Health Promotion International 21 (S1), 75–83.

Kolbe, L.J., 2005. A framework for school health programs in the 21st century. Journal of School Health 75 (6), 226–228.

Labonte, R., 1992. Heart health inequalities in Canada: modules theory and planning. Health Promotion International 7 (2), 119–128.

Lister-Sharp, D., Chapman, S., Stewart-Brown, S., et al., 1999. Health promoting schools and health promotion in schools: two systematic reviews. Health Technology Assessment 3 (22), 1–7.

McFarlane, M., Kachur, R., Klausner, J., et al., 2005. Internet-based health promotion and disease control in the 8 cities: successes, barriers, and future plans. Sexually Transmitted Disease 32 (10), S60–S64.

McKinlay, J., Marceau, L., 2000. US public health and the 21st century: diabetes mellitus. Lancet 356 (9231), 757–761.

Marmot, M.G., 2003. Understanding social inequalities in health. Perspectives in Biology and Medicine 46, S9–S23.

National Aboriginal Community Controlled Health Organisation (NACCHO) website. Online. Available: <http://www.naccho.org.au/about-us/> (19 Feb 2014).

National Health Performance Authority, 2013. inFocus: Healthy Communities—Tobacco smoking rates across Australia, 2011–12. Online. Available: <http://www.nhpa.gov.au/internet/nhpa/publishing.nsf/Content/Our-reports> (20 Feb 2013).

National Health Strategy Unit, 1993. Pathways to Better Health. Issues Paper No. 7. National Health Strategy Unit, Melbourne.

Neiger, B.L., Thackeray, R., Van Wagenen, S.A., et al., 2012. Use of social media in health promotion, purposes, key performance indicators, and evaluation metrics. Health Promotion Practice 13 (2), 159–164.

Nutbeam, D., 2000. Health literacy as a public health goal: a challenge for contemporary health education and communication strategies into the 21st century. Health Promotion International 15 (3), 259–267.

Nutbeam, D., 2008a. What would the Ottawa Charter look like if it were written today? Commentary. Critical Public Health 18 (4), 435–441.

Nutbeam, D., 2008b. The evolving concept of health literacy. Social Science and Medicine 67 (12), 2072–2078.

Nutbeam, D., Harris, E., Wise, M., 2010. Theory in a Nutshell: A Practical Guide to Health Promotion Theories, third ed. McGraw-Hill, Sydney.

Oldenburg, B., Burton, N., Parker, E., 2004. Health promotion and environmental health. In: Cromar, N., Cameron, S., Fallowfield, H. (Eds.), Environmental Health in Australia and New Zealand. Oxford University Press, Melbourne.

Olver, I., 2014. Extreme caution needed on electronic cigarettes. Cancer Council Australia. Online. Available: <http://www.cancer.org.au/news/blog/prevention/extreme-caution-needed-on-electronic-cigarettes.html> (14 Nov 2014).

PACT website. E-cigarettes. Online. Available: <http://www.pelhampact.org/e-cigarettes> (17 Nov 2014).

Panaretto, K., 2007. Mums and Babies Program. Australians for Native Title and Reconciliation, Success stories in Indigenous health: a showcase of successful Aboriginal and Torres Strait Islander health projects. Morprint, Rydalmere, pp 8–9.

Panaretto, K., Mitchell, M., Anderson, L., et al., 2007. Sustainable antenatal care services in an urban Indigenous community; the Townsville experience. Medical Journal of Australia 187 (1), 18–22.

Ritchie, J., 1991. From health education to education for health in Australia: a historical perspective. Health Promotion International 6 (2), 157–163.

Rollnick, S., Mason, P., Butler, C., 1999. Health Behavior Change: A Guide for Practitioners. Churchill Livingstone, London.

Samdal, O., Rowling, L., 2013. The Implementation of Health Promotion Schools—Exploring the Theories of What, Why and How. Routledge, London.

Shanahan, M., 2010. Townsville Mums and Babies Program: an actualization of Indigenous self-determination and women's empowerment. The University of Western Australia. Outskirts online journal 23.

Therapeutic Goods Administration, 2014. Electronic cigarettes. Online. Available: <http://www.tga.gov.au/community-qa/electronic-cigarettes> (17 Nov 2014).

Trust for America's Health, 2008. Prevention for a healthier America: investments in disease prevention yield significant savings, stronger communities. In: Catford, J., 2009. Advancing the 'science of delivery' of health promotion: not just the 'science of discovery'. Health Promotion International 24 (1), 1–5. doi:10.1093/heapro/dap003; Editorial.

Vartianen, E., Jousilahti, P., Alfthan, G., et al., 2000. Cardiovascular risk factor changes in Finland, 1972–1997. International Journal of Epidemiology 29, 49–56.

Vos, T., Carter, R., Barendregt, J., et al., 2010. Assessing Cost-Effectiveness in Prevention (ACE–Prevention): Final Report. University of Queensland, Brisbane, and Deakin University, Melbourne.

Wenzel, E., 1997. A comment on settings in health promotion. Internet Journal of Health Promotion. Online. Available: <http://ldb.org/setting.htm> (24 Feb 2014).

World Health Organization, 1978. Declaration of Alma-Ata. International Conference on Primary Health Care, Alma-Ata, USSR, 6–12 September 1978. WHO, Geneva. Online. Available: <http://www.who.int/publications/almaata_declaration_en.pdf> (20 Mar 2014).

World Health Organization, 1984. Health promotion: concepts and principles: report of a working group. Online. Available: <http://whqlibdoc.who.int/euro/-1993/ICP_HSR_602__m01.pdf> (24 Feb 2014).

World Health Organization, 1986. The Ottawa Charter for Health Promotion. 1st International Conference on Health Promotion, Ottawa, 21 November 1986. WHO, Geneva. Online. Available: <http://www.who.int/healthpromotion/conferences/previous/ottawa/en/> (25 Feb 2014).

World Health Organization, 1988. Adelaide Recommendations on Healthy Public Policy. Second International Conference on Health Promotion, Adelaide, South Australia, 5–9 April 1988. WHO, Geneva. Online. Available: <http://www.who.int/healthpromotion/conferences/previous/adelaide/en/index1.html> (24 Feb 2014).

World Health Organization, 1991. Sundsvall Statement on Supportive Environments for Health. 3rd International Conference on Health Promotion, Sundsvall, Sweden, 9–15 June 1991. WHO, Geneva. Online. Available: <http://www.who.int/healthpromotion/conferences/previous/sundsvall/en/> (23 Feb 2014).

World Health Organization, 1997. Jakarta Statement on Healthy Workplaces. Symposium on Healthy Workplaces at the 4th International Conference on Health Promotion (Jakarta, July 1997). WHO, Geneva. Online. Available: <http://www.who.int/healthpromotion/conferences/previous/jakarta/statements/workplaces/en/> (24 Feb 2014).

World Health Organization, 1998. Health Promotion Glossary. WHO, Geneva. Online. Available: <http://whqlibdoc.who.int/hq/1998/WHO_HPR_HEP_98.1.pdf> (19 Sep 2014).

World Health Organization, 2000. The Fifth Global Conference on Health Promotion Health Promotion: Bridging the Equity Gap 5–9th June 2000, Mexico City. WHO, Geneva. Online. Available: <http://www.who.int/healthpromotion/conferences/previous/mexico/en/> (25 Feb 2014).

World Health Organization, 2005. The Bangkok Charter for Health Promotion in a Globalized World. WHO, Geneva. Online. Available: <http://www.who.int/healthpromotion/conferences/6gchp/bangkok_charter/en/> (25 Feb 2014).

World Health Organization, 2009. The 7th Global Conference on Health Promotion Promoting Health and Development: Closing the Implementation Gap. 26–30 October 2009, Nairobi, Kenya. WHO, Geneva. Online. Available: <http://www.who.int/healthpromotion/conferences/7gchp/en/index.html> (25 Feb 2014).

World Health Organization, 2013. The 8th Global Conference on Health Promotion. Health in All Policies (HiAP). WHO, Geneva. Online. Available: <http://www.who.int/healthpromotion/conferences/8gchp/en/> (21 Feb 2014).

World Health Organisation Commission on Social Determinants of Health, 2007. Final Report. WHO, Geneva. Online. Available: <http://www.who.int/social_determinants/thecommission/finalreport/en/> (19 March 2014).

World Health Organization School and youth health website. What is a health promoting school? Online. Available: <http://www.who.int/school_youth_health/gshi/hps/en/index.html> (20 Mar 2014).

World Health Organization Tobacco Free Initiative website, 2011. WHO Report on the Global Tobacco Epidemic, 2009. WHO, Geneva. Online. Available: <http://www.who.int/tobacco/mpower/2009/appendix_viii/en/> (25 Feb 2014).

World Lung Foundation, American Cancer Society, The tobacco atlas. Online. Available: <http://www.tobaccoatlas.org/topic/prices> (20 Apr 2015).

Ybarra, M., Bull, S., 2007. Current trends in internet-and cell phone-based HIV prevention and intervention. HIV/AIDS Reports 4 (4), 201–207.

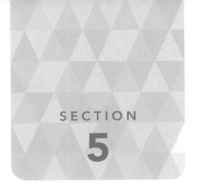

CONTEMPORARY ISSUES

Introduction

- **An understanding of** the impact of globalisation on population health is essential for a public health practitioner in the twenty-first century. How is globalisation defined and what public health strategies might we put in place to deal with the impact of globalisation on health? Authors like Koplan and his colleagues (2009 p 1995) define *global health* as being 'an area for study, research, and practice that places a priority on improving health and achieving equity in health for all people worldwide'. In their article, they proposed several distinctions between public, international and global health, and derived the above-mentioned definition from the geographical reach, level of cooperation, object and orientation of the different fields (Koplan et al. 2009). The authors pose questions that are key to an understanding and conceptualisation of global health. Bozorgmehr (2010) carries this debate further by attempting to define the 'global' in global health.

- **Chapter 15 addresses this** question as well as introducing you to the concept of a global burden of disease in developing and developed countries. The chapter is divided into four major sections: an introduction to globalisation; globalisation and its impact on population health; the global burden of disease; and the global response from the public health community. Increasingly, the way in which the planet has become relatively easy to traverse in short periods of time poses real challenges for public health. In addition, refugee health is a large and growing issue for public health consideration. Globalisation is here to stay, and Chapter 15 provides us with an opportunity to see how it impacts on the population's health and how public health might respond.

- **We also explore** in detail Aboriginal and Torres Strait Islander health in Chapter 16. The life expectancy of Aboriginal and Torres Strait Islander Australians continues to lag substantially behind other population groups in Australia. Late in 2007 the Council of Australian Governments (COAG) agreed on six specific targets to reduce disadvantage among Indigenous Australians. These targets focus on reducing the gap in levels of health and improving the social determinants of health, and have timelines for achievement attached to each. They include: closing the life expectancy gap within a generation (by 2030); halving the gap in mortality rates for Indigenous children within a decade (by 2018); ensuring that all Indigenous four-year-olds in remote communities have access to early childhood education within five years (by 2013); halving the gap for Indigenous students in reading, writing and numeracy within a decade (by 2018); halving the gap for Indigenous students in Year 12 attainment by 2020; and halving the gap in employment levels within a decade (by 2018). The National Indigenous Reform Agreement (see website in References) has been established to outline the task of closing the gap in Indigenous disadvantage. The Australian Government and states and territories will work in partnership to: achieve the agreed targets; develop, progress and review the national objectives and outcomes for Indigenous reform; and ensure that their data are of high quality and available for reporting. Fundamental to this is a respectful and collaborative partnership with Aboriginal and Torres Strait Islander Australians. This approach draws on the strengths of Indigenous cultures, and is considered particularly important in creating lasting change in the lives of Indigenous Australians (Australian Institute of Health and Welfare 2010 p 230).

- **The final chapter** in Section 5 focuses on grand challenges for public health. Chapter 17 looks at identifying the major challenges facing public health in the twenty-first century, and in particular it focuses on new and ongoing challenges, such as globalisation and health impacts, sustainable ecological public health, the re-emergence of infectious diseases, genetics, biotechnology and information technology, and their impact on public health. The chapter emphasises the importance of politics in decision-making about public health resources, infrastructure and strategies. It discusses the varying roles of the public health worker in light of the re-emergence of infectious diseases and the development of a range of chronic illnesses. It addresses a new paradigm for public health activity that is trans-disciplinary in nature. It also tackles the important issue of an ageing population and the public health implications. Chapter 17 discusses the relevance of a well-structured and comprehensive translational research agenda for public health.

References

Australian Institute of Health and Welfare, 2010. Australia's Health 2010. Cat. No. AUS 122. AIHW, Canberra.

Bozorgmehr, K., 2010. Rethinking the 'global' in global health: a dialectic approach. Globalization and Health 6, 19.

Koplan, J.P., Bond, T.C., Merson, M.N., et al., 2009. Towards a common definition of global health. Lancet 373 (9679), 1993–1995.

National Indigenous Reform Agreement. Online. Available: <http://www .federalfinancialrelations.gov.au/content/npa/health_indigenous/ indigenous-reform/national-agreement_sept_12.pdf> (13 June 2014).

CHAPTER 15

The impact of globalisation on health

Xiang-Yu Hou

Learning objectives

After reading this chapter, you should be able to:

- understand the concept of globalisation, and appreciate its complexity

- identify the significant impacts of globalisation on population health, particularly infectious and chronic diseases

- understand the distribution of the global burden of disease in high-, middle- and low-income countries

- critically evaluate the factors contributing to the major causes of death in low-income countries

- understand some of the achievements of the global public health community, and appreciate the challenges it faces.

Introduction

Globalisation affects what we eat and what we drink, what we use for transport and home entertainment, and so many other activities in our lives. An understanding of the impact of globalisation on population health is vital for any twenty-first-century health professional. This chapter is organised into four sections: an introduction to globalisation; globalisation in population health; the global burden of disease; and the global public health community.

'"Globalisation" is a relatively new term used to describe a very old process', and has only been in use for about three decades. Globalisation is 'a historical process that began with our human ancestors moving out of Africa' (YaleGlobal online 2015)—there were no national borders then—to the Mediterranean about 100,000 years ago, and a second migration to Asia about 50,000 years ago (Chanda 2002). In the historical era, most of those people moving from country to country were traders, preachers, explorers and soldiers (Chanda 2002). (See Activity 15.1.)

Global communication

The increase in globalisation is associated with technological developments, mainly in transportation and communication, which have significantly reduced the 'size' of the world. The speed of communication is now faster than we could ever have imagined. For example, 'in the late nineteenth century it took Queen Victoria 16.5 hours to send a greeting to the American President' via a transatlantic cable (Chanda 2002). Today we can communicate with each other via mobile phone, email, Twitter, Facebook, Instagram and videoconferencing almost instantaneously.

This increased speed and decreased cost of communication has effectively connected the world. The decreasing cost of telecommunications, and enhanced technology, have greatly increased accessibility for most people worldwide, thus facilitating communications. Mobile phones were introduced into Australia in February 1987. As of May 2013, Australia, with a population of over 23 million people (Australian Bureau of Statistics 2013), had 11.19 million smart phone users (Australian Communications and Media Authority 2013).

Internet usage is another sign of globalisation in communication. Among the 2.8 billion internet users in the world, about 45% are from Asia, 20% from Europe, 10% from North America, 11% from Latin America, 8.6% from Africa, 3.7% from the Middle East and 1% from Australia/Oceania (Miniwatts Marketing Group 2014). Globally, internet usage increased by 676% over the period 2000 to 2014. Australia had 6.6 million internet users in 2000, 14.7 million in 2007 and 19.6 million in 2014 (respectively, about 34%, 70% and 80% of the population) (Miniwatts Marketing Group 2014). No other communication technology has seen such an increase in uptake in such a short timeframe.

> **BOX 15.1**
>
> ### DEFINING 'GLOBALISATION'
>
> *Globalisation* is the movement across national boundaries of people, ideas, money, goods and services, which results in the world becoming politically, economically and culturally interconnected and interdependent.

National and international air travel

Air travel contributes to local economic development itself, but in combination with related services, such as hotels, local transport and food, it is an important contributor to the overall economy. Internationally, the most significant impact of increased air travel is that it has made the world a face-to-face meeting place, thus greatly enhancing global interconnectedness and interdependence. It has also meant that illness and disease spread rapidly across the globe as people move from country to country in a relatively short amount of time. Around 15.1 million Australian residents and 12.6 million overseas visitors passed through Australian airports in 2010–11 (Bureau of Infrastructure, Transport and Regional Economics 2012 p 9).

Globalisation has positive as well as negative impacts; supporters claim it increases economic prosperity and development opportunities. Globalisation can also support the development of civil liberties. Another aspect of globalisation—the movement of money, goods and services—can initiate a more efficient distribution of resources, which can then enhance employment prospects, reduce the cost of goods and services, and thus increase the standard of living globally.

Research has shown that poverty rates have dropped significantly in globalised countries such as China, compared with less globalised regions, such as sub-Saharan Africa, where poverty rates are still high (The World Bank 2014). According to Rees and Riezman (2012), 'the effect of globalization on fertility, human capital, and growth' depends on whether increased market opportunities created by globalisation are available for men or women (Rees & Riezman 2012 p 107). If women benefit from these opportunities, then fertility decreases and 'human capital formation' is enhanced, while if men profit, 'then fertility increases and human capital formation falls' (Rees & Riezman 2012 p 107).

Critics of globalisation claim that the rapid flow of capital and consumer goods has caused damage to the planet and increased poverty, socioeconomic inequality, injustice and the erosion of traditional cultures. Many organisations in developed countries involved in globalisation have failed to consider the welfare of underprivileged countries and people of low socioeconomic status, or the interests of the natural world (Institute of Medicine 2012).

How many people around the world do you think support globalisation? In 2006, people from 56% of the world's population territories were asked about their perceptions of globalisation (University of Maryland 2007). Table 15.1 presents the results of that study.

Support for globalisation is remarkably strong throughout the world. The question, '[G]lobalisation, especially increasing connections of our economy with others around the world, is mostly good or mostly bad' was asked (University of Maryland 2007).

TABLE 15.1 The view of globalisation by country		
Country	Mostly good (%)	Mostly bad (%)
Australia	65	27
China	87	6
France	51	42
Iran	63	31
India	54	30
Israel	83	10
Mexico	41	22
Philippines	49	32
Russia	41	24
South Korea	86	12
United States	60	35

(Source: University of Maryland 2007 www.worldpublicopinion.org)

In every country, positive responses outweighed negative ones. The level of support may be related to the extent of the countries' export economies. For example, respondents in China, South Korea and Israel expressed strong support for globalisation, while the greatest scepticism about globalisation was found in Mexico, Russia and the Philippines (University of Maryland 2007).

In Australia, the same survey was conducted by the Lowy Institute in July 2006 (University of Maryland 2007); it showed that most Australians viewed globalisation favourably. About 65% of Australians considered globalisation to be 'mostly good' for the country, while 27% said that it is 'mostly bad'. Explore your own perceptions of 'globalisation' by completing Activity 15.2.

Globalisation in population health

Globalisation affects population health by changing the ways in which people interact across boundaries (Chirico 2014). For example, global trade has led to increased spatial and temporal exposure to infectious disease through the rapid cross-border transmission of infectious diseases—for example, Ebola virus disease (EVD) and avian influenza. Similarly, global trade increases the risk of chronic diseases through the marketing of unhealthy products and risk behaviours, such as tobacco smoking and the consumption

ACTIVITY 15.2 Is globalisation good?

- Do you think that globalisation is good, especially with regard to increasing the connections of our economy with others around the world?
- What information would you use to answer the question?
- Make a table, with one column for the positive aspects and another for the negative aspects.

REFLECTION 15.2

It is likely that your answer reflects your personal circumstances, including your educational level, economic status, country of birth, cultural background and personal beliefs. What do you consider to be some of the positive aspects of globalisation? Would you include easier access to information, a broader range of opportunities, and an understanding of different cultures and the issues they face? Could the negative aspects of globalisation include unwanted economic and cultural influences, which may negatively impact on some cultures?

of fast food (Smith 2006). In addition, the global distribution of health-related goods (e.g. pharmaceutical products, medical equipment) and people (both patients and health professionals) is another example of how the health of the population might be affected. An example is 'medical tourists'—patients who travel to other countries for clinical treatment, mainly surgery. Medical tourism is now a rapidly growing industry.

Patients become medical tourists for two main reasons: finance and technology. In the United States the lack of health insurance makes many treatments unaffordable. A single heart-valve replacement in 2006 cost US$9,500 in India but US$273,395 in the United States. In the United Kingdom, long waiting lists and the high cost of private care motivate patients to become medical tourists. Patients from the Middle East and Africa travel long distances for surgery because the medical technology or expertise is lacking in their countries (Shetty 2010).

However, there is a disparity between issues such as the duty of care and accountability among those cross-border healthcare facilities. Additional issues are the effects of medical tourism on local healthcare systems.

In this section of the chapter, we will discuss two of the main effects of globalisation on population health. We will consider the impact of globalisation with regard first to the increased exposure to infectious diseases, and second to the increased risk of chronic diseases. The background to infectious diseases and chronic diseases and the strategies directed towards their control and management are outlined in Chapter 11.

Globalisation of infectious diseases

Arguably, infectious diseases cause the greatest threat to population health, because of the potential for such diseases to rapidly spread to large numbers of people across the world. The potential for geographical spread is particularly apparent if you consider that most infectious diseases have an incubation period exceeding 36 hours, and that any part of the world can now be reached within 36 hours (Kawachi & Wamala 2007b). The rapid increase in Ebola virus disease (EVD) demonstrates the spread of infectious pathogens around the globe.

The 'Ebola virus disease, formerly known as Ebola haemorrhagic fever, is a severe, often fatal illness in humans' (World Health Organization (WHO) 2014). The virus spreads in the 'human population through human-to-human transmission' with a case fatality rate of approximately 50%, but rates have varied from 25% to 90% (WHO 2014). The most recent outbreak in West Africa involves both urban and rural communities (WHO 2014). The only way to successfully control outbreaks is via the community and having good case management, surveillance and contact tracing, a good laboratory service, safe burials and social mobilisation (WHO 2014). (See Activity 15.3.)

The EVD example demonstrates the need for a worldwide collaborative approach. Research has shown that global resources to counter emerging infectious diseases (EIDs) are 'poorly allocated, with the majority of the scientific and surveillance effort

ACTIVITY 15.3 Globalisation and the spread of infectious diseases

- List your ideas about how globalisation impacts on the spread of infectious diseases such as Ebola virus disease (EVD).
- Group the ideas into different categories, such as political, economic, educational, research, tourism, cultural and policy.

REFLECTION 15.3

Did you think about the links between this activity and the content of Chapters 6 and 7, to clarify some of the potential factors that could either promote or impede the spread of EVD? Did you consider the contribution of research to understanding the nature of the disease, policies related to travel, social gathering or social distancing, and the possible cultural differences in managing the media and public panic?

Australia's response to Ebola

Ebola virus disease (EVD) has been described as the greatest humanitarian challenge globally at the moment by Burnet Institute Deputy Director Mike Toole (Australian Council for International Development media release 2014). The media release goes on to say:

> … the Australian Government can play an essential role in averting a further escalation of this global public health crisis. We welcome the government's $18 million contribution, and acknowledge that Australia has been one of the quickest countries to disburse funds. Rapid funding allows UN agencies and NGOs to immediately get on with the work required to halt the spread of this disease. … We strongly urge the government to continue to accelerate bilateral negotiations with key partner countries and when formal arrangements are reached, support the deployment of appropriate personnel.

Australia has established a super-committee encompassing senior members of several public service departments to help tackle the spread of the EVD outbreak. '"This is a priority for the government … [This] is a significant outbreak and Australia wishes to do its part in helping to deal with it," the Head of DFAT [Department of Foreign Affairs and Trade], Peter Varghese, told a senate estimates committee …' (Medhora 2014).

The *Sydney Morning Herald* (October 30 2014) referred to an opinion poll that said:

> Seven out of 10 Australians support sending Australian health workers to West Africa to help tackle the deadly Ebola virus … The Morgan telephone poll of 647 people this week showed 70 per cent of Australians support deploying Australian doctors and nurses to the source of the outbreak, 23 per cent were opposed and 7 per cent could not say. The poll comes as the United States is set to open an Ebola hospital in West Africa that could treat infected Australian health workers, helping clear the way for the government to aid the ravaged region.

focused on countries from where the next important EID is least likely to originate' (Jones et al. 2008 p 990). Case study 15.1 deals with Australia's initial response to EVD.

This case study is an example of how some good things have been done, such as Australia giving financial support; but it also challenges a first world country like Australia where potential medical and nursing support at the source of the outbreaks has been bureaucratic and slow to occur. Therefore, the international investment needs to be targeted at developing countries for capacity-building to detect, identify and monitor infectious diseases. As shown in the most recent EVD example, emerging infectious diseases are every country's problem.

Globalisation and chronic diseases

The main global chronic diseases today are heart disease, stroke, cancer, chronic respiratory diseases and diabetes (WHO 2011). These are generally the consequences of intermediate risk factors, such as raised blood pressure, raised glucose levels, abnormal blood lipids (particularly low-density lipoprotein and cholesterol) and overweight (body mass index (BMI) $\geq$ 25) and obesity (BMI $\geq$ 30). The most important modifiable risk factors are unhealthy diet, physical inactivity and tobacco use. These risk factors, in conjunction with the non-modifiable risk factors of age and heredity, explain the majority of new cases of heart disease, stroke, chronic respiratory diseases and some cancers (WHO 2011). To explore the effects of globalisation on the modifiable risk factors, the next sections discuss tobacco use and unhealthy diets.

TOBACCO USE

Globalisation processes, including trade liberalisation, foreign direct investment and marketing, have shifted the focus of the tobacco-using population in the world.

While cigarette consumption in most high-income countries has declined, it increased threefold, from 1.1 billion to 3.3 billion cigarettes in total per year, in low- and middle-income countries between 1997 and 2000 (Kawachi & Wamala 2007a). According to the 2013 WHO report on the global tobacco epidemic, nearly 80% of the world's 1 billion smokers live in low- and middle-income countries (WHO 2013).

Tobacco-related diseases were responsible for nearly 4.8 million premature deaths in 2000 (Ezzati & Lopez 2003). By 2015, tobacco is projected to be responsible for 10% of all deaths globally (see Table 15.2), and by 2030 will be responsible for 8.3 million deaths (Mathers & Loncar 2006b). Globalisation has led to this increase in cigarette consumption in middle- and low-income countries. Let us consider tobacco consumption in China as an example.

TABLE 15.2 Projected global tobacco-caused deaths by 2015—adapted from baseline scenario

	Cause	Number of tobacco-caused deaths (million)
All causes		6.43
	Tuberculosis	0.09
	Lower respiratory infections	0.15
Malignant neoplasms		2.12
	Trachea, bronchus, lung cancers	1.18
	Mouth and oropharynx cancers	0.18
	Oesophagus cancer	0.17
	Stomach cancer	0.12
	Liver cancer	0.10
	Other malignant neoplasms	0.34
Diabetes mellitus		0.13
Cardiovascular disease		1.86
	Ischaemic heart disease	0.93
	Cerebrovascular disease	0.52
	Other cardiovascular disease	0.24
Respiratory disease		1.87
	Chronic obstructive pulmonary disease (COPD)	1.76
Digestive disease		0.20

(Source: Mathers & Loncar 2006a)

In China, chronic diseases account for an estimated 80% of deaths and 70% of disability-adjusted life years (DALYs) lost (Wang et al. 2005). Cardiovascular diseases and cancer are the leading causes of both death and the burden of disease. More than 300 million men smoke cigarettes, and, if current smoking patterns persist, 2 million out of the 7 million deaths related to smoking worldwide will occur in China (Wang et al. 2005). This estimate does not include passive smokers.

Yin et al. (2007) demonstrated that exposure to passive smoking is associated with an increased prevalence of chronic obstructive pulmonary disease (COPD) and respiratory symptoms (sample size >20,000). It was estimated that 1.9 million excess deaths from COPD among those who had never smoked could be attributed to passive smoking in the current population in China (Yin et al. 2007).

In addition to the direct health effects of smoking, indirect consequences include the financial cost, especially in developing countries. In some rural areas in China, expenditure on tobacco occurs at the expense of education, medical care, insurance and investments in farming (Wang et al. 2006). The excessive medical spending attributable to smoking and consumption spending on cigarettes combined are estimated to be responsible for impoverishing 30.5 million urban residents and 23.7 million rural residents in China (Liu et al. 2006).

Since the late 1990s, multinational tobacco companies have signed numerous cooperation agreements with China to modernise manufacturing facilities, improve crop yields, and build crop-processing plants (Kawachi & Wamala 2007b). China now produces the largest amount of tobacco in the world, whereas previously it was an agrarian, subsistence economy. It is critical that the Chinese central government, including the ministries of health, finance and foreign affairs, work together to address this serious problem (see Activity 15.4).

OVERWEIGHT AND OBESITY

Globalisation has contributed to a worldwide epidemic of overweight and obesity. Hawkes et al. (2010) refer to the concept of *nutrition transition*, a term that depicts the globalisation of poor-quality, energy-dense diets that lead to obesity and chronic disease. Prevalence rates for overweight and obesity are very different in each region, with the Middle East, central and Eastern Europe and North America having higher prevalence rates than Asia and Northern Europe (James 2004). Table 15.3 demonstrates

---

ACTIVITY 15.4 Tobacco— health and economic issues

- Assign the following roles to a group of seven fellow students: a representative from a global tobacco company, a Department of Health (DoH) spokesperson, an economist, a spokesperson for the Department of Foreign Affairs and Trade (DFAT), a sports commentator, a media representative, and a tobacco consumer.

- Multinational tobacco companies are approaching populations in developing countries, using mass-media campaigns and sponsorship of popular sports. Are these tactics going to produce a large proportion of people who smoke, which then requires that these countries develop interventions to reduce the number of smokers? Or could a developing country effectively develop national strategies to promote non-smoking? What challenges would a country face in taking this approach?

- Give each group 15 minutes to consider the strategies for and against tobacco importation. Each group should do their role-play for the class, and then everyone can discuss the issues.

REFLECTION 15.4

Did the DoH representatives develop and implement a non-tobacco import/use policy for the population? Did the DFAT representatives try to justify a free trade policy (e.g. tobacco) between countries? Did the economists focus on the income brought into the country by exporting tobacco? Did the sports commentators and media representatives—who may owe their jobs to tobacco company sponsorship of sports events—support the tobacco companies? Lastly, did the tobacco consumers argue that they have the right to decide whether or not they use tobacco? This role-play should help you to understand the process of globalisation, and its potential negative impacts on population health.

TABLE 15.3 Prevalence of pre-obese (overweight) and obese in the world	
Country	Prevalence rate of pre-obese and obese
United States in 2000 (Sturm & Wells 2001)	59% (36% pre-obese 23% obese)
WHO European region—percentage of pre-obese or obese men, 2007	
Bulgaria (urban), Ireland, Malta and Slovenia	70%
Cyprus, the Czech Republic and Germany	75%
Albania (urban), Croatia and Slovakia (urban)	80%
WHO European region—percentage of pre-obese or obese women, 2007	
Croatia, Hungary, Ireland, Latvia and Spain	50%
Czech Republic, Cyprus, Scotland and Turkey	60%
Malta	70%
Slovakia (rural) and Albania (rural)	80%

(Sources: Adapted from Knai et al. 2007, Sturm & Wells 2001)

the prevalence of overweight and obesity in the United States and in the WHO European regions. It shows that in some countries in the WHO European regions, a high percentage of both men and women are pre-obese (i.e. overweight) or obese.

Some nations, such as the United States, are almost completely globalised in their food and activity patterns for all social strata. Other countries, for example China, are currently less globalised, with primarily higher socioeconomic status individuals becoming incorporated into global systems, and consequently, members of this group being more likely to become obese (Hawkes et al. 2010). As developing countries catch up with developed countries in the prevalence rates of overweight and obesity, the number of obese people (currently more than 400 million people worldwide) could double by the year 2025 (Formiguera & Canton 2004, Hawkes et al. 2010).

The process of globalisation, and its influence on the social system, changes in the food system, international food trade and global food advertising and promotion, have all played a role in shaping the nutrition transition (Hawkes et al. 2010).

Children and adolescents tend to assimilate global culture more quickly than their parents. Therefore, their eating and activity levels, and consequently their body weight, are more rapidly modified (Sobal 2001). In China, the prevalence of childhood overweight/obesity in 2000 was similar to that of Great Britain and the United States in the 1980s (Liu et al. 2007). While China is catching up with the West, studies show that, within China, rural areas are fast approaching the prevalence of overweight and obesity of urban areas (Table 15.4) (Wang et al. 2005). A study in Shenzhen (Hui & Bell 2003), a relatively wealthy city in China, found that 19% of boys and 11% of girls were overweight or obese.

To fully understand the global epidemic of obesity, especially in developing countries, we need to move beyond individual physiology and personal characteristics to examine collective social, economic and political structures, and cultural changes (Hawkes et al. 2010, Sobal 2001). These include factors such as urbanisation, technological shifts, economic forces and cultural factors (Kawachi & Wamala 2007a).

TABLE 15.4 Prevalence of overweight and obesity in Chinese children aged 7–17 years old in 2002

	Prevalence of overweight (%)	Prevalence of obesity (%)
Large city	13.1	8.1
Middle-sized city	7.1	3.2
Wealthy rural areas	4.1	1.9
Poor rural areas	2.3	0.7

(Source: Wang et al. 2005)

TABLE 15.5 Factors contributing to global epidemic of obesity

	Factors	Contribution (%)
Cultural factors	Modern advertising Other elements affecting food choice and dietary patterns	25%
Economic forces	Food and price changes	30%
Technological shifts	Energy expenditure decreases at work, travel, home production and leisure	30%
Urbanisation	Urbanisation and others	15%

(Source: Kawachi & Wamala 2007a)

Table 15.5 outlines the factors contributing to the global epidemic of obesity. Among the cultural factors which have changed people's food choices and dietary patterns in many developing countries, we will examine two aspects: large shifts in food imports and modern advertising.

Large changes in food imports are evident. For example, between 1989 and 1998, sales by US-owned food-processing affiliates in South America grew from US$5 billion to US$15 billion, and sales in Asia increased from US$5 billion to US$20 billion (Bolling & Somwaru 2001). In China in 2004, there were more than 1000 KFC restaurants, and they were increasing at a rate of 200 each year (China Daily 2004). The most common expressions for this phenomenon are the 'burgerisation', 'coca-colonisation' or 'McDonaldisation' of food culture (Lang 1998, Zimmet 2000).

The marketing of brands and shifts in cultural norms can actually influence people's tastes (Chopra et al. 2002, Hawkes et al. 2010). This particularly applies to young people and populations longing for a Western lifestyle. Marketing and product branding have the ability to transform food culture in surprisingly short periods of time (Labonte et al. 2010). This has enormous implications both for state budgets and for health inequalities. How can a government with a limited budget hope to influence a population with a health education message when a transnational company can spend almost unlimited amounts of money on advertising to promote brand recognition and consumption

---

ACTIVITY 15.5 Promoting a healthy diet

- As a health professional, how would you promote a healthy diet among school students in a developing country, where fast-food restaurants are emerging as a major source of their dietary intake?
- Are there other professionals with whom you would consider it important to collaborate?
- How might you use the school curriculum to help you?

REFLECTION 15.5

Did you think about the role a country's food policy plays in promoting a healthy diet or, conversely, how it might make it more difficult to adopt a healthy lifestyle? Did you consider the food industry's contribution to choices and opportunities? Did you consider using health education and school health promotion activities to support healthy dietary messages?

(Labonte et al. 2010; Lang 1998)? (Activity 15.5 will help you to understand these issues better.)

A transformation in food cultures, including an increase in meat consumption, also has a negative effect on our environment. Worldwide, agriculture, particularly livestock production, comprises approximately 20% of total greenhouse gas emissions, thus contributing to global climate change (McMichael et al. 2007). Worldwide, current average meat consumption is about 100 g per person per day, with about a tenfold difference between high- and low-consuming populations. To prevent increased greenhouse gas emissions from this production sector, '90 g per day is proposed as a working global target, shared more evenly, with no more than 50 g per day being red meat from ruminants (i.e. cattle, sheep and goats)' (McMichael et al. 2007 p 1253). Reducing the consumption of meat will benefit not only population health, but also the natural environment.

Globalisation is a two-way street. While Western food cultures are imported into developing countries, Eastern food cultures are also exported from developing countries, but mainly as raw and unprocessed foods. For example, exports of poultry to Japan from China almost quadrupled during the period 1988–1993 (McMichael 2000). The quality of food exports is of potential national public health concern. For example, in 2007 low levels of banned antibiotics were identified in one-third of the samples of prawns, fish, crabs and eels imported from Thailand, Indonesia, China and Vietnam into Australia (Mitchell & Wilson 2007). This was a major concern for Australia, because it imported around 70% of its annual seafood consumption in 2005–06 (Mitchell & Wilson 2007).

Globalisation is a complex and multifaceted issue that influences, and is influenced by, social, cultural, economic and health factors. The effects of globalisation are an important multisectoral focus for modern public health practice.

Refugee health

It is important to discuss refugee health when investigating the impact of globalisation on population health. This is because the refugee crisis affects Australia and many other countries. The 1951 Convention relating to the Status of Refugees defines a refugee as:

> Any person who owing to a well founded fear of being persecuted for reasons of race, religion, nationality, membership of a particular social group or political opinion, is outside the country of his/her nationality and is unable, or owing to such fear, is unwilling to avail himself/herself of the protection of that country. (United Nations High Commissioner for Refugees 1951)

The United Nations High Commissioner for Refugees (UNHCR) is responsible for protecting refugees and overseeing adherence to the Convention. The UNHCR plays a leadership role in managing refugee issues worldwide, and estimates that global resettlement needs in 2011 were around 805,500 persons (UNHCR 2010). However, the annual quotas set by nations offering to resettle refugees have remained unchanged at 80,000

(UNHCR 2011). Therefore, only 10% of all refugees are resettled. Among those, 90% are accepted by the United States, Canada and Australia, while only 6% go to Europe (UNHCR 2011). As a signatory to the 1951 Convention, if a person is found to be a refugee, Australia is obliged under international law to offer support and to ensure that the person is not sent back unwillingly to the country of origin (Refugee Council of Australia 2011). In January 2010, Australia had 22,548 refugees and 2350 asylum seekers residing in Australia (UNHCR 2011).

There are clearly misunderstandings among the general population about refugee resettlement in Australia. So let us consider three myths about refugees. The first is that 'most refugees want to be resettled'. The truth is that most refugees want to return home and live in their own country in peace and safety. A person may adopt another culture or identity, but the original self has been shattered and torn (Dugan 2007). So resettlement is for refugees who have no other solution. The second myth is that resettlement leads to a 'brain drain'. On the contrary, many resettled refugees contribute their knowledge and skills to improving the society. The third myth is that 'resettlement costs too much'. However, human life, human dignity and human protection are priceless, and the human, financial and security costs to keep refugees in camps for generations are much higher than the costs of resettlement (UNHCR 2010).

In Australia, asylum-seekers on bridging visas who live in the community experience extreme poverty, as they do not have the right to work (UNHCR 2013). Thus, they are unable to afford decent housing or other necessities, and must rely on charitable groups for their basic needs (UNHCR 2013).

Having the right attitudes towards refugees is the first step in protecting and promoting their health. It is widely recognised that refugees usually have different health problems from the general population. For example, the most common health problems among the African refugees attending four health services in metropolitan Melbourne in 2005 were inadequate vaccination status, nutritional deficiencies (vitamin D and iron), infectious diseases (gastrointestinal infections, schistosomiasis, and latent tuberculosis) and dental disease (Tiong et al. 2006).

Inadequate vaccination is a major concern among refugees. A community survey of immigrants and refugees from East Africa showed inadequate immunity against at least one of tetanus (67%), hepatitis B (41%), diphtheria (34%) or measles (3%) for 81% of the participants (Skull et al. 2008).

Other health professionals face similar challenges in serving refugees. Refugee and migrant young people in Western Sydney have poor levels of primary care utilisation (general practitioners—GPs) relative to their needs (Thomas et al. 2007). There are many factors contributing to this under-use of GP services. For example, it is not clear how many GPs would have adequate listening skills for the complex care needs of many refugees (Gardiner & Walker 2010). In addition, the physical and psychosocial effects of the traumatisation of refugees can affect presenting symptoms, so that a 'strong therapeutic relationship built by patient-led, sensitive assessment over time is the foundation to care' (Gardiner & Walker 2010 p 198). Unquestionably, an education program for health service providers is required to improve the interaction between primary care workers in the health system and refugees.

Furthermore, having spent time in a refugee camp could mean that a refugee is at risk of a decline in mental health status after arrival in Australia (Maximova & Krahn 2010); and the length of time taken for refugee assessment procedures is the strongest predictor for a low quality of life (Laban et al. 2008). Professor and psychiatrist Patrick McGorry (2010 Australian of the Year) described detention centres as 'factories for producing mental illness and mental disorder' (Anonymous 2010).

In summary, refugees have to be resettled in foreign countries because they have no other options. There are many challenges to protecting and promoting the health of refugees, including different health problems, and language and cultural barriers.

The global public health community

The global public health community has a 160-year history of working together to deal with international health problems. In this section, we will briefly describe the current international health organisations, their programs, and their contributions to global public health.

The first international meeting of the public health community was held in 1851 in Paris. In the mid-twentieth century the collaboration was formalised through the United Nations and its various agents, including the WHO (Walt 1998). During that meeting, it was agreed that resources for health development would be channelled through multilateral (global system) and bilateral (government-to-government) organisations, and non-government organisations (NGOs). In addition to the WHO, the World Bank has been a significant contributor to the global public health community, through providing financial and technical support. Private sector organisations, such as non-government foundations (e.g. the Rockefeller Foundation, and the Bill and Melinda Gates Foundation) and for-profit organisations (e.g. pharmaceutical and insurance companies) have been very active as well. Some of the main international players in the global public health community are introduced below.

The United Nations (UN) is a multilateral organisation that was officially established on 24 October 1945 with 50 member countries (UN 2008). The five purposes of the UN articulated at that time were:

- 'to maintain international peace and security
- to develop friendly relations among nations
- to cooperate in solving international economic, social, cultural and humanitarian problems
- to cooperate in promoting respect for human rights and fundamental freedoms
- to be a centre for harmonizing the actions of nations in attaining these ends' (UN 2008).

Through its agencies, the UN has been an active and effective player in numerous aspects of international politics and health. In September 2000, at the *Millennium Summit*, member states of the UN (including Australia) reaffirmed their commitment to eliminate global poverty and hunger, to improve health, gender equality, education and environmental sustainability, and to create a global partnership for development (UN 2008). One of the outcomes of this historic assembly was the announcement of eight Millennium Development Goals (MDGs—introduced in Chapter 1), which are listed in Table 15.6 (Wamala et al. 2007, UN website).

The UN has collaborated with member states to achieve the eight goals listed in Table 15.6. For example, climate change: 187 countries were present at the *United Nations Climate Change Conference* in Bali, Indonesia, in December 2007. The purpose of the conference was to try to reach a consensus on a new international climate change agreement, which would contribute to achieving the MDG goal of 'ensuring environmental sustainability'.

This new agreement, with a new global emissions reduction objective, will help to achieve the targets. However, it will require the major carbon emitters, such as the United States and China, to make a commitment.

TABLE 15.6 The UN Millennium Development Goals

	Goal	Targets	Status of targets, 2014
1	Eradicate extreme poverty and hunger	Between 1990 and 2015, halve the proportion of people whose income is less than $1 a day and who suffer from hunger	'poverty rates have been halved between 1990 and 2010, but 1.2 billion people still live in extreme poverty'
2	Achieve universal primary education	By 2015, every child (boy or girl) will complete a full course of primary schooling	'Too many children are still denied their right to primary education, if current trends continue the world will not meet the goal of universal primary education by 2015'
3	Promote gender equality and empower women	Eliminate gender disparity in all levels of education by 2015	'Women are assuming more power in the world's parliaments, boosted by quota systems' 'Globally, 123 million youth (aged 15 to 24) lack basic reading and writing skills; 61 per cent of them are young women'
4	Reduce child mortality	Between 1990 and 2015, reduce mortality by two-thirds in children under five years of age	'Big gains have been made in child survival, but efforts must be redoubled to meet the global target'
5	Improve maternal health	Between 1990 and 2015, reduce maternal mortality by 75%	'Maternal mortality has declined by nearly half since 1990, but falls far short of the MDG target'

TABLE 15.6 Continued

	Goal	Targets	Status of targets, 2014
6	Combat HIV/AIDS, malaria, and other diseases	By 2015, have halved and begun to reverse the spread of HIV/AIDS. By 2015, have halved and begun to reverse the incidence of malaria and other diseases	'The incidence of HIV is declining steadily in most regions; but 2.5 million people are still newly infected each year'
7	Ensure environmental sustainability	For example: integrate the principles of sustainable development into country policies and programs, and reverse the loss of environment resources	'More than 2.1 billion people and almost 1.9 billon people, respectively, have gained access to improved water sources and sanitation facilities since 1990' 'Global emissions of carbon dioxide (CO_2) have increased by more than 46 per cent since 1990'
8	Develop a global partnership for development	For example: develop further an open, rule-based, predictable, non-discriminatory trading and financial system, including a commitment to good governance, development, and poverty reduction—both nationally and internationally	'There is less aid money overall, with the poorest countries most adversely affected'

(Sources: United Nations Development Programme 2015. The 8 UN Millennium Development Goals. (Available: <http://www.un.org/millenniumgoals/>.) © 2015 United Nations. Reprinted with permission of the United Nations)

Within the UN system, there is a wide range of agencies that undertake work directly or indirectly to support international health. These include the WHO, the World Bank, UNICEF, the UN Development Programme, the UN Educational, Scientific and Cultural Organization (UNESCO), the Food and Agriculture Organization, the UNHCR, the International Labour Organization, the UN Environment Programme, the UN Fund for Drug Abuse Control, and the World Trade Organization. Some of the activities of these agencies are directly related to public health. For example, the World Bank provides funds to fight HIV/AIDS, tuberculosis and malaria (Aidspan 2002–2014).

Other UN programs have indirect links to health. For example, UNESCO works to promote pride and engagement in cultural activities, and to preserve cultural heritage, which also contributes to improving the wellbeing of both the individual and the population.

National governments are essential participants in this global public health community. Under the initiative on global health and foreign policy, launched in New York in September 2006, the foreign affairs ministers of Brazil, France, Indonesia, Norway, Senegal, South Africa and Thailand issued an official statement in Oslo on 20 March 2007 (Ministers of Foreign Affairs 2007). These ministers agreed to work towards greater links and recognising the influence of foreign policy decisions on health. Box 15.2 describes the major areas of commonality identified by the group.

The *Oslo Statement of Ministers of Foreign Affairs* clearly articulates the importance of policy decisions with regard to population health:

> In today's era of globalisation and interdependence there is an urgent need to broaden the scope of foreign policy … We believe that health is one of the most important, yet still broadly neglected, long-term foreign policy issues of our time … We have therefore agreed to make

---

BOX 15.2

MAJOR AREAS OF COMMONALITY IDENTIFIED IN THE OSLO STATEMENT

'Increase awareness of our common vulnerability in the face of health threats by bringing health issues more strongly into the arenas of foreign policy discussions and decisions, in order to strengthen our commitment to concerted action at the global level.'

'Build bilateral, regional and multilateral cooperation for global health security by strengthening the case for collaboration and brokering broad agreement, accountability, and action.'

'Reinforce health as a key element in strategies for development and for fighting poverty, in order to reach the Millennium Development Goals; ensure that a higher priority is given to health in dealing with trade issues and in conforming to the Doha principles [referring to the Doha Declaration on the Trade-Related Aspects of Intellectual Property Rights and Agreement on Public Health], affirming the right of each country to make full use of TRIPS (Trade-Related Aspects of Intellectual Property Rights) flexibilities in order to ensure universal access to medicines.'

'Strengthen the place of health measures in conflict and crisis management and in reconstruction efforts' (Ministers of Foreign Affairs 2007 p 1373).

impact on health a point of departure and a defining lens that each of our countries will use to examine key elements of foreign policy and development strategies, and to engage in a dialogue on how to deal with policy options from this perspective. (Ministers of Foreign Affairs 2007 p 1373)

Another example of foreign policy deliberations that have an impact on health is Australia's foreign aid programs. The Australian Government's new development policy *Australian aid: promoting prosperity, reducing poverty, enhancing stability* and new performance framework *Making Performance Count: enhancing the accountability and effectiveness of Australian aid* build an aid program that is effective in promoting economic growth and reducing poverty, and that projects and protects Australia's broader interests in the Indo-Pacific region (Australian Government Department of Foreign Affairs and Trade 2014). On average, every week, every Australian contributes around $2.40 to pay for the aid program, which is less than the cost of a loaf of bread.

Why do Australians give aid? Whether or not people give aid is influenced by their beliefs, knowledge, experiences and motivations, as well as by their perceptions about their financial status. Many individuals believe that giving aid is the right thing to do because it makes a real difference to the lives of less fortunate people. Conversely, the Australian Government's aid program is now focused on innovation, and leveraging other drivers of development, such as private sector investment and domestic finance. It supports economic growth as the most sustainable way to reduce poverty and lift living standards, and it improves Australia's own economic and security interests by helping to build stronger communities and more stable governments in the region (Australian Government Department of Foreign Affairs and Trade 2014). How could you help to improve the health status of people in a developing country? Activity 15.6 explores the option of working in a developing country.

ACTIVITY 15.6 Working in developing countries

- Would you like to work in a developing country to improve the population's health status, even if this meant earning less income than a person working in a developed country?
- Make a list of the reasons for and against working in a developing country to improve the health of the population.
- Add all the lists together and then discuss with the whole class.

REFLECTION 15.6

What factors would motivate you to work in a health-related position in a developing country? One of the obvious reasons would be the satisfaction gained from trying to make a difference, no matter how small, to people's wellbeing.

Philanthropic organisations also play significant roles in the global public health community, such as the Bill and Melinda Gates Foundation (Gates Foundation). The Gates Foundation focuses on two main areas: improving access to existing vaccines, drugs and other tools to fight diseases common in developing countries; and research to develop health solutions that are effective, affordable and practical (Gates Foundation 2014). For example, for the year ended 31 December 2012, the Gates Foundation donated US$892,868,000 for global health and US$1,559,545,000 for global development (Gates Foundation 2014).

In addition to non-government organisations, such as philanthropic agencies, government international aid organisations, and multilateral organisations such as the UN, the WHO and the World Bank, there are also professional organisations working together to address specific health issues. One of these is the International Society for the Prevention of Child Abuse and Neglect (ISPCAN 2008) (see Activity 15.7).

Currently, there is insufficient direction for global public health from organisations such as the WHO, and limited consistency in policies and programs, which lowers the likelihood of sustainable health improvements in developing countries (Kruk 2012).

While there are examples of immense achievements, there are still challenges ahead, and some clear shortcomings in activity and focus. It has been suggested that some essential functions had been neglected by international public health agencies, such as the creation of comprehensive information systems to promote cooperation in health policy development, at both the national and international levels, and the sharing of experiences in health reforms between countries (Frenk et al. 1997).

Others have suggested that the WHO needs to move from traditional disease governance approaches to new public health governance approaches, which would include global leadership in public health education and interventions. It has also been suggested that the WHO should use data from a range of resources, including treaties, regulations, recommendations and travel advisories, to provide for global public health security (Aginam 2006). However, the WHO faces many challenges to implement the above ideas, including insufficient funding.

Investigations have shown 'that national autonomy over health policy is not preserved under' the World Trade Organization's *General Agreement on Trade in Services* (GATS), 'and that accordingly, there is a role for international standards that protect public services from the adverse effect of trade and market forces' (Pollock & Price 2003 p 1072). Sustainability, an issue for any international aid program, needs to be appropriately addressed. To provide support for sustainability, Edwards and Roelofs (2006) recommend: the 'development of strong and transparent partnerships'; the management of 'planned transition points'; and the use of 'local champions who led integration efforts' (Edwards & Roelofs 2006 pp 47–48).

Looking to the future of the global public health community, it has been predicted that global cooperation will be:

- likely to focus on global public health governance and regulations, such as environmental issues and cross-national trade of health products and services
- likely to have a public–private partnership as an increasing characteristic
- unlikely to be dominated by the UN or its agencies, such as the WHO, but will be represented by a more diverse set of actors, including private sectors, NGOs, consumer and professional groups, environmental groups, and civil society organisations (Merson et al. 2006 p 675).

ACTIVITY 15.7 International Society for Prevention of Child Abuse and Neglect

Go to the website of the International Society for the Prevention of Child Abuse and Neglect (ISPCAN) and answer the following questions:

- How many members are there, and how many countries are represented?
- What professional activities are undertaken?
- How is the society supported financially?

REFLECTION 15.7

Consider the effort required for health professionals to form a global organisation like ISPCAN, especially organising funding and developing professional activities. Then you should be able to appreciate the achievements of this organisation, and its potential to improve the health status of children.

A final word

This chapter has introduced the concept of globalisation and its impacts on population health, particularly on infectious and chronic diseases. We discussed the distribution of the global burden of diseases in high-, middle- and low-income countries, and introduced the role of the global public health community by describing some of their achievements and current challenges.

REVIEW QUESTIONS

1 What is 'globalisation', and how can it be defined?

2 How does globalisation impact on population health—for example, with reference to infectious diseases, tobacco use and unhealthy diets?

3 What are the main factors contributing to the differences in the leading causes of death between high- and low-income countries?

4 What are the major challenges for the global public health community in responding to globalisation?

5 Review the status of the Millennium Development Goals (MDGs). Which, if any, of the goals have been achieved or are on track? What are some of the factors that may impede reaching the MDGs? Is the progress towards achieving the MDGs the same in different countries?

6 How do you think multinational companies—for example, tobacco companies— will respond to increasingly strict laws in developed countries regarding their ability to market their products, and what impact will this have on developing countries?

7 In Australia, what is the difference between a refugee and an asylum seeker? What are Australia's obligations to both groups of people, and how does refugee or asylum seeker status impact on a person's health?

8 Why do relatively wealthy, developed countries, such as Australia, give aid to developing countries, such as Papua New Guinea and the Solomon Islands? If you are not sure, go to *Australia's aid program*, http://aid.dfat.gov.au/makediff/Pages/default.aspx#where

9 Do you think medical tourism is a positive or negative phenomenon, and what do you think are the impacts on the counties that offer such services?

10 Explain how globalisation may impact differentially on populations, depending on whether globalisation creates opportunities for men or for women.

Acknowledgement

The author would like to thank Professor Michael Dunne and Professor Mary Louise Fleming of the School of Public Health and Social Work, QUT.

References

Aginam, O., 2006. Globalization of health insecurity: the World Health Organization and the new International Health Regulations. Medicine and Law 25 (4), 663–672.

Aidspan, 2002–2014. Global Fund and US Government top external financiers of AIDS, TB and malaria: report. Online. Available: <http://www.aidspan.org/gfo_article/global-fund-and-us-government-top-external-financiers-aids-tb-and-malaria-report> (10 Sep 2014).

Anonymous, 2010. Mental illness in Australian immigration detention centres. Lancet 375 (9713), 434.

Australian Bureau of Statistics, 2013. 3101.0—Australian demographic statistics, Sep 2013. Online. Available: <http://www.abs.gov.au/ausstats/abs@.nsf/mf/3101.0/> (17 May 2014).

Australian Communications and Media Authority, 2013. Australia's mobile digital economy— ACMA confirms usage, choice, mobility and intensity on the rise. Australian Government, Canberra. Online. Available: <http://www.acma.gov.au/theACMA/Library/Corporate -library/Corporate-publications/australia-mobile-digital-economy> (9 Jun 2014).

Australian Council for International Development, 2014. Australian humanitarian agencies issue joint call to action for the Australian Government on Ebola. Media release 22 Oct 2014. Online Available: <http://www.burnet.edu.au/news/443_australian_humanitarian _agencies_issue_joint_call_to_action_on_ebola> (13 Nov 2014).

Australian Government Department of Foreign Affairs and Trade, 2014. Australia's new development policy and performance framework: a summary. DFAT, Canberra. Online. Available: <http://aid.dfat.gov.au/Publications/Documents/aid-policy-summary-doc.pdf> (8 Sep 2014).

Bolling, C., Somwaru, A., 2001. US food companies access foreign markets through investment. Economic Research Service Food Review 24 (3), 23–28.

Bureau of Infrastructure, Transport and Regional Economics (BITRE), 2012. Air passenger movements through capital and non-capital city airports to 2030–31. Report 133. BITRE, Canberra. Online. Available: <http://www.bitre.gov.au/publications/2012/files/ report_133.pdf> (28 Aug 2014).

Chanda, N., 2002. Coming together: globalization means reconnecting the human community. Online. Available: <http://yaleglobal.yale.edu/about/essay.jsp> (17 May 2014).

China Daily, 2004. KFC and McDonald's—a model of blended culture. China Daily Beijing, 1 June 2004. Online. Available: <http://www.chinadaily.com.cn/english/doc/2004-06/01/ content_335488.htm> (17 May 2014).

Chirico, J.A., 2014. Globalisation: Prospects and Problems. Sage, Los Angeles.

Chopra, M., Galbraith, S., Darnton-Hill, I., 2002. A global response to a global problem: the epidemic of overnutrition. Bulletin of the World Health Organization 80, 952–958.

Dugan, B., 2007. Loss of identity in disaster: how do you say goodbye to home? Perspectives in Psychiatric Care 43 (1), 41–46.

Edwards, N.C., Roelofs, S.M., 2006. Sustainability: the elusive dimension of international health projects. Canadian Journal of Public Health 97 (1), 45–49.

Ezzati, M., Lopez, A.D., 2003. Estimates of global mortality attributable to smoking in 2000. Lancet 362 (9387), 847–852.

Formiguera, X., Canton, A., 2004. Obesity: epidemiology and clinical aspects. Best Practice and Research: Clinical Gastroenterology 18 (6), 1125–1146.

Frenk, J., Sepúlveda, J., GómezDantés, O., et al., 1997. The future of world health: the new world order and international health. BMJ (Clinical Research Ed.) 314, 1404–1407.

Gardiner, J., Walker, K., 2010. Compassionate listening: managing psychological trauma in refugees. Australian Family Physician 39 (4), 198–203.

Gates Foundation, 2014. Global Health Program. Bill and Melinda Gates Foundation. Online. Available: <http://www.gatesfoundation.org> (13 Feb 2014).

Hawkes, C., Chopra, M., Friel, S., 2010. Globalization, trade and the nutrition transition. In: Harrison, D., Wroe, D., Poll backs Ebola action by Australian health workers. The Sydney Morning Herald, 30 Oct 2014. Online. Available: <http://www.smh.com.au/ federal-politics/political-news/poll-backs-ebola-action-by-australian-health-workers -20141030-11eh34.html> (4 Nov 2014).

Hui, L., Bell, A.C., 2003. Overweight and obesity in children from Shenzhen Peoples Republic of China. Health and Place 9 (4), 371–376.

Institute of Medicine, 2012. Promoting Cardiovascular Health in the Developing World: A Critical Challenge to Achieve Global Health. National Academies Press, Washington, DC.

International Society for the Prevention of Child Abuse and Neglect, 2008. ISPCAN celebrates 30 years. Online. Available: <http://www.ispcan.org/> (17 May 2014).

James, P.T., 2004. Obesity: the worldwide epidemic. Clinics in Dermatology 22 (4), 276–280.

Jones, K.E., Patel, N.G., Levy, M.A., et al., 2008. Global trends in emerging infectious diseases. Nature 451, 990–994.

Kawachi, I., Wamala, S., 2007a. Globalization and health: challenges and prospects. In: Kawachi, I., Wamala, S. (Eds.), Globalization and Health. Oxford University Press, New York, pp. 3–15.

Kawachi, I., Wamala, S., 2007b. Globalization and Health. Oxford University Press, New York.

Knai, C., Suhrcke, M., Lobstein, T., 2007. Obesity in Eastern Europe: an overview of its health and economic implications. Economics and Human Biology 5 (3), 392–408.

Kruk, M.E., 2012. Globalisation and global health governance: implications for public health. Global Public Health 7 (Suppl. 1), S54–S62.

Laban, C.J., Komproe, I.H., Gernatt, H.B.P.E., et al., 2008. The impact of a long asylum procedure on quality of life, disability and physical health in Iraqi asylum seekers in the Netherlands. Social Psychiatry and Psychiatric Epidemiology 43 (7), 507–515.

Labonte, R., Schrecker, T., Packer, C., et al., 2010. Globalization and Health: Pathways, Evidence and Policy. Taylor and Francis, Hoboken.

Lang, T., 1998. The new globalisation food and health: is public health receiving its due emphasis? Journal of Epidemiology and Community Health 52 (9), 538–539.

Liu, J.-M., Ye, R., Li, S., et al., 2007. Prevalence of overweight/obesity in Chinese children. Archives of Medical Research 38 (8), 882–886.

Liu, Y., Raob, K., Huc, T., et al., 2006. Cigarette smoking and poverty in China. Social Science and Medicine 63 (11), 2784–2790.

Mathers, C., Loncar, D., 2006a. Projections of global mortality and burden of disease from 2002 to 2030. PLoS Medicine 3 (11), e442. This material is licensed under Creative Commons Attribution 3.0 Unported license, <http://creativecommons.org/licenses/by/3.0/>.

Mathers, C.D., Loncar, D., 2006b. Updated Projections of Global Mortality and Burden of Disease, 2002–2030: Data Sources, Methods and Results. Evidence and Information for Policy Working Paper. WHO, Geneva, pp. 1–12.

Maximova, K., Krahn, H., 2010. Health status of refugees settled in Alberta: changes since arrival. Canadian Journal of Public Health 101 (4), 322–326.

McMichael, A.J., 2013. Globalization, climate change, and human health. New England Journal of Medicine 368, 1335–1343.

McMichael, A.J., Powles, J.W., Butler, C.D., et al., 2007. Food livestock production energy climate change and health. Lancet 370 (9594), 1253–1263.

McMichael, P., 2000. A global interpretation of the rise of the East Asian food import complex. World Development 28 (3), 409–424.

Medhora, S., 2014. Australia tackles Ebola outbreak with super-committee of public servants. The Guardian, Thursday, 23 Oct 2014. Online. Available: <http://www.theguardian.com/world/2014/oct/23/australia-tackles-ebola-outbreak-with-super-committee-of-public-servants> (4 Nov 2014).

Merson, M.H., Black, R.E., Mills, A., 2006. International Public Health: Diseases, Programs, Systems and Policies, 2nd ed. Jones and Bartlett Learning, Sudbury, MA.

Ministers of Foreign Affairs, 2007. Oslo Ministerial Declaration—global health: a pressing foreign policy issue of our time. Lancet 369 (9570), 1373–1378.

Miniwatts Marketing Group, 2014. Internet world stats: usage and population statistics. Online. Available: <http://www.internetworldstats.com/stats.htm> (7 Sep 2014).

Mitchell, S., Wilson, L., 2007. Fish bans raise poison risk. The Australian, 4 Aug 2007. Online. Available: <http://www.theaustralian.com.au/news/fish-bans-raise-poison-risk/story-e6frg6n6-1111114106484> (19 May 2014).

Pollock, A., Price, D., 2003. The public health implications of world trade negotiations on the general agreement on trade in services and public services. Lancet 362 (9389), 1072–1075.

Rees, R., Riezman, R., 2012. Globalization, gender, and growth. Review of Income and Wealth 58 (1), 107–117.

Refugee Council of Australia, 2011. Australia's refugee program. Online. Available: <http://www.refugeecouncil.org.au/fact-sheets/who-are-refugees/definitions/> and <http://www.refugeecouncil.org.au/fact-sheets/who-are-refugees/refugee-convention/> (19 May 2014).

Shetty, P., 2010. Medical tourism booms in India, but at what cost? Lancet 376 (9742), 671–672.

Skull, S.A., Ngeow, J.Y.Y., Hogg, G., et al., 2008. Incomplete immunity and missed vaccination opportunities in East African immigrants settling in Australia. Journal of Immigrant and Minority Health 10 (3), 263–268.

Smith, R.D., 2006. Trade and public health: facing the challenges of globalisation. Journal of Epidemiology and Community Health 60 (8), 650–651.

Sobal, J., 2001. Globalization and the epidemiology of obesity. Commentary. International Journal of Epidemiology 30 (5), 1136–1137.

Sturm, R., Wells, K.B., 2001. Does obesity contribute as much to morbidity as poverty or smoking? Public Health 115 (3), 229–235.

Thomas, P., Milne, B., Raman, S., et al., 2007. Refugee youth—immunisation status and GP attendance. Australian Family Physician 36 (7), 568–570.

Tiong, A.C.D., Patel, M.S., Gardiner, J., et al., 2006. Health issues in newly arrived African refugees attending general practice clinics in Melbourne. Medical Journal of Australia 185 (11/12), 602–606.

United Nations, 2008. About the UN: introduction to the structure and work of the UN. Online. Available: <http://www.un.org/en/about-un/index.html> (19 May 2014).

United Nations Development Programme, 2014. Online. Available: <http://www.undp.org/content/undp/en/home/mdgoverview/mdg_goals/progress/> (9 Jun 2014).

United Nations Development Programme, 2015. The 8 UN Millennium Development Goals. Online. Available: <http://www.un.org/millenniumgoals/>.

United Nations High Commissioner for Refugees, 1951. Convention and Protocol Relating to the Status of Refugees. UNHCR, Geneva.

United Nations High Commissioner for Refugees, 2010. UNHCR Projected Global Resettlement Needs 2011. Resettlement Service. Division of International Protection, UNHCR Geneva.

United Nations High Commissioner for Refugees, 2011. 2011 regional operations profile—East Asia and the Pacific. UNHCR Geneva.

United Nations High Commissioner for Refugees, 2013. Report on asylum-seekers on bridging visas in Australia: Protection Gaps. UNHCR Geneva. Online. Available: <http://unhcr.org.au/unhcr/index.php?option=com_content&view=article&id=361&catid=37&Itemid=61> (18 May 2014).

University of Maryland, 2007. World public favors globalization and trade but wants to protect environment and jobs: a publication of the Program on International Policy Attitudes at the University of Maryland. Online. Available: <http://worldpublicopinion.org/pipa/articles/btglobalizationtradera/349.php?lb=btgl&pnt=349&nid=&id=.> (19 May 2014).

Walt, G., 1998. Globalisation of international health. Lancet 351 (9100), 434–437.

Wamala, S., Kawachi, I., Mpepo, B.P., 2007. Poverty reduction strategy papers: bold new approach to poverty eradication, or old wine in new bottles? In: Wamala, S., Kawachi, I. (Eds.), Globalization and Health. Oxford University Press, New York, pp. 234–249.

Wang, H., Sindelar, J.L., Busch, S.H., 2006. The impact of tobacco expenditure on household consumption patterns in rural China. Social Science and Medicine 62 (6), 1414–1426.

Wang, L., Kong, L., Wu, F., et al., 2005. Preventing chronic diseases in China. Lancet 366 (9499), 1821–1824.

The World Bank, 2014. Working for a world free of poverty: data. Online. Available: <http://data.worldbank.org/topic/poverty> (8 Sep 2014).

World Health Organisation, 2011. Noncommunicable Diseases Country Profiles 2011: WHO Global Report. WHO, Geneva.

World Health Organization, 2013. WHO Report on the Global Tobacco Epidemic, 2013. WHO, Geneva. Online. Available: <http://www.who.int/tobacco/global_report/2013/en/> (17 May 2014).

World Health Organization, 2014. Ebola virus disease. Fact Sheet No. 103. Updated September 2014. Online. Available: <http://www.who.int/mediacentre/factsheets/fs103/en/> (4 Nov 2014).

YaleGlobal online, 2015. What is globalization? Online. Available: <http://yaleglobal.yale.edu/content/about-globalization> (20 Apr 2015).

Yin, P., Jiang, C.Q., Cheng, K.K., et al., 2007. Passive smoking exposure and risk of COPD among adults in China: the Guangzhou Biobank Cohort Study. Lancet 370 (9589), 751–757.

Zimmet, P., 2000. Globalization, coca-colonization and the chronic disease epidemic: can the doomsday scenario be averted? Journal of Internal Medicine 247, 301–310.

Aboriginal and Torres Strait Islander health

CHAPTER 16

Bronwyn Fredericks, Vanessa Lee, Mick Adams & Ray Mahoney

Learning objectives

After reading this chapter, you should be able to:

- describe why Aboriginal and Torres Strait Islander Australians experience poorer health status than other Australians

- outline the role and importance of Aboriginal and Torres Strait Islander community-controlled health organisations

- provide an overview of the issues associated with research with Aboriginal and Torres Strait Islander peoples

- discuss some of the public health strategies being utilised to address health disparities in Australia

- advocate for extra emphasis and effort in improving the health of Aboriginal and Torres Strait Islander peoples.

Introduction

Australia ranks lowest among the first-world wealthy nations working to improve the health and life expectancy of Indigenous people (Australian Health Ministers Advisory Council 2006). Life expectancy for Australia's Aboriginal and Torres Strait Islander peoples is estimated to be 10.6 years less for men than for non-Indigenous males, and 9.5 years less for women than for non-Indigenous females (Australian Bureau of Statistics (ABS) 2013a). There are similar disparities across all social, economic and health indicators. Specific public health approaches are needed to address these disparities and improve both the health status and the wellbeing of Aboriginal and Torres Strait Islander peoples. This chapter focuses on Aboriginal and Torres Strait

Islander health within Australia. It complements the content relating to Aboriginal and Torres Strait Islander peoples found in the other chapters in this book.

Who are Aboriginal and Torres Strait Islander peoples?

Aboriginal and Torres Strait Islander peoples are the Indigenous peoples of Australia. Aboriginal peoples are indigenous to mainland Australia; Torres Strait Islanders are indigenous to the islands between the Australian mainland and New Guinea. Australia and New Guinea annexed the Torres Strait Islands in the 1800s. While Aboriginal and Torres Strait Islander peoples are generally grouped under one banner, it is important to understand that there are significant differences in social, cultural and linguistic customs between different clan groups. It is estimated that before European settlement there were 250–300 languages, with 600 dialects, spoken by Aboriginal and Torres Strait Islander peoples (Australian Institute of Aboriginal and Torres Strait Islander Studies 1994).

Archaeological evidence demonstrates that Aboriginal people have lived in Australia for at least 50,000 years (some historians suggest 125,000 years). Aboriginal peoples belonged (and still belong) to specific geographical areas, known as 'Country'. Country refers to a specific clan, tribal group or nation of Aboriginal people, and encompasses all the knowledge, cultural norms, values, stories and resources within that area. The notion of Country is central to Australian Aboriginal identity, and contributes to overall health and wellbeing. Torres Strait Islander people identify particular islands or island groups as the areas to which they belong.

Prior to colonisation, Aboriginal and Torres Strait Islander peoples had complex societies and self-determining lives, with control over all of life's aspects, including ceremony, spiritual practices, medicine, birthing, child-rearing, relationships, management of land, and organisational systems and law. People had a healthy diet of protein and plants that contained adequate minerals and vitamins. They ate very little fat, sugar and salt (Flood 2006 p 122). They looked after their individual, family and community health and wellbeing, with most treatment provided by traditional spiritual healers and self-care, using traditional remedies (Couzos & Murray 2008). Aboriginal people kept on the move, with activities such as fishing, hunting, food-gathering, land management, ceremonies and visiting other nations on their Country. They were physically fit (Flood 2006 p 122). Torres Strait Islander people were active, with fishing, food-gathering and ceremonies.

Accounts from early colonisers present evidence that, at the time of colonisation, Aboriginal people who survived infancy were fairly disease-free, fit and healthy. For example, James Cook outlined on several occasions the health and physical status of the Aboriginal peoples he observed. Cook stated that they were 'of middle Stature straight bodied slender-limb'd the Colour of Wood soot or of dark chocolate ... Their features are far from disagreeable' (Cook in Clark 1966 p 51). Eyre, an early European explorer writing on the Murray River area, described the Aboriginal people of that area as 'almost free from diseases and well-shaped in body and limb' (quoted in Cleland 1928). Prior to the arrival of the British in 1788, Aboriginal Australian peoples experienced a relatively healthy lifestyle and quality of life (Saggers & Gray 1991 p 59). Thomson claims that Aboriginal Australians were 'physically, socially and emotionally healthier than most Europeans of that time' (1984 p 939). This is reiterated in the Strategy, Consultation Draft of the National Aboriginal and Torres Strait Islander Health Council (NATSIHC) (NATSIHC 2001 p 5) and in Engles (1892/1973 pp 130–133).

Colonisation had a profound impact on Australia's Aboriginal and Torres Strait Islander peoples. The establishment of the British penal colony at Botany Bay began a parallel destruction of Aboriginal lifestyles and cultures. It involved massacres and the removal of children from their mothers, families, peoples and lands (Blainey 1994, Evans et al. 1975, Rintoul 1993). Colonisation also brought with it infectious diseases, such as smallpox, to which Aboriginal people had little immunity. Today, 'the ill health of Aboriginal and Torres Strait Islander peoples exceeds that of any other sector of Australian society and the causes can be partly attributed to the impact of colonisation on the health of Aboriginal and Torres Strait Islander peoples' (NATSIHC 2001 p 5). The NATSIHC strategy document (2001) continues: 'acts of dispossession, introduced diseases, loss of traditional foods and lifestyle, forced resettlement, loss of social cohesion, separation of children and the actions of health and welfare services reflect this impact' (NATSIHC 2001 p 5).

Aboriginal and Torres Strait Islander peoples today understand the impact that colonisation has had on their health and wellbeing. They live daily with seeing family and community members who are ill and need healthcare. They attend the funerals of those who have passed away. They are the relatives and friends of the Aboriginal and Torres Strait Islander people counted in the statistics. It is a testament to Aboriginal and Torres Strait Islander peoples' strength and endurance that cultural, social and spiritual practices have survived in many communities, and that they continue to be maintained and revived.

ACTIVITY 16.1 Aboriginal pre- and post-colonisation experience

- Aboriginal people in Australia are often referred to as 'the oldest living culture on the planet'. Why do you think this is said?
- What do you think would be the kind of knowledge that Aboriginal people would have needed to sustain their health and wellbeing for such a long time?
- Why did colonisation have such an impact on the health and wellbeing of Aboriginal and Torres Strait Islander peoples? How might some of these events and issues from the past affect the health and wellbeing of Aboriginal and Torres Strait Islander peoples today?

REFLECTION 16.1

Reflect on your own background and your family's history. What is your culture? Where is your family from? What has been your family's history over the past 200 years? How have government and institutional policies directed, and impacted on, your family's health and wellbeing? How can you draw on your own family's history and culture to gain an understanding of how Aboriginal and Torres Strait Islander peoples might feel about their experiences?

Government policy

From the time of colonisation, policy decisions made about Aboriginal and Torres Strait Islander peoples have influenced their health and wellbeing. The modern history of Aboriginal and Torres Strait Islander peoples is one of control. Policies were (and are) made by federal, state and territory governments, by churches and other institutions. A range of people, including health professionals, police officers, and church and government administrators, have helped to implement the policies (and in some instances carried out questionable practices). Phillips (2003 p 93) explains that a range of people 'operated in concert to suppress local Aboriginal sovereignty, steal their lands, and destroy their languages, cultures and social cohesion'. An obvious example is the practice of removing children from their families. This continued through the 1950s and 1960s under child welfare legislation in most states, and allowed missionaries, government officials and others to restrict contact between Aboriginal children and their parents and culture (Beresford & Omaji 1998 p 96). Other government polices prevented Aboriginal and Torres Strait Islander peoples from enjoying the rights that other

Australians exercised, such as buying a home, voting, moving from one town to another, receiving wages for work, and going to school or university. These policies were implemented in the living memories of today's Aboriginal and Torres Strait Islander peoples, families and communities. They contribute to the attitudes towards health professionals, healthcare delivery, religious people, teachers, law and order workers, and government officials held today by Aboriginal and Torres Strait Islander peoples. Some of the practices resulted in *situational traumatisation*, which has 'produced cumulative trauma as a result of shame and self-hate, and intergenerational trauma as a result of unresolved and unaddressed grief and loss' (Phillips 2003 p 23).

The National Aboriginal Health Strategy

In recent times, a concerted effort has been made by governments and institutions to address the poor health of Aboriginal and Torres Strait Islander peoples. The National Aboriginal Health Strategy Working Party was established in 1987, and it produced the *National Aboriginal Health Strategy* (NAHS 1989). The NAHS was an important milestone, as it was the first time that representatives from Aboriginal and Torres Strait Islander communities, the Commonwealth and the state and territory governments collaborated on a national policy for Aboriginal and Torres Strait Islander peoples. The NAHS recognised the need for separate women's and men's meetings, and for joint meetings. The NAHS was the first time that an Aboriginal and Torres Strait Islander concept of health was embedded in a national document:

> Health is not just the physical well-being of the individual but the social, emotional, and cultural well-being of the whole community. This is a whole-of-life view and it also includes the cyclical concept of life–death–life (NAHS 1989 p ix)

This statement has been widely adopted by Aboriginal and Torres Strait Islander peoples themselves, and in various government and academic documents. It has been used by Aboriginal and Torres Strait Islander peoples to work with governments to deliver more comprehensive health services and primary healthcare services. However, despite the efforts of many people, the NAHS was never fully funded. The NAHS is still considered a living document by many Aboriginal and Torres Strait Islander health groups, and it is still referenced in meetings and gatherings by Indigenous peoples due to the significance of the document itself. It is important to understand the significance of this document in relation to the history of Indigenous health, including public health, in Australia.

Close the Gap

Close the Gap is a human-rights-based campaign for Aboriginal and Torres Strait Islander health equality, publicly launched in April 2007 and initiated following the Aboriginal and Torres Strait Islander Social Justice Commissioner's *Social Justice Report 2005*. Australia's peak Aboriginal and Torres Strait Islander and non-Indigenous health bodies, non-government organisations (NGOs) and human rights organisations first met as the Close the Gap Steering Committee in March 2006. Close the Gap campaign activities work outside of government and are completely self-funded, with Oxfam Australia being the major contributor (National Aboriginal Community Controlled Health Organisation (NACCHO) & Oxfam 2007). The steering committee is led by its Aboriginal and Torres Strait Islander members.

The campaign's goal is to close the gap by 2030: to raise the health and life expectancy of Aboriginal and Torres Strait Islander peoples so that within one generation they are on par with those of the non-Indigenous population. Each year since 2007, 24 March is celebrated as the national Close the Gap day. Coordinated by Oxfam Australia, events are conducted across Australia to continue to promote the campaign goal, increase participation through encouraging more Australians to sign the pledge, and support community and workplace events (Close the Gap Campaign Steering Committee (CTGSC) 2011 p 2, Human Rights and Equal Opportunity Commission (HREOC) 2008a p 5).

The Close the Gap campaign has been an effective policy driver. In 2014, almost 200,000 Australians had signed the Close the Gap pledge, which calls on government to take action, and approximately 140,000 Australians participated in the 2013 National Close the Gap Day (Oxfam Australia Close the Gap website). High-profile ambassadors advocate for and promote the campaign. The Close the Gap campaign has provided a compelling evidence base about Aboriginal and Torres Strait Islander health.

Following the election of the Labor Government in November 2007, the Council of Australian Governments (COAG) agreed that the then 17-year gap in life expectancy between Indigenous and non-Indigenous Australians must be closed. Prime Minister Kevin Rudd gave an official apology to the Stolen Generations in the first session of Federal Parliament on 13 February 2008 (Rudd 2008). On 20 March 2008, at the Indigenous Health Equity Summit organised by the Close the Gap campaign, the Prime Minister signed the Statement of Intent to Close the Gap. Later that year, the *National Partnership Agreement on Closing the Gap in Indigenous Health Outcomes* was developed and endorsed by Government through COAG. 'Closing the Gap' was the name adopted for the Government policy and for funding initiatives under the COAG commitments (HREOC 2008a; Rudd 2008).

The terms 'Close the Gap' and 'Closing the Gap' are used interchangeably to describe a wide range of events and initiatives aiming to reduce the health and life expectancy gap between Aboriginal and Torres Strait Islander peoples and non-Indigenous peoples in Australia. However, the Close the Gap Campaign Steering Committee is specific in its terms, and points out that Closing the Gap is an Australian Government initiative that does not necessarily reflect the human rights-based approach of the Close the Gap campaign. Closing the Gap policies are not necessarily endorsed by the CTGSC (2011 p 2).

Each state and territory partner has supported the need to address the social and cultural factors that influence the gap, including housing, community safety and security, justice, education, culture, language, community development, and other issues that influence the health and wellbeing of Aboriginal and Torres Strait Islander peoples. These issues are often referred to as the *social determinants of health* (discussed in Chapter 7), and they have specific relevance in addressing the health of Aboriginal and Torres Strait Islander peoples (Carson et al. 2007, Mowbray 2007, World Health Organization (WHO) 2007). Key Closing the Gap targets relevant to the social determinants of health include measures for improved housing, reduced smoking, and the availability of fresh food, which will work to significantly reduce the rates of Indigenous death and illness from infectious and chronic diseases.

The Australian Human Rights Commission (AHRC 2009) and Calma (2009) state that Aboriginal and Torres Strait Islander peoples themselves must be involved in decision-making about their health, and involved in developing policies to address inequalities.

Each year since 2009, in the Federal Parliament the Prime Minister has reported to Parliament on progress on Closing the Gap. In 2014, Prime Minister Tony Abbott presented a report that had a different style and a different outlook. According to the

Prime Minister, '... Government is shifting the focus of this yearly report from what the Government is doing, to how our people are living' (Commonwealth of Australia 2014 p 1). Reports previously presented were approximately 150 pages, containing extensive information and Government-produced evidence about the progress towards achieving targets (Commonwealth of Australia 2014). The report as presented in 2014 was a brief snapshot of individual and/or community examples of success and improvement as a result of the Closing the Gap policy.

The Prime Minister also states that 'One of the first acts of the new Government was to bring the administration of more than 150 Indigenous programs and services, from eight different government departments, into the Department of the Prime Minister and Cabinet' (Commonwealth of Australia 2014 p 4). This represented a major policy shift. Another significant change introduced after the Coalition won the 2013 federal election was the introduction of The Prime Minister's Indigenous Advisory Council, chaired by Mr Warren Mundine. This group has been formed to focus on practical changes to improve people's lives. It is hoped, by many, that these changes, along with other initiatives of Government, will ensure that initiatives already supported and funded will be maintained and where necessary expanded to address the health needs of Indigenous people (Commonwealth of Australia 2014 p 1).

Each year since 2010 the AHRC has published a 'shadow' report that is an assessment of the Australian Government's progress, including assessment of its implementation of the Statement of Intent. At times this report has been a useful mechanism to see beyond the Government-reported achievements to identify areas that may not be a priority for the Closing the Gap policy and/or that need additional attention. Up until 2013, the AHRC report was titled the 'Shadow Report', and contained a cautiously optimistic tone, and, while not providing outright endorsement of the Closing the Gap policy, there has been a willingness to give credit where it is due but also to remind readers that there is still a long way to go. For example, the report states that 'there is no room for complacency. As has been discussed, at this critical juncture we are faced with significant challenges. But these are challenges of political will only. None are insurmountable if we hold to the vision of what could be achieved, and allow ourselves as a nation to be inspired by it: Aboriginal and Torres Strait Islander health equality within our lifetimes, within a generation' (Close the Gap Campaign Steering Committee for Indigenous Health Equality 2014 p 39).

In 2014, the AHRC issued its *Progress and priorities report 2014*, and, while evident that it is still maintaining the goal to achieve health equality by 2030, the report states that 'it is clear that the Australian public demand that government, in partnership with Aboriginal and Torres Strait Islander peoples and their representatives, build on the close the gap platform to meet this challenge' (Close the Gap Campaign Steering Committee for Indigenous Health Equality 2014 p 2).

The Northern Territory Intervention

On 21 June 2007, the Australian Government announced the Northern Territory Emergency Response (NTER), commonly referred to as the 'Intervention'. This introduced a series of broad-ranging measures in Aboriginal communities across the Northern Territory, and received bipartisan support from the then Leader of the Opposition, Kevin Rudd. The Australian Government stated that the Intervention was a response to the national emergency confronting the welfare of Aboriginal children in the Northern Territory, and went on to justify the immediate action as a response to the first recommendation of the report *Little children are sacred: report into the protection of Aboriginal children from child abuse in the Northern Territory* (Brough 2007, Commonwealth of Australia 2008 p 66).

The Intervention was categorised into seven measures: welfare and employment; law and order; enhancing education; supporting families; improving child and family health; housing and land reform; and coordination (Commonwealth of Australia 2008 p 64). Most of the measures required the Australian Government to enact new legislation before proceeding. The legislative process was concluded within 10 days of the Bills being introduced to Parliament, which provided limited time for consideration and analysis, despite the complexity and potential implications of the legislation (HREOC 2008b).

At the time, opinions were divided about the Intervention, its justification, objectives and implementation; and they are still divided (AHRC 2011, Aboriginal Medical Services Alliance of the Northern Territory (AMSANT) 2009 p 4, Australian Indigenous Doctors' Association (AIDA) 2010, Commonwealth of Australia 2008 pp 9–10). Debate has continued about the implementation process, benefits, impact and outcomes of the Intervention, which has now become known as the 'Stronger Futures' federal government initiative for the Northern Territory (Australians for Native Title and Reconciliation (ANTaR) 2012, Commonwealth of Australia 2011a, 2011b). Over its lifetime, the NTER and now the Stronger Futures initiative have resulted in a plethora of reports and evaluations that continue to highlight the amount of resources used for the implementation process (Commonwealth of Australia 2011a, 2011b). However, what continues to be missing in the equation is the lack of community engagement between government and the Indigenous communities, which has been highlighted as an important process when connecting with Indigenous people (AHRC 2011, AIDA 2010, Viswanathan et al. 2011). At this time, it appears that the interventionary measures will be broadened and not scaled back. Moreover, they will be rolled out by the Australian Government in other geographical localities.

Aboriginal and Torres Strait Islander peoples today

In 2011, Australia's Aboriginal and Torres Strait Islander population was approximately 669,900 people, or about 3% of the total Australian population (ABS 2013b). While most identify as Aboriginal people, 6% identify as being Torres Strait Islander and 4% identify as both Aboriginal and Torres Strait Islander (ABS 2013b). Of the total Aboriginal and Torres Strait Islander population, 79% live in major cities and non-remote regional areas (ABS 2013b). This is in contrast to perceptions held by many Australians, and the images shown by the Australian media. There are large urban populations in some areas. For example, the 2011

ACTIVITY 16.2 Close the Gap and the Intervention

- Go to http://www.oxfam.org.au/explore/indigenous-australia.
- How many organisations signed the Close the Gap pledge in March 2008? Why do you think they would sign such a document? What are these individual organisations doing with regard to the Close the Gap campaign?
- Find the National Aboriginal Community Controlled Health Organisation (NACCHO) and Oxfam Australia's 'Close the Gap: solutions to the Indigenous health crisis facing Australia' at http://bahsl.com.au/old/pdf/CloseTheGap.Report.pdf. Look at the sections titled 'Solutions to the Aboriginal and Torres Strait Islander health crisis in Australia' and 'Recommendations', pp 7–13.
- Go to http://www.whatsworking.com.au/aboutus/history-of-women-for-wik/, which is monitoring the Northern Territory Emergency Response (the Intervention). What do you notice about this site?
- Do a brief search on the 'Northern Territory Emergency Response'. What are some of the ongoing debates with regard to the Intervention now? Keep in mind that it has now been going for some time. What are your thoughts about this for the future?

REFLECTION 16.2

How would you feel if you knew your family members might not live as long as other Australians, and that this was not because they had a genetic disorder or a form of childhood illness? How do you feel knowing that the Close the Gap campaign might be just another policy response, like all the other policies since the National Aboriginal Health Strategy (1989)?

census data indicate that 188,954 Aboriginal and Torres Strait Islander peoples (or 28.2% of Australia's total Indigenous population) live in Queensland (ABS 2013b). Some Aboriginal and Torres Strait Islander peoples are now second-, third- or multi-generation urban dwellers, while others may travel to and from cities and big urban centres and their home communities. When Indigenous Australians migrate into capital cities, they tend to move to areas where there are already concentrations of Indigenous people—generally areas of low socioeconomic status (Taylor 2006).

Living in urban areas is as much a part of reality for Aboriginal and Torres Strait Islander peoples as living in discrete Aboriginal rural, regional or isolated communities, or on one of the Torres Strait Islands (Fredericks 2004, Rowse 2006). Their urban living is varied, and includes a diversity of experience, needs and prospects that are shaped by gender, education, religion, age and security (Fredericks 2004; Tripcony 1995; Watson 1981). Their urban reality includes: choosing accommodation (houses, flats, caravans, renting, buying, or living on the streets or in parks); buying goods and services; finding a job; participating in sporting groups, clubs and organisations; and sharing and interacting with people from a diverse range of backgrounds, with their own languages and cultures. Living in urban environments also includes trying to find or make space within the city or regional centre for Aboriginal and Torres Strait Islander cultures, languages and individual and collective expression. Urban areas have witnessed the establishment and maintenance of Aboriginal and Torres Strait Islander organisations, programs, services and other structures. There is no single urban Indigenous experience or identity, nor is there a single urban Indigenous community in cities and regional areas. The multifaceted nature of urban Indigenous people and communities presents researchers, planners and government officers with a range of issues (Scrimgeour & Scrimgeour 2008).

Regardless of where they live, some statistics describing Aboriginal and Torres Strait Islander peoples as a group are useful. Overall, Aboriginal and Torres Strait Islander Australians have the poorest health status of any group in Australia. The Aboriginal and Torres Strait Islander population is also much younger than the non-Indigenous Australian population. In 2011, the median age of Aboriginal and Torres Strait Islander people was 21.8 years, compared with 37.6 years for the non-Indigenous population (ABS 2013b). These young people try to find a path for themselves like any other Australian young person, but they often experience greater difficulties in finding appropriate education or training, securing a job or housing, and living without racism. These issues are exacerbated by ill health—all measures of health status indicate poorer health outcomes for Aboriginal and Torres Strait Islander peoples (ABS 2013c). People who work in health, human services, housing, education, childcare, justice, and numerous other sectors witness the human face of these statistics

---

ACTIVITY 16.3 Profile and culture of Aboriginal and Torres Strait Islander peoples

- How many Aboriginal and Torres Strait Islander peoples live in the area in which you live?
- What are some of the Aboriginal and Torres Strait Islander organisations in your area or region? What do they do? Who goes there? Who works there? Have you noticed them before? Why/why not?
- Look at the newspapers in your city or regional area, and analyse how Aboriginal and Torres Strait Islander peoples and cultures are written about.

REFLECTION 16.3

What might be some of the stressors you might experience being an Aboriginal or Torres Strait Islander person living in the city? How would you cope?

and the toll it takes on the people who access their services. These support workers can suffer social and emotional wellbeing issues and burn-out as a result of dealing with such issues every day.

Community and gendered health

Prior to colonisation, Aboriginal and Torres Strait Islander men and women held diverse gendered realities. Traditional ways of understanding gender were lost during colonisation, including: traditional approaches to reproduction, mothering and child-rearing; the recognition of developmental milestones and the attainment of male and female adulthood; and all that included the economic, political, social, spiritual and ceremonial domains of life (Bell 1983). Today, Aboriginal and Torres Strait Islander men's and women's cultural and spiritual practices continue to varying degrees. In some places, they demonstrate Aboriginal and Torres Strait Islander men's and women's relationships to land, children, men and women, each other, law, ceremony, what is secret and sacred, and responsibilities within Country.

Aboriginal and Torres Strait Islander women's health

In 2010–2012, life expectancy at birth for Aboriginal and Torres Strait Islander women was 73.7, compared with 83.2 for all Australian women (ABS 2013a). This is a life expectancy gap of 9.5 years.

Aboriginal and Torres Strait Islander families include more one-parent families with dependent children (30% compared with 10% for non-Indigenous, with most of these having the mother as the head of the family), fewer one-parent families without dependants (about 33% compared with 53%), and a similar percentage of families comprising couples with dependent children (about 37%) (ABS 2006). Aboriginal and Torres Strait Islander households are larger than other Australian households, with an average of 3.3 people per household (compared with 2.5).

Aboriginal and Torres Strait Islander women have more children than non-Indigenous women, 2.8 compared with 2.0 (ABS 2008), and are considerably younger than non-Indigenous women when they have their first child—in 2011, 25.3 and 30.2 years, respectively (Li et al. 2013). In 2009, 5% of all births in Australia were Aboriginal or Torres Strait Islander, with the median age of Indigenous mothers 24.5 years (6 years lower than the median age for all mothers) (ABS 2010). Babies born to Aboriginal and Torres Strait Islander women were twice as likely to be of low birth weight (see the *Mums and Babies Program* featured in Case Study 14.1), and were more likely to die in their first year than those born to non-Indigenous women (ABS 2008, 2010). Aboriginal and Torres Strait Islander babies are more likely to be unwell than non-Indigenous babies (Kennedy & McGill 2009).

Specific maternal and child health services have become a critical component in the delivery of comprehensive primary healthcare for Aboriginal and Torres Strait Islander women. Most services are based in community-controlled health services, and are staffed by midwives and specially trained Aboriginal health workers and, where possible, general practitioners. They often operate in partnership with mainstream services. Each state and territory coordinates a network of Indigenous maternal and child health services, with policies and professional support coordinated through a central site. Two examples are the *Koori Maternity Service* in Victoria and the *Aboriginal and Maternal Infant Health Strategy* in New South Wales.

Aboriginal and Torres Strait Islander women experience much poorer health than non-Indigenous women. They are 10 times more likely to have kidney disease, 4 times more likely to have diabetes, and almost twice as likely to have asthma (ABS 2007). They report higher levels of chronic disease, and many experience multiple conditions (comorbidities). The most common health conditions reported by Aboriginal and Torres Strait Islander women are eye/sight problems (54%), back pain/symptoms (23%), heart/circulatory diseases (23%) and asthma (22%). Aboriginal and Torres Strait Islander women with chronic diseases and disabilities are more likely to report high/very high levels of psychological distress (34% compared with 21% for Australian women without chronic diseases) (ABS 2007). In addition, Aboriginal and Torres Strait Islander women earn lower incomes than non-Indigenous women and men.

In the past, Australian women's health services have varied according to different state and territory government policies. Initiatives have included women's health centres, mobile women's health programs, sexual assault programs, reproductive services, same-sex services, women's cancer prevention programs, and alternative birthing programs. Overall, the Australian women's health sector has varied in its ability to incorporate the health and wellbeing needs of Aboriginal and Torres Strait Islander women into its wider agenda. Aboriginal and Torres Strait Islander women have benefited through advocacy undertaken by the women's health movement—particularly strategies related to control over their bodies and the inappropriateness of the biomedical model of health for women (Wass 1998, Weeks 1994). However, Aboriginal and Torres Strait Islander women had limited access to funding and, when they did, it was mostly for birthing programs and birthing centres (Dorman 1997, Harrison 1991), sexual assault programs and shelters. While these services are important, other areas of priority were identified in the NAHS document under *Women's business* (NAHS 1989 p 179–190). When the NAHS was being developed, Aboriginal and Torres Strait Islander women were extensively engaged in developing the community-controlled health movement and delivering services based on a comprehensive primary healthcare approach (NACCHO 1993, NAHS Working Party 1989).

To develop the new National Women's Health Policy, the Australian Government undertook a range of consultations with women, community groups, health service providers, and state and territory governments. In 2009, the Australian Women's Health Network received funding from the then Department of Health and Ageing (Gender and Reproductive Health Branch) for consultation with Aboriginal and Torres Strait Islander women, and to provide input into the new National Women's Health Policy. The Australian Women's Health Network Talking Circle was established to develop the National Aboriginal and Torres Strait Islander Women's Health Strategy (Fredericks et al. 2010).

Around the time the strategy was released, other data were released which showed that there had been little improvement in Indigenous women's health, and in fact in some areas it had become worse. Since 2011, a group of Indigenous and non-Indigenous women—including academics, community advocates, health professionals, representatives from peak body organisations and others—have been working together at a national level with the view to establishing a national Indigenous women's health alliance to specifically address and advocate for Indigenous women's health concerns. They held a national forum in 2013, and while they have

---

ACTIVITY 16.4 Aboriginal and Torres Strait Islander women's health

- View the National Aboriginal and Torres Strait Islander Women's Health Strategy at http://www.naccho.org.au/download/aboriginal-health/National_Aboriginal_and_Torres_Strait_Islander_Womens_Strategy_May_2010.pdf.
- What do you notice about the action areas and recommendations? How could you use these within your public health practice?
- What changes might you need to make in order to specifically address your practice?

sought funding to continue their work, this has not been forthcoming. The group still refers to itself as the Indigenous Women's Health Alliance, and is still meeting and continuing to undertake advocacy, using monies from individual women's personal donations and through limited organisational and institutional support.

Aboriginal and Torres Strait Islander men's health

While there is an abundance of literature about the health and wellbeing of women, literature about men's health tends to emphasise the negative consequences of male social behaviour (Brown 2004). The literature typically describes Aboriginal and Torres Strait Islander men as experiencing the worst in health and social statistics. They are rarely recognised as being dynamic, essential parts of families, communities and societies (Brown 2004).

> **REFLECTION 16.4**
>
> If you are a woman, have you ever used a woman-specific service? Think about what that was like: why did you go there, how did it feel, did you get what you needed or wanted from the service? If you are male, do you know any women who have used a woman-centred service? What are your thoughts about these kinds of services? Why might a woman use a service just for women?
>
> How do you think your family would cope with a sick baby or child? What if there were several sick children in your family or extended family? What would be some of the struggles? What would you do?

The health of Aboriginal and Torres Strait Islander men needs to be understood within the context of the historical, cultural, physiological, psychosocial, economic, environmental and political contexts they face (Adams et al. 2003, Brown 2004, Hayman 1999, Wenitong 2002, 2006). Their health also needs to be understood from their perspectives, in terms of their own gendered reality and their relations to other men. Aboriginal and Torres Strait Islander men are extremely diverse; some have been able to maintain strong connections to their cultural practices, while others have had little choice about losing their culture and language. Different Aboriginal and Torres Strait Islander communities have varied understandings of men's health, and of sexuality and sexual preferences.

The social and emotional wellbeing of many Aboriginal and Torres Strait Islander people has been undermined by trauma, grief or loss. For men, this is reflected in their mental health, displacement, high rates of suicide, alcohol and substance misuse, community disorder, family violence and abuse, and incarceration. These behaviours are not traditional parts of Aboriginal and Torres Strait Islander cultures. They arise from: cultural dispossession and disempowerment; poor health, poverty and insecure food supply; difficulties accessing employment, education or training; and difficulties accessing appropriate housing (Cronin 2007, Walter 2009). While many causes of ill health within Aboriginal and Torres Strait Islander communities may be preventable with lifestyle changes, the issues that cause ill health are highly complex. Political will and appropriate levels of government funding are also the core ingredients required to produce improvements.

The major killers of Aboriginal and Torres Strait Islander men are diseases of the circulatory system (heart attacks and strokes), injury and poisoning, respiratory diseases, cancers, and endocrine disorders (predominately diabetes) (ABS 2008, Australian Institute of Health and Welfare (AIHW) 2010). Several risk factors contribute to the overall ill health of Aboriginal and Torres Strait Islander peoples, including lack of access to healthy, affordable food and food preparation areas, poor nutrition, and using harmful substances (e.g. smoking and alcohol abuse). Other issues that are significant for men include: intergenerational trauma; loss of cultural practices and roles through colonisation; lack of health education; language, gender and cultural barriers; and difficulty in accessing health services (Adams 2007, Adams et al. 2003, Adams & McCoy 2011, Andrology Australia 2001, Hayman 1999). Aboriginal and Torres Strait Islander men are far less likely than non-Indigenous men to have completed Year 12 or equivalent. The difference in education affects health literacy, with clear impacts on their ability to understand general health and medicine information, and their commitment to taking prescribed medication.

Many of the chronic health problems facing Aboriginal and Torres Strait Islander men could be readily treated if they were diagnosed early. However, evidence shows that the men are reluctant to seek medical attention (Adams et al. 2003, Andrology Australia 2001, Hayman 1999, Wenitong 2002, 2006). Usually, Aboriginal and Torres Strait Islander men only seek healthcare when they are seriously ill. Even then, they may not reveal the real symptoms to a doctor (Hayman 1999). Brown (2004) has suggested that Aboriginal and Torres Strait Islander men tend to present for medical intervention when they can no longer bear the inconvenience or disability of their illness. Unfortunately, these presentations seem to occur at a time of physical, emotional or psychological crisis, when little prevention can transpire.

> ### ACTIVITY 16.5 Aboriginal and Torres Strait Islander men's health
>
> - List some of the settings in which to talk with Aboriginal and Torres Strait Islander men about their health.
> - What kind of empowerment and advocacy strategies might you need to utilise in working with Aboriginal and Torres Strait Islander men? To gain some ideas, see Chapter 14, on health promotion.

> ### REFLECTION 16.5
>
> One of the ways to connect with Aboriginal and Torres Strait Islander men in a health-promoting way may be through an Aboriginal and Torres Strait Islander organisation or specific men's group. You will need to think creatively. If you are a woman, you will also need to consider whether it is appropriate for you, depending on the issue, to work with Aboriginal and Torres Strait Islander men.

Community-controlled health service sector

Aboriginal and Torres Strait Islander community-controlled health services are now found in every state and territory of Australia. They may be referred to as Aboriginal medical services (AMSs—commonly found in New South Wales), Aboriginal community-controlled health services (ACCHSs), or Aboriginal community-controlled health organisations (ACCHOs—commonly found in Victoria). The first service in Australia was established in 1971 in Redfern, New South Wales. Redfern AMS was established as a community response to the poor health services that Aboriginal people received. The service was set up by Aboriginal people to deliver holistic, comprehensive and culturally appropriate healthcare (NATSIHC 2001). There are now over 150 Aboriginal and Torres Strait Islander health services in Australia, within urban, regional, rural and remote communities (NACCHO website).

Community-controlled health services diagnose and treat illness, provide referrals to specialists and other providers, refer to allied health services (sometimes with visiting programs, such as optometry and podiatry), provide counselling and support, and undertake broader community advocacy. They may also undertake research, support the development of culturally appropriate materials, and provide training for health professionals. Numerous nursing and medical programs offer placements in Aboriginal and Torres Strait Islander health organisations.

Around 70% of the staff in the ACCHS sector are Aboriginal and Torres Strait Islander people. Aboriginal and Torres Strait Islander health workers (AHWs) form a core component of the staff, and are vital within community-controlled health services. Eckerman et al. state that 'relevance, appropriateness and acceptability of health care within an Aboriginal group can only be achieved through Aboriginal Health Workers' (2006 p 162). They are not only 'the most appropriate health professionals to be dealing with their own people, but often they are also the cultural brokers guiding and protecting non-Aboriginal peoples in their own community' (Eckerman et al. 2006 p 163). Generally, AHWs are permanently based within health services, while nurses, doctors and allied health professionals tended to come and go. In time we may see the functions of health workers change, as these health environments change, although their role in supporting Indigenous peoples may remain the same. Similarly, as the workforce has matured and as the ACCHSs have become more corporatised in their approach, health workers have been able to seek out a broader range of professional development opportunities, including the opportunity to undertake studies at TAFE or university to become a nurse, general practitioner or allied health worker.

ACCHSs usually receive government grants and other funding to run services, but they are not government services and their employees are not government workers. Most ACCHSs are run by a board of directors or management committee which is elected by its members. The local Aboriginal and Torres Strait Islander population become members of the ACCHS. Accountability is through the board, annual general meetings (AGMs), annual reports, and reports to funding bodies (NATSIHC 2001). The board sets the overall direction of the ACCHS and formally employs the staff.

The ACCHSs have a national representative organisation—NACCHO. There are also state- and territory-based representative organisations. NACCHO and its state- and territory-based affiliates provide a representative voice for Aboriginal and Torres Strait Islander communities in health-related issues. They also have work areas that specifically focus on public health and research.

ACCHOs play an important role in providing primary healthcare services for Aboriginal and Torres Strait Islander people that are planned and managed by the communities themselves. They aim to deliver high-quality, holistic and culturally appropriate healthcare. While ACCHOs are committed to the reasons why they were established, in this current political and economic climate they are also having to explore how they operate and explore issues of sustainability for the future.

ACTIVITY 16.6 Aboriginal and Torres Strait Islander health services

- Access a few of the following organisational websites:
  - The Victorian Aboriginal Health Service: http://www.vahs.org.au/
  - The Aboriginal and Torres Strait Islander Community Health Service Brisbane Ltd: http://www.atsichsbrisbane.org.au/
  - Wuchopperen Health Service: http://www.wuchopperen.com/
  - The Victorian Aboriginal Community Controlled Health Organisation (VACCHO): http://www.vaccho.org.au/
  - The Queensland Aboriginal and Islander Health Council (QAIHC): http://www.qaihc.com.au/
  - The National Aboriginal Community Controlled Health Organisation (NACCHO): http://www.naccho.org.au/
- What are their aims? What kind of services do they offer? Who are the websites designed for? What is reflected?
- What are five key messages you have gained about the community-controlled health service sector?
- What are some of the issues they might face in the future?

REFLECTION 16.6

Think about why Aboriginal and Torres Strait Islander peoples established their own health services, and why they still exist today. A number of them have been going for over 40 years, showing great sustainability and strength in organisational management. Think about the changes in policy they have experienced along the way. Try to imagine what some of the challenges and benefits might be in working in an Aboriginal community-controlled health organisation on a day-to-day, week-to-week basis.

Research

There is a long history of research conducted on Aboriginal and Torres Strait Islander peoples, and on Indigenous peoples throughout the world. Tuhiwai Smith (1999 p 3) suggests that Indigenous people 'are the most researched people in the world'. Historically, the vast majority of this research was carried out by non-Indigenous people. Often, research intrudes into Aboriginal and Torres Strait Islander peoples' lives and communities. For many years, Aboriginal and Torres Strait Islander peoples questioned research: how non-Indigenous people have wrongfully assumed ownership of Indigenous knowledge; how museums and libraries have misappropriated precious objects and ancestral remains; and why numerous non-Indigenous people have gained qualifications, assumed 'expert' status over and above Indigenous people, and secured career advancement and increased salaries, while the communities that are 'researched' have been left with very little.

Over the past 20 years there have been considerable changes in the way research is conducted with Aboriginal and Torres Strait Islander populations. Several publications on ethics and protocols in Aboriginal and Torres Strait Islander research have been developed since the 1990s. One of the most recent documents is the National Health and Medical Research Council's *The NHMRC Road Map II: A strategic framework for improving the health of Aboriginal and Torres Strait Islander peoples through research* (NHMRC 2010). This document sets out criteria for health and medical research with, and for, Aboriginal and Torres Strait Islander Australians, which all research proposals and funding applications must address. Road Map II (NHMRC 2010 p 6) identifies seven action areas:

1 improving the participation of Aboriginal and Torres Strait Islander peoples in NHMRC programs
2 capacity exchange
3 promotion of the NHMRC's role in Aboriginal and Torres Strait Islander health
4 Close the Gap
5 evaluation research
6 intervention research
7 priority-driven research.

Some examples of research that embraces these principles include work undertaken at the Onemda VicHealth Koori Health Unit (University of Melbourne), the Indigenous Health Unit (James Cook University), the Lowitja Institute (formerly the Cooperative Research Centre of Aboriginal Health), and within the community-controlled health service sector (such as the Public Health and Research Unit at the Victorian Aboriginal Community Controlled Health Organisation (VACCHO)). Case Study 16.1 describes one example.

ACTIVITY 16.7 Research with Aboriginal and Torres Strait Islander peoples

- From Case Study 16.1, what might have been some of the first steps in commencing this research project? List the steps in the order that you would undertake them.
- Go back to the first part of this section, where the principles of research with Aboriginal and Torres Strait Islander peoples are outlined (NHMRC 2010). Review the case study and explain how it has met the principles.
- Visit the following websites and explore the variety of research programs and public health programs currently underway:
  ○ The Australian HealthInfoNet: http://www.healthinfonet.ecu.edu.au
  ○ The Lowitja Institute: http://www.crcah.org.au/
  ○ The Australian Institute of Aboriginal and Torres Strait Islander Studies: http://www.aiatsis.gov.au/main.html

REFLECTION 16.7

When exploring research with Aboriginal and Torres Strait Islander peoples, what are some of the issues you might need to consider with regards to your own skills, abilities and experience? How could you address these?

The Victorian Aboriginal Community Controlled Health Organisation

The Victorian Aboriginal Community Controlled Health Organisation (VACCHO) sought to address poor health from smoking through a three-year research project (2009–2011) titled *Goreen Narrkwarren Ngrn-toura—Healthy Family Air*. VACCHO represents a collective of 24 Aboriginal community-controlled health organisations (ACCHOs) around Victoria, and is well placed to facilitate such a project within the sector, working with the Koori Maternity Services. The project was funded by the former Victorian Department of Human Services (now the Department of Health). VACCHO is the grant recipient, and it is through VACCHO that all project activities are driven.

It is well established that smoking tobacco is a major cause and contributor to heart disease, stroke, lung diseases, some cancers and a variety of other illnesses and conditions (Centre for Excellence in Indigenous Tobacco Control (CEITC) 2009). Within Australia, cigarette smoking is responsible for at least 20% of all deaths in Aboriginal communities (CEITC 2008). The Goreen Narrkwarren Ngrn-toura—Healthy Family Air project aimed to increase the understanding and knowledge of smoking cessation, create supportive environments with Aboriginal health organisations, support Aboriginal women to quit smoking in pregnancy, and support young mothers not to take up smoking. Engagement was a key component of this project, which meant the involvement of individuals, key stakeholders and multiple organisational partners (such as QUIT Victoria, the Women's Alcohol and Drug Service (WADS) and the Aboriginal Women's Business Unit at the Royal Women's Hospital). Three individual ACCHOs participated in the project, along with VACCHO as the pilot site. The ACCHOs self-selected into the project—that is, they expressed their interest in being involved and were engaged based on their interest. The project was led by Aboriginal people, and also sought strong working relationships with other projects (both non-Indigenous, and Aboriginal and Torres Strait Islander) that had the objective of reducing smoking in pregnancy.

This project was not based on a clinical trial, nor was it designed to measure only program success or failure. It used an action research approach to develop, implement and evaluate a community-based holistic intervention aimed at reducing smoking among Aboriginal women during pregnancy. Action research means that people had opportunities to talk about the research processes throughout the project, and were able to have a say and influence the research within their organisation and within their community. The project sought to address the following research questions:

- Does strengthening the capacity of Aboriginal health workers (AHWs), Koori Maternity Services (KMS) workers and in-home support (HIS) workers regarding smoking cessation contribute in the long term to a reduction in smoking for pregnant Aboriginal women?

- Does strengthening the capacity of ACCHOs to deliver personal support and smoking reduction programs to young Aboriginal mothers and Aboriginal women who are pregnant contribute in the long term to a reduction in smoking for pregnant Aboriginal women?

The project undertook a literature review (van der Sterren et al. 2009) centred on the questions posed, and found that the project needed to include:

- strategies that denormalise smoking in Aboriginal communities, and provide skills and supportive environments for pregnant women to quit
- interventions provided in the primary healthcare setting to advise and support the women to quit—such interventions may include brief interventions and behavioural counselling (e.g. nicotine replacement therapy (NRT) and Quit courses)
- training provided to AHWs to improve their confidence and capacity to deliver individual clinic-based interventions, and community-based tobacco control activities
- strategies for AHWs to support and encourage their members to quit smoking themselves, including the development of supportive work environments
- multicomponent family- and community-focused programs that take a broad-based and holistic approach to tobacco control, and incorporate components that target families and communities, not just pregnant women
- the development of policies and protocols in Aboriginal organisations (such as smoke-free workplaces and cars) to provide supportive environments in which to deliver smoking cessation programs.

The literature review can be found on the Australian Indigenous Health *InfoNet* http://www.healthinfonet.ecu.edu.au/key-resources/programs-projects?pid=572. Copies of other resources and documents from the project will also be available on the website as work is published.

The project has already resulted in a number of outcomes, including new and innovative health promotion resources for services in Victoria to use, individual organisational policy change, and training and support for smoking cessation programs. These outcomes are the result of Aboriginal people being engaged in all aspects of the research project, from conception to development, ethics, implementation and evaluation. This could be said to also be an outcome of the project. The project has had ongoing activities since its conclusion in 2011.

Acknowledgement is offered to VACCHO for allowing us to use the Goreen Narrkwarren Ngrn-toura—Healthy Family Air project as a case study within this chapter.

Indigenous people in other parts of the world

Australia ranks at the bottom in a league table of first-world, wealthy nations working to improve the health and life expectancy of Indigenous people. The gap in health status between Aboriginal and Torres Strait Islander peoples and non-Indigenous Australians is still far greater than that of other Indigenous and non-Indigenous populations from similar countries—such as Canada, New Zealand and the United States (AIHW 2011). While the life expectancy gap for Australia's Aboriginal and Torres Strait Islander peoples is now about 10 years (ABS 2013a), it is difficult to know whether this reflects a genuine health improvement (because the 2008 estimate of a life expectancy gap of 17 years was based on 2001 statistics) (Kennedy & McGill 2009). It is possible that the methods now used by the ABS to measure the life expectancy gap have reduced the apparent disparity. The AIHW suggests that the new method means we cannot conclude that there has been a sudden improvement in Aboriginal and Torres Strait Islander peoples' life expectancy (AIHW 2010 p 234). It is uncertain what method Canada, New Zealand and the United States use to measure the gap in life expectancy for their Indigenous peoples. Even though they report disparities, the disparity in Australia remains 5 to 10 years more. Regardless of the way the gap is measured or its size, what is important is that there is still a significant gap between the life expectancy of Aboriginal and Torres Strait Islander Australians and non-Indigenous Australians.

A final word

Within the Australian population, Aboriginal and Torres Strait Islander peoples have the poorest health status and are considered the most socially and economically disadvantaged. The reasons for this are complex, as there is a range of factors that influence health and wellbeing, such as housing, community safety and security, justice, education, culture, language, employment and income, locality and community development. In order for public health to make a difference to the health and wellbeing of Aboriginal and Torres Strait Islander peoples, it needs to recognise, understand and work across the historical, cultural, social, physiological, psychosocial, economic, environmental and political contexts of individuals, groups and communities (Carson et al. 2007, Mowbray 2007, WHO 2007). The Australian Indigenous HealthInfoNet (2009 p 12) recognises this when it states that 'without substantial reductions in the overall disadvantages experienced by many Indigenous people, even fully committed approaches within the health sector will have a limited impact on achieving major improvements in Indigenous health status'. The poor health and wellbeing of Aboriginal and Torres Strait Islander peoples presents many challenges for public health workers. As the sub-population with the greatest need, it is also the area where you can make the greatest difference.

REVIEW QUESTIONS

1 How has colonisation impacted on Aboriginal and Torres Strait Islander peoples' health and wellbeing?

2 What are some of the present-day health and wellbeing concerns of Aboriginal and Torres Strait Islander peoples?

3 What might you need to consider when working with Aboriginal and Torres Strait Islander peoples in improving their health and wellbeing?

4 What do you understand to be the social determinants of health, and how do they impact on the health and wellbeing of Aboriginal and Torres Strait Islander peoples?

5 How is the Northern Territory Intervention impacting on Aboriginal and Torres Strait Islander peoples living in the areas where it is imposed? What are the advantages and disadvantages of this initiative?

6 What are the differences between Close the Gap and Closing the Gap?

7 What is meant by a 'gendered reality'?

8 What motivated the policies made by federal, state and territory governments, churches and other institutions that controlled the lives of Aboriginal and Torres Strait Islander peoples?

9 What is meant by 'Country', and how do Aboriginal and Torres Strait Islander peoples' spiritual, social and historical links to Country contribute to their health and wellbeing?

10 What do you think are some of the factors that have facilitated the survival and revitalisation of many Aboriginal and Torres Strait Islander cultures?

References

Aboriginal Medical Services Alliance of the Northern Territory, 2009. AMSANT Annual Report 2009–2010. AMSANT, Darwin. Online. Available: <http://www.amsant.org.au> (4 June 2014).

Adams, M., 2007. Sexual and Reproductive Health Problems among Aboriginal and Torres Strait Islander Males. (PhD thesis.) Institute of Health and Biomedical Innovation, School of Public Health, Queensland University of Technology, Brisbane.

Adams, M., De Kretser, D., Holden, C., 2003. Male sexual and reproductive health among the Aboriginal and Torres Strait Islander population. Rural and Remote Health 3 (2), Article 153. Online. Available: <http://www.rrh.org.au/articles/subviewnew.asp?ArticleID=153> (15 Apr 2015).

Adams, M., McCoy, B., 2011. Lives of Indigenous Australian men. In: Thackrah, R., Scott, K.Winch, J. (Eds.), Indigenous Australian health and cultures: an introduction for health professionals. Pearson Australia, Frenchs Forest, pp. 127–151.

Andrology Australia (The Australian Centre of Excellence in Male Reproductive Health), 2001. Annual Report 2001. Monash Institute of Reproduction and Development, Monash Medical Centre, Melbourne.

Australian Bureau of Statistics, 2006. National Aboriginal and Torres Strait Islander Health Survey, Australia 2004–2005. ABS Cat. No. 4715.0. ABS, Canberra.

Australian Bureau of Statistics, 2007. Population distribution, Aboriginal and Torres Strait Islander Australians, 2006. ABS Cat. No. 4705.0. 2006, ABS, Canberra. Online. Available: <http://www.abs.gov.au/ausstats/abs@.nsf/mf/4705.0> (4 Jun 2014).

Australian Bureau of Statistics, 2008. The health and welfare of Australia's Aboriginal and Torres Strait Islander peoples. ABS, Canberra.

Australian Bureau of Statistics, 2010. The health and welfare of Australia's Aboriginal and Torres Strait Islander peoples. ABS, Canberra. Online. Available: <http://www.abs.gov.au/ausstats/abs@.nsf/mf/4704.0/> (15 Feb 2014).

Australian Bureau of Statistics, 2013a. Life tables for Aboriginal and Torres Strait Islander Australians, 2010–2012. ABS Cat. No. 3302.0.55.003. ABS, Canberra. Online. Available: <http://www.abs.gov.au/ausstats/abs@.nsf/latestProducts/3302.0.55.003Media%20 Release12010-2012> (4 Jun 2014).

Australian Bureau of Statistics, 2013b. Estimates of Aboriginal and Torres Strait Islander Australians, June 2011. ABS Cat. No. 3238.0.55.001. ABS, Canberra. Online. Available: <http://www.abs.gov.au/ausstats/abs@.nsf/mf/3238.0.55.001> (27 May 2014).

Australian Bureau of Statistics, 2013c. Australian Aboriginal and Torres Strait Islander Health Survey: first results, Australia, 2012–13. ABS Cat. No. 4727.0.55.001. ABS, Canberra. Online. Available: <www.abs.gov.au/ausstats/abs@.nsf/Latestproducts/4727.0.55 .001Main%20Features99992012-13?opendocument&tabname=Summary&prodno =4727.0.55.001&issue=2012-13&num=&view=> (14 Jan 2014).

Australian Health Ministers Advisory Council, 2006. Aboriginal and Torres Strait Islander Health Performance: framework report. AHMAC, Canberra.

Australian Human Rights Commission, 2009. Will COAG deliver on Indigenous health? Media release, 01 July 2009. Online. Available: <https://www.humanrights.gov.au/news/media -releases/2009-media-release-will-coag-deliver-indigenous-health> (22 Sep 2014).

Australian Human Rights Commission, 2011. The suspension and reinstatement of the RDA and special measures in the NTER. AHRC, Sydney. Online. Available: <https:// www.humanrights.gov.au/publications/suspension-and-reinstatement-rda-and-special -measures-nter> (22 Sep 2014).

Australian Indigenous Doctors' Association and Centre for Health Equity Training, Research and Evaluation, University of New South Wales, 2010. Health Impact Assessment of the Northern Territory Emergency Response. AIDA, Canberra.

Australian Indigenous HealthInfoNet, 2009. Summary of Australian Indigenous health 2009. Available: <http://www.healthinfonet.ecu.edu.au/summary> (4 Jun 2014).

Australian Institute of Aboriginal and Torres Strait Islander Studies, 1994. Encyclopaedia of Aboriginal Australia. Aboriginal Studies Press, Canberra.

Australian Institute of Health and Welfare, 2010. Australia's Health 2010. AIHW Cat. No. AUS 122. AIHW, Canberra.

Australian Institute of Health and Welfare, 2011. Comparing Life Expectancy of Indigenous People in Australia, New Zealand, Canada and the United States: Conceptual, Methodological and Data Issues. AIHW Cat. No. IHW 47. AIHW, Canberra.

Australians for Native Title and Reconciliation, 2012. Submission to the Senate and Community Affairs Committee. Inquiry into Stronger Futures in the Northern Territory Bill 2011 and two related Bills. Australians for Native Title and Reconciliation, Sydney.

Bell, D., 1983. Daughters of the Dreaming. George Allen and Unwin, Sydney.

Beresford, Q., Omaji, P., 1998. Our State of Mind: Racial Planning and the Stolen Generations. Fremantle Arts Centre Press, South Freemantle.

Blainey, G., 1994. Triumph of the Nomads: A History of Ancient Australia. MacMillan, South Melbourne.

Brough, M., 2007. National emergency response to protect children in the NT. Media release, 21 June 2007. Online. Available: <http://parlinfo.aph.gov.au/parlInfo/search/display/ display.w3p;query=Id%3A%22media%2Fpressrel%2F8ZFN6%22> (22 Sep 2014).

Brown, A., 2004. Building on the Strengths: A Review of Male Health in the Anangu Pitjantjatjara Lands. Nganampa Health Council, Alice Springs.

Calma, T., 2009. Report highlights need for things to be done differently. Media statement. Online. Available: <http://www.humanrights.gov.au/news/media-releases/2009-media -release-report-highlights-need-things-be-done-differently> (22 Sep 2014).

Carson, B., Dunbar, T., Chenhall, D., et al., 2007. Social Determinants of Indigenous Health. Menzies School of Health Research. Allen and Unwin, Crows Nest.

Centre for Excellence in Indigenous Tobacco Control, 2008. Indigenous Tobacco Control in Australia: Everybody's Business. National Indigenous Tobacco Control Research Roundtable Report, Brisbane. CEITC, University of Melbourne, Melbourne.

Centre for Excellence in Indigenous Tobacco Control, 2009. Reducing Tobacco Dependency in Aboriginal and Torres Strait Islander Communities: A Review of the Evidence. CEITC, University of Melbourne, Melbourne.

Clark, M., 1966. Sources of Australian History. Mentor, New York.

Cleland, J.B., 1928. Disease amongst the Australian Aborigines. Journal of Tropical Medicine and Hygiene 31, 53–70, 125–130, 141–145, 157–160, 173–177, 196–198, 202–206, 216–220, 232–235, 262–266, 281–282, 290–294, 307–313, 326–330. (series of articles across same volume, different editions, available at University of Queensland).

Close the Gap Campaign Steering Committee for Indigenous Health Equality, 2011. Shadow report: on Australian government's progress towards closing the gap in life expectancy between Indigenous and non-Indigenous Australians. Close the Gap Campaign Steering Committee for Indigenous Health Equality.

Close the Gap Campaign Steering Committee for Indigenous Health Equality, 2014. Progress and priorities report 2014. Close the Gap Campaign Steering Committee for Indigenous Health Equality. Online. Available: <https://www.humanrights.gov.au/publications/close-gap-progress-and-priorities-report-2014> (24 Sep 2014).

Commonwealth of Australia, 2008. Report of the NTER Review Board—October 2008. Australian Government, Canberra.

Commonwealth of Australia, 2011a. Northern Territory Emergency Response Evaluation Report 2011. Department of Families, Housing, Community Services and Indigenous Affairs. Australian Government, Canberra.

Commonwealth of Australia, 2011b. Stronger Futures in the Northern Territory. Discussion paper June 2011. Department of Families, Housing, Community Services and Indigenous Affairs.

Commonwealth of Australia, 2014. Closing the Gap Prime Minister's Report 2014. Australian Government, Canberra.

Couzos, S., Murray, R., 2008. Aboriginal Primary Health Care: An Evidence-Based Approach. Oxford University Press, South Melbourne.

Cronin, D., 2007. Welfare dependency and mutual obligation: negotiating Indigenous sovereignty. In: Moreton-Robinson, A. (Ed.), Sovereign Subjects Indigenous Sovereignty Matters. Allen and Unwin, Sydney, pp. 179–200.

Dorman, R., 1997. Ngua Gundi (mother and child) program. Aboriginal and Islander Health Worker Journal 21 (5), 2–6.

Eckerman, A., Dowd, T., Martin, M., et al., 2006. Binan Goonj: Bridging Cultures in Aboriginal Health. University of New England Press, Armidale.

Engles, F., 1892/1973. The Condition of the Working-Class in England. Progress Publishers, Moscow.

Evans, R., Cronin, K., Saunders, K. (Eds.), 1975. Exclusion, Exploitation and Extermination: Race Relations in Colonial Queensland. Australia and New Zealand Book Company, Sydney.

Flood, J., 2006. The Original Australians: Story of the Aboriginal People. Allen and Unwin, Sydney.

Fredericks, B., 2004. Urban identity. Eureka Street 14 (10), 30–31.

Fredericks, B., Adams, K., Angus, S., 2010. The Australian Women's Health Network Talking Circle. National Aboriginal and Torres Strait Islander Women's Health Strategy. Australian Women's Health Network, Melbourne.

Harrison, J., 1991. Tjitji Tjuta Atunymanama Kamiku Tjukurpawanangku—looking after children grandmothers' way. Nagaanyatjarra, Pitantjatjara Yankunytatjara Women's Council, Alice Springs.

Hayman, N., 1999. Medical and clinical issues for Aboriginal men. In: Proceedings, 1st National Indigenous Male Health Convention, Ross River, N.T. Aboriginal Men's Health Policy Unit, Territory Health Service, Darwin.

Human Rights and Equal Opportunity Commission, 2008a. Close the Gap: National Indigenous Health Equality Targets. Human Rights Equal Opportunity Commission, Sydney.

Human Rights and Equal Opportunity Commission, 2008b. Social Justice Report 2007. Aboriginal and Torres Strait Islander Social Justice Commissioner, Sydney.

Kennedy, B., McGill, K., 2009. Indigenous and non-Indigenous life expectancy at birth in Queensland and Australia. Queensland Health Statbite 17. Online. Available: <http://www.health.qld.gov.au/hsu/pdf/statbite/statbite17.pdf> (22 Sep 2014).

Li, Z., Zeki, R., Hilder, L., et al., 2013. Australia's Mothers and Babies 2011. Perinatal Statistics Series No. 28. Cat. No. PER 59. AIHW National Perinatal Epidemiology and Statistics Unit, Canberra.

Mowbray, M., 2007. Social determinants and Indigenous health: the international experience and its policy implications. Report on specially prepared documents, presentations and discussions at the International Symposium on the Social Determinants of Indigenous Health. Adelaide, 29–30 April 2007 for the Commission on Social Determinants of Health (CSDH). RMIT University, Melbourne.

National Aboriginal Community Controlled Health Organisation (NACCHO) website, Online. Available: <http://www.naccho.org.au/aboriginal-health/naccho-healthy-futures -plan-2013-2030/> (22 Sep 2014).

National Aboriginal Community Controlled Health Organisation, 1993. Manifesto on Aboriginal well-being and specific health areas; position paper. NACCHO, Canberra.

National Aboriginal Community Controlled Health Organisation, Oxfam Australia, 2007. Close the Gap: Solutions to the Indigenous Health Crisis Facing Australia. NACCHO and Oxfam Australia, Braddon.

National Aboriginal Health Strategy Working Party, 1989. A National Aboriginal Health Strategy. AGPS, Canberra.

National Aboriginal and Torres Strait Islander Health Council, 2001. National Aboriginal and Torres Strait Islander Health Strategy: consultation draft. National Aboriginal and Torres Strait Islander Health Council, Canberra.

National Health and Medical Research Council, 2010. The NHMRC Road Map II: a strategic framework for improving the health of Aboriginal and Torres Strait Islander people through research. NHMRC, Canberra.

Oxfam Australia Close the Gap website. Online. Available: <https://www.oxfam.org.au/explore/indigenous-australia/close-the-gap/get-involved-with-close-the-gap/> (22 Sep 2014).

Phillips, G., 2003. Addictions and Healing in Aboriginal Country. Aboriginal Studies Press, Canberra.

Rintoul, S., 1993. The Wailing: A National Black Oral History. William Heinmann, Port Mlebourne.

Rowse, T., 2006. Transforming the notion of the urban Aborigine. Urban Policy and Research 18 (2), 171–190.

Rudd, K., 2008. Apology to Australia's Indigenous peoples, 13 February 2008. Online. Available: <http://www.dfat.gov.au/indigenous/apology-to-stolen-generations/rudd _speech.html> (22 Sep 2014).

Saggers, S., Gray, D., 1991. Aboriginal Health and Society: The Traditional and Contemporary Aboriginal Struggle for Better Health. Allen and Unwin, Sydney.

Scrimgeour, M., Scrimgeour, D., 2008. Health care access for Aboriginal and Torres Strait Islander people living in urban areas, and related research issues: a review of the literature. Co-operative Research Centre for Aboriginal Health, Darwin.

Smith, L.T., 1999. Decolonising Methodologies Research and Indigenous Peoples. Zed Books, London.

Taylor, J., 2006. Population and diversity: policy implications of emerging Indigenous demographic trends. Discussion Paper No 283/2006. Centre for Aboriginal Economic Research, Canberra.

Thomson, N., 1984. Australian Aboriginal health and health-care. Social Science and Medicine 18, 939–948.

Tripcony, P., 1995. Teaching to difference: working with Aboriginal and Torres Strait Islander students in urban schools. Aboriginal Child at School 23 (3), 35–43.

van der Sterren, A., Goreen Narrkwarren Ngrn-toura (reducing smoking amongst pregnant Aboriginal women in Victoria: an holistic approach) Project Team, 2009. Goreen Narrkwarren Ngrn-toura—Healthy Family Air: a literature review to inform the VACCHO Smoking in Pregnant Aboriginal Women Research Project. Victorian Aboriginal Community Controlled Health Organisation, Melbourne.

Viswanathan, R., Franklin, E., Phillips, J., 2011. A better way: building healthy, safe and sustainable communities in the Northern Territory through a community development approach. Australians for Native Title and Reconciliation (ANTaR): Sydney.

Walter, M., 2009. An economy of poverty? Power and the domain of Aboriginality. International Journal of Critical Indigenous Studies 2 (1), 2–14.

Wass, A., 1998. Promoting Health: The Primary Health Care Approach, 2nd ed. Harcourt Saunders, Sydney.

Watson, L.J., 1981. A report on a week of activities with Aboriginal street kids in the Brisbane area, St. Lucia, Brisbane. Held in the Australian Institute of Aboriginal and Torres Strait Islander Studies (AIATSIS) collection, Canberra.

Weeks, W., 1994. Women Working Together: Lessons from Feminist Women's Services. Longman Cheshire, Melbourne.

Wenitong, M., 2002. Indigenous male health: a report for Indigenous males, their families and communities, and those committed to improving Indigenous male health. The Office of Aboriginal and Torres Strait Islander Health, Commonwealth Department of Health and Ageing, Canberra.

Wenitong, M., 2006. Aboriginal and Torres Strait Islander male health, wellbeing and leadership. Medical Journal of Australia 185 (8), 466–467.

World Health Organization, 2007. Social determinants and Aboriginal Torres Strait Islander health: the international experience and its policy implications. WHO, Geneva. Online. Available: <www.who.int/social_determinants/resources/indigenous_health_adelaide _report_07.pdf> (22 Sep 2014).

CHAPTER 17

Grand challenges for public health

Mary Louise Fleming

Learning objectives

After reading this chapter, you should be able to:

- identify and describe the grand challenges facing public health in the twenty-first century

- critique the relationship between grand challenges for public health and the capacity of the workforce to meet these challenges

- analyse the importance of ecological sustainability to the survival of the planet, and its impact on public health activity in the future

- discuss the varying roles of the public health worker in the future in the light of emerging infectious diseases and the development of a range of chronic illnesses

- consider the important place of politics in decision-making about public health resources, infrastructure and strategies, and learn about effective advocacy at various levels of government for public health

- critique the issues that have influenced the globalisation of health and the impact of this development on public health in Australia.

Introduction

What is the future for public health in the twenty-first century? Can we glean an idea about the future of public health from its past? As Winston Churchill once said: '[T]he further backward you look, the further forward you can see.' What can we see in the history of public health that gives us an idea of where public health might be headed in the future? (Gruszin et al. 2012).

In the twentieth century there was substantial progress in public health in Australia. These improvements were brought about through a number of factors. In part, improvements were due to increasing knowledge about the natural history of disease and its treatment. Added to this knowledge was a shifting focus from legislative measures for protecting health to the emergence of improved promotion and prevention strategies, and a general improvement in social and economic conditions for people living in countries such as Australia. Gruszin et al. (2012) consider the range of social and economic reforms of the twentieth century as the most important determinants of the public's health at the start of the twenty-first century (Gruszin et al. 2012 p 201). The same could not, however, be said for second or third world countries, many of which have the most fundamental of sanitary and health protection issues still to deal with. For example, in sub-Saharan Africa and in Russia the decline in life expectancy can be said to be related to a range of interconnected factors. In Russia, issues such as alcoholism, violence, suicide, accidents and cardiovascular disease could be contributing to the falling life expectancy (McMichael & Butler 2007). In sub-Saharan Africa, a range of factors, such as HIV/AIDS, poverty, malaria, tuberculosis, undernutrition, totally inadequate infrastructure, gender inequality, conflict and violence, political taboos and a complete lack of political will, have all contributed to a dramatic drop in life expectancy (McMichael & Butler 2007).

Within Australia, subpopulations still suffer adverse health effects. For Aboriginal and Torres Strait Islander peoples, mortality rates are higher for almost all causes of death. The major risk factors for poor health in this population include low birth weight, obesity, poor nutrition, high levels of alcohol and other drug use, substandard housing and living conditions, and inadequate access to healthcare (Australian Bureau of Statistics 2013a). These issues have been canvassed extensively in Section 2 of the book and, in particular, in Chapter 16.

The multidisciplinary nature of contemporary public health is evident in the range of developments that have advanced public health during the twentieth century. Biomedical scientists identified many of the disease-causing organisms and developed methods to manage them. Epidemiologists identified the determinants that underpin many chronic diseases, enabling this information to be used to reduce people's risk of illness. Efforts to provide clean air and water have resulted in some successes when compared with the situation 50 years ago (Schneider 2011).

Improvements such as these have advanced the health of Australians and meant that life expectancy has also increased substantially; to some degree, improvements have been attributed to public health interventions. The 10 great American public health achievements in the twentieth century are listed in Box 17.1. It is interesting to note that none of these achievements had a focus on the ecosystem or ecological sustainability. However, these latter issues are now firmly on the world stage, and on the public health agenda, for action in the twenty-first century.

We can clearly see the re-emergence of infectious diseases as a major challenge for public health in the twenty-first century. The challenge of HIV/AIDS has been with the community for 30 years, but newer diseases such as swine flu, severe acute respiratory syndrome (SARS), avian influenza ('bird flu'), Australian bat lyssavirus (ABLV) and Hendra virus have also emerged as major diseases that may affect the

---

BOX 17.1

TEN GREAT PUBLIC HEALTH ACHIEVEMENTS— UNITED STATES, 1900–1999

1 Vaccination
2 Motor vehicle safety
3 Safer workplaces
4 Control of infectious diseases
5 Decline in deaths from coronary heart disease and stroke
6 Safer and healthier foods
7 Healthier mothers and babies
8 Family planning
9 Fluoridation of drinking water
10 Recognition of tobacco use as a health hazard

(Source: CDC MMWR Weekly 1999)

---

public's health in the future. All of these diseases underscore the importance of surveillance and monitoring strategies in public health. In the late 1990s, the National Public Health Partnership (National Public Health Partnership (NPHP) 1998) produced an overview of the public health system and its activities. In that document, a section outlined recent key achievements for public health. Many of these achievements are similar to those of the United States listed in Box 17.1. Countries such as Australia and the United States have a similar set of public health successes, in which they have demonstrated improvements in mortality and morbidity over the past century. Others on the Australian list have a more contemporary flavour, as shown in Box 17.2.

New health challenges require a changing set of strategies for public health action into the future. This is an ambitious agenda of growing urgency, with daunting challenges. Since the 1986 *Ottawa Charter for Health Promotion* (World Health Organization (WHO) 1986), globalisation, new patterns of consumption and communication, urbanisation, environmental changes and public health emergencies, along with accelerating social and demographic changes to work, learning, family and community life, have become critical factors influencing health (Kawachi et al. 2013). Baum (2008) argues for public health strategies in the future that have the development of supportive societies and communities as their central plank (Baum 2008). She goes on to state:

> Social support, high self-esteem and a sense of personal control are important determinants of health, best achieved in societies and communities that are relatively equal and that have reasonable levels of social solidarity. (Baum 2008 p 576)

BOX 17.2

KEY ACHIEVEMENTS WITHIN THE AUSTRALIAN PUBLIC HEALTH SECTOR

Recent achievements in the Australian public health sector include:

- increasing community awareness, behaviour change and early detection in relation to risk factors for tobacco-related cancer, skin cancers and breast cancer
- developing infectious disease control and reducing communicable disease transmission
- reducing mortality and morbidity from motor vehicle crashes
- providing communities with evidence-based practice through public health information and innovative techniques in the social marketing of public health policy
- improving data analysis by applying epidemiological principles to statistical analysis

(Source: National Public Health Partnership 1998; AIHW 2000)

Other researchers (Friel & Marmot 2011, Gostin 2010, Magnusson 2009) point out that there are several interrelated global developments that continue to have a profound effect on public health. These include: relationship differences between wealthy and poor countries; prevailing ideology that stresses the role of the free market and individualism; global threats to the environment; the globalisation of chronic disease; and health inequalities.

Grand challenges in the twenty-first century

Over a decade into the twenty-first century, public health faces new challenges, yet it also needs to remember its roots. While we have discussed some of these issues in Sections 2, 4 and 5, the challenges into the future are complex and bring together the importance of fundamental public health with the emergence of large global issues, such as climate change. In some countries, basic sanitation is still a major challenge for public health. There are renewed threats from infectious diseases, food-borne pathogens, and ecological issues that threaten the planet, such as climate change. An ageing population brings its own issues, including the associated increased costs of healthcare. The emergence of health issues associated with physical inactivity and unhealthy diets has contributed to increasing levels of overweight and obesity, and a range of associated chronic conditions in the Australian population and many other developed countries.

In the twenty-first century, one of the major challenges for health systems and governments around the world will be the increasing cost of health and medical care. Advances in the medical model and a focus on curing health problems, rather than preventing them, have meant that more resources have been expended on medical care and treatment. And, as that type of care has become more sophisticated, the costs have also increased.

In 2012, the Institute of Medicine (IOM), in their report titled *For the public's health: investing in a healthier future*, noted that the United States spends extensively on clinical care, but meagerly on other types of population-based actions that influence health more profoundly than medical services. The health system's failure to develop and deliver effective preventive strategies continues to take a growing toll on the economy and society (IOM 2012).

A health system for the future needs to shift its attention from funding high-tech infrastructure that supports a small percentage of the population to a continuum of care that enhances health promotion; and to comprehensive primary healthcare strategies that recognise the major contributions of social, economic and cultural factors outside of the individual, and the provision of health services, to health outcomes (Baum et al. 2013 p 503).

Twenty-first-century solutions

Several authors (Hanlon et al. 2012, Kelly 2011) have begun to argue that public health requires new and more appropriate strategies to deal with a complex present and an unknown future. Table 17.1 summarises some of the issues presented by a range of authors in the past decade (Beaglehole & Bonita 2004, Hancock 2007, Hanlon et al. 2012, Kelly 2011, McMichael 2006, McMichael & Butler 2007), who articulate future developments that will impact on public health. It is amazing how similar the lists from many different authors are. The focus is clearly on the big social, environmental and economic issues that have both a direct and an indirect effect on the health of the population. Consider the range of issues presented and the implications for public health, and complete Activity 17.1 and Reflection 17.1.

Gostin (2010) argues for a global plan for justice for the world's least healthy people based on three core components: essential vaccines and medicines; basic survival needs; and adaption to climate change. Similarly, Friel and Marmot (2011) discuss the need to reduce inequities in health through attention to the unfair distribution of power, money and resources, and the influences of everyday life. Others have argued for more recognition of the important role of population in environmental impact (Butler

---

ACTIVITY 17.1 Health challenges for the twenty-first century

- Consider the health issues raised in Table 17.1. What do you think are the three major challenges for public health in the twenty-first century?
- How prepared do you think the public health workforce needs to be, and what skills would you identify as important for a public health worker in the twenty-first century?
- Can you, as a health professional in Australia, have an impact on these global issues? What impact do you think you can have in your environment, in your country, and/or globally? Why do you think that? Try to justify your answer.

REFLECTION 17.1

You might like to consider: the impact of globalisation on health; the issues of social and economic inequalities and their impact on health; or the advances in science and technology that might lead health systems further down the pathway of specialised technologies that are enormously expensive with limited population health returns. Possibly your impact can be at a local level, which in turn impacts with others at a national level, which may impact beyond a national level to a more global strategy for change. Read on further as we start to add additional issues for your consideration in dealing with twenty-first-century public health problems.

We have discussed the public health workforce and its development in Section 1, as well as in this chapter. Reflect back on what you have read, and think about the skills that a public health worker might need to meet the challenges of the twenty-first century.

Public health workers will probably need to specialise more as public health practice becomes more complex. What other health professionals have moved in this direction? The catch-cry of 'think global, act local' is already in our vocabulary, but what does that really mean for health workers? Does it mean that, no matter how small your actions, you can have an impact if others in the profession are working in similar ways to you? Describe some local actions that might have a greater impact on the community.

TABLE 17.1 Future issues impacting on public health activity in the twenty-first century

Future issues	Implications for public health
Influence of globalisation (markets, technology and communications)	Epidemics, terrorism and environmental concerns have expanded to have international as well as domestic implications for population health
Global issues—poverty, urbanisation, globalisation, and social and economic inequalities	Obstacles to sustainability impact on the level and equity of population health
Global environmental changes	Depletion and degradation of natural capital is not sustainable; need to focus on dependence on maintaining Earth's life support system; population wellbeing and health are the real bottom line of sustainability
Risk management—necessary to predict, influence and minimise risks in major systems on which society depends	Protect and improve population health through mitigation and management of risk
Social factors—values, demography, education, housing, mobility, migration, social inequality, literacy, health status	Social determinants influence patterns of health, access to health, understanding of health issues and healthcare
Technological factors—developments in information technology and telecommunications, and medical technology	Information technology developments enhance knowledge and analysis of health patterns to enable health management and care; costs, however, mean that society will not be able to support the increasing technological sophistication
Economic factors—employment, income, inflation, consumer spending on health resources, demand and supply issues	Socioeconomic gradients and health, unemployment and associated health consequences, social isolation, increasing costs for consumers and sophistication of healthcare

TABLE 17.1 Continued

Future issues	Implications for public health
Resource factors —use of resources, particularly energy, and impact	Maintaining viable ecosystem for sustainable development, renewable energy sources, implication of current systems on long-term sustainability
Political factors—government stability, ideological climate, policy priorities	Level of investment in public health, and the focus of that investment, priority issues, state–federal collaboration and divisions
Re-emergence of infectious diseases	Need for public health researchers and practitioners to transmit to the public information about the risks inherent in current modes of social and economic development, and the resultant large-scale environmental changes, and to find ecologically attuned ways of managing social change to minimise health risk Surveillance and monitoring of new diseases and ways of preventing widespread mortality will need to be an important part of public health activity in the future
Decline in life expectancy in several regions	After some gains, declines in life expectancy in poor countries as a result of the re-emergence of infectious diseases, new infectious diseases, poor basic health services, poverty, malnutrition, lack of affordable drug therapies, lack of political support and will

(Sources: Beaglehole & Bonita 2004, Hancock 2007, Hanlon et al. 2012, Kelly 2011, McMichael 2006, McMichael & Butler 2007)

& McMichael 2010). Regardless of the health issue under consideration, one of the salient themes in public health in the twenty-first century is the notion of global impacts and global responses. This leads us into one of our first contemporary public health challenges: a global perspective on health and its inequitable distribution.

Globalisation and health

A global agenda for public health is a major challenge for health practitioners, public health advocacy groups, and governments, both nationally and internationally. Issues such as free trade, modern economic theory (which asserts 'that increased per capita income will offset the non-costed losses'), mobility of capital, and the deregulation of labour conditions all contribute to social and economic inequalities and environmental risk (McMichael & Butler 2007 pp 21–22). There needs to be a focus on creating sustainable environments and social conditions that result in equitable and enduring improvements in population health. How might public health actions make a difference to sustainable environments, equity and population health improvements?

As discussed in Chapter 15, there are a number of international organisations involved in global health advances. Sometimes, however, these roles overlap and there is a serious lack of coordination between agencies and their activities.

The World Bank acknowledges that inequalities are a substantial barrier to prosperity and growth, and that there is a need for strong government leadership, an active trade union movement, and greater equality in poor countries. However, these messages are not always consistent. Similarly, the influence and success of the WHO has varied considerably. Pressures from vested interests, such as the tobacco industry, and more recently the food industry in the United States, have always had an impact on the policies and actions of international agencies such as the WHO, by pressuring them to modify their positions on contentious issues (Magnusson 2009).

Balancing the important global public health challenges against the needs of member countries and the pressure from vested interest groups will always be a struggle for the WHO. Strong and consistent leadership will be required for the WHO in the twenty-first century.

The UN is working with governments, civil society and other partners to build on the momentum generated by the Millennium Development Goals (MDGs) and to carry on with an ambitious post-2015 sustainable development agenda that is expected to be adopted by UN member states at a summit in September 2015 (United Nations 2014).

Public health will have to be global to be effective, and take on a strong advocacy role in order to deal with global inequalities, and inequities within countries. In particular, Friel and Marmot (2011) argue that chronic disease and its social determinants should be at the forefront of global action to improve health (see Chapter 11). A number of factors have contributed to the increase in chronic diseases, including population ageing, reasonable success in controlling infectious diseases, and the globalisation of chronic disease risk factors (Gostin 2010, Magnusson 2009). Tackling the global burden of chronic disease constitutes one of the major challenges for twenty-first-century development.

Dietary imbalance, physical inactivity and sedentary behaviour

In the past two decades there has been a striking increase in the prevalence of obesity observed in many countries. Decreasing levels of physical activity and a high intake of kilojoules have made significant contributions to the epidemic of overweight and obesity. It is interesting to note that, while health workers in wealthy countries are concerned about the health effects of over-nutrition, from a global perspective hunger still remains a much more important problem (Beaglehole & Bonita 2004). Participation in physical activity is an important protective factor for health; furthermore, physical inactivity (AIHW 2012) is second only to tobacco smoking in terms of its contribution to the burden of disease. Recent evidence suggests that having a high level of sedentary behaviour negatively impacts on health independently of other factors, including body weight, diet and physical activity (Katzmarzyk 2010) (see also the Department of Health website on sedentary behaviour).

One of the major concerns for health professionals in countries such as Australia is that the contribution of both the lack of physical activity and the overconsumption of food has a strong association with cardiovascular risk factors, obesity and diabetes. It also compounds the risks when associated with smoking, alcohol consumption and poor nutrition (AIHW 2010).

Many of the factors that contribute to overweight and obesity in wealthy countries are social and economic factors, including an explosion of fast-food outlets, longer working hours, limited leisure time and appropriate facilities, and a range of labour-saving devices that have reduced our opportunities to engage in adequate physical activity. The challenge for public health is not only about reorienting the health system, but also about working in concert with other sectors to promote a balance between work and leisure. In addition, it is important to ensure that people have the opportunities to achieve such a balance, and an understanding of the health implications of long working hours or having limited opportunities for physical activity. It means that health professionals, working in collaboration with governments, architects and builders, need to reorganise living spaces to facilitate physical activity. True multisector collaboration for enhancing health is likely to be a central strategy for public health into the future.

Population ageing

Older Australians are people aged 65 years or over (AIHW 2012), and this group makes up 14% of the population (3.22 million people in June 2012) (ABS 2013b). During the past several decades, the number and proportion of the population aged 65 years or over have increased rapidly in Australia. The increase in the population aged 85 years or over has been even more marked (AIHW 2010).

Maintaining good health among older Australians helps to moderate the demand for health and aged-care services, which is important as Australia's population ages over the coming decades. In response to population ageing, Australia has made improving older people's health a national research priority (AIHW 2012). One area of special interest is adopting a healthy lifestyle at older ages, because its benefits include preventing disease and functional decline, extending longevity and enhancing quality of life (AIHW 2012).

At age 65, Australia's males now expect to live for a further 17.8 years and females for another 21.1 years, which is about 6 years more than their counterparts at the beginning of the twentieth century (AIHW 2010). Males and females aged 85 years can expect to live for a further 5.7 and 6.9 years, respectively, which is about 2 years more than for the early 1900s.

Maintaining good health for older people in Australia is essential, not only for their own quality of life but also because the costs of curative and long-term care for an ever-increasing subpopulation will not be sustainable into the future. As we mentioned earlier in this chapter, the public health workforce needs to work towards maintaining the health of our ageing population through fundamental promotion strategies, such as good nutrition, moderate physical activity, and enhanced mental health and wellbeing.

Sustainable ecological public health

Accomplishing sustainable social, economic and environmental conditions underpins achieving population health. However, environmental changes—including climate change, loss of biodiversity, productivity downturns in land and oceans, and freshwater depletion—have all contributed to the potential of serious health risks to current and future human societies (Butler & McMichael 2010).

Reflecting on 20 years since the Ottawa Charter (WHO 1986), Hancock (2007) commented that he would strengthen four major areas for debate and discussion if he was to present now on the role of public health and health promotion into the future. These areas are:

1   An explicit link between human health and ecosystem health: '[G]lobal environmental change, including climate and atmospheric change, resource depletion, ecotoxicity, habitat destruction and species extinction, is the ultimate threat to health …' (Hancock 2007 p 7).

2   More emphasis on the built environment, and how we design, build and operate our built environments is of major importance to our health, and it also has a profound impact on the natural environment.

3   A broadening of the focus on social capital to include *formal* social capital, such as the system of social programs and institutions, as well as *invisible* social capital, which includes the legal, political and constitutional infrastructure that underpins our societies and communities.

4   A focus on a new economics based on human wellbeing—as Hancock states, 'real capitalists in the twenty-first century will be those who simultaneously build all four forms of capital—natural, social and human as well as economic capital' (Hancock 2007 p 8).

In addition, Friel (2010) discusses the importance of the link between food, population health and climate stabilisation agendas, concluding that 'food security is no longer just about making food available, accessible and affordable', but that 'climate change means that sustainability must be placed at the heart of the food system' (Friel 2010 p 129). And this means making judgements about 'food production and consumption' for their environmental impact, 'health, quality and social values' (Friel 2010 p 132).

Further, McMichael (2006) says that health researchers have been slow to engage with the issue of 'ecological sustainability' and its impact on health, and a decade on this is still the case. He suggests that the reason for this is the reluctance of scientists to look beyond defined professional boundaries and paradigms, and the enormity of a task that asks researchers to examine how changes in whole natural systems can affect health (McMichael 2006 p 580). Nevertheless, these are issues which must be addressed if we are to be able to sustain a way of life that is based on the recognition of the centrality of maintaining viable ecosystems for a sustainable world future.

Emerging and re-emerging infections

Infectious diseases have re-emerged in recent years, associated with mobility, shifts in the ecology of human living, technologies and economic activity. This has required public health researchers to undertake 'study and surveillance of infectious disease transmission patterns' (McMichael 2006 p 580). A recent upturn in the range, burden and risk of infectious diseases has been produced by a variety of factors, including increased population density, persistent poverty, and the vulnerability of younger population groups, as well as many environmental, political and social factors. These causes are compounded by gender, economic and structural inequalities, by political denial, vaccine obstacles, and the mismatch between health resource distribution and major causes of illness (Friel & Marmot 2011).

Effectively managing infectious diseases in society is reliant on a range of complementary strategies, which together aim to prevent, monitor or treat disease. This approach is equivalent to primary, secondary and tertiary prevention. Accordingly, the three key aspects of managing infectious diseases are: (1) disease prevention; (2) surveillance, early recognition and early intervention; and (3) managing a disease outbreak.

Genetics, biotechnology and information technology

Molecular and genetic approaches to controlling disease are well underway. Supporters of such approaches argue that money will be well spent because of the potential that understanding genes and molecular structures have for promoting health and improving life expectancy (Baum 2008). Baum (2008) argues that public health practitioners will have to take a critical and sceptical view of genetic technology, questioning its potential for impact on population health status and the impact its availability would have on equity.

Technology has a number of possibilities that raise both ethical and legal issues, and these will need to be resolved through public debate and difficult policy choices. Included in this list are genetic engineering, cloning, stem cell research, and slowing the ageing process. The bottom line with respect to biotechnology is not that these advances might occur—the ultimate challenge to public health in the twenty-first century is the *cost* of these innovations, and the limited resources available to pay for them (Schneider 2011).

Advances in information technology have led to improvements in public health surveillance capabilities. However, as technology has improved, ethical and legal questions have arisen about the need to be able to keep information private, as well as ensuring that information that should be made public is available in the public domain. The rise of the internet as a source of information and commerce also poses many challenges for consumers with regard to how to evaluate the information, and for governments and policymakers about how to protect consumers from inappropriate advice and information (Schneider 2011).

The public health workforce: skills for a complex future

The public health workforce is an important consideration in advancing public health activity into the twenty-first century. In Australia, a wide range of universities offer Master of Public Health degrees with a range of specialisations, such as environmental health, epidemiology, health promotion, health management, and occupational health and safety. A key focus for public health education is the link between the processes of education and the practice of public health. There is a gap between academic and practical public health, which does not well serve either the public health workforce or the public health academic community, and ultimately, the public. Clearly, what we need is strong institutional support and leadership for public health education and training, to ensure that students understand and adopt the fundamental values of public health.

Health professionals need an understanding of the core competencies of practice, and a clear appreciation of the complexity of the task and the multiple drivers of population health patterns. The development of competencies for public health and health promotion have been well researched in Australia, including the work of Rotem et al. (1995), and research from Western Australia (Shilton et al. 2006) to update health promotion competencies. In 2009, Genat et al. (2009) produced *Foundation competencies for Master of Public Health graduates in Australia*. This work reinforces the importance of the public health professional who understands the complexity of the task. These competencies are currently being reviewed.

People working to promote population health need to have a focus on equity and equality, and values that acknowledge the Indigenous population's right to self-determination. However, they also need to understand that public health now has a global perspective to consider, and, importantly, must acknowledge and act on the issues that impact on ecological sustainability.

Strategic planning for public health: political will and action

The need for planning and coordination of public health activities is, as ever, the underlying priority for advancing a national public health agenda in Australia.

Public health is as much about democracy, empowerment, accountability, transparency and communication as it is about professional skill sets. In many developed countries, governments focus on medical research and treating disease rather than promoting the health of the public. The Millennium Development Goals (2014) contain three specific *health* goals: reduce child mortality; improve maternal health; and combat HIV/AIDS, malaria and other diseases. Together, these account for 32% of global mortality, while chronic disease accounts for 59% (Magnusson 2009). In addition, where public health has taken a front seat in debate and discussion, it has often been focused on lifestyle approaches to health rather than life circumstance approaches (Watterson 2003 p 11).

In addition, several authors (Hanlon et al. 2012; Kelly 2011) argue that current public health science requires consideration of emergent sciences that, for example, reflect the need to be engaged in ecological forms of public health in order to respond to the threats posed by global ecological hazards to human health.

Leadership and public health: establishing a research agenda

Internationally, both the World Bank and the WHO have already identified the major public health research challenges; these are presented in Box 17.3.

Public health needs research that focuses on the health risks posed by global environmental changes. Three types of research have been proposed: first, empirical studies that are designed to describe how variations in environmental and ecological systems affect health risks; secondly, evidence about whether global environmental changes already affect health; and thirdly, the need to make 'credible estimates of future changes in the health risks due to plausible scenarios of ongoing changes in large-scale environmental systems' (McMichael 2006 p 580).

BOX 17.3

MAJOR PUBLIC HEALTH RESEARCH CHALLENGES

These have been identified as:

1 continuing epidemics of preventable childhood infectious diseases, which are aggravated by poverty and under-nutrition

2 economic, social and environmental changes, which lead to emerging and re-emerging infectious diseases

3 growing epidemics of chronic diseases and injuries

4 assessing the effectiveness and efficiency of public health programs

5 wider impacts on health that influence patterns of health inequalities

6 acknowledging different levels of analysis that are involved in what we do, and that take a trans-disciplinary approach.

(Sources: Beaglehole & Bonita 2004, Gruszin et al. 2012, Hanlon et al. 2012)

Most recently, there has been increased international attention given to translating public health research into practice. The type of research we are talking about is related to the application and dissemination of basic science research into community practice and health policy (Spaulding 2014). There are a number of factors that limit the translation of research evidence into practice and the ability of practice to inform the evidence base. These include: the lack of an evaluation culture; ethical and programmatic difficulties in designing evaluations, selection of appropriate outcome measures, poor design and implementation of current interventions; and the fact that policymaking is based on more than evidence (Bauman & Nutbeam 2014). There is limited research on the development and testing of interventions to improve public health. The challenge for researchers, practitioners and advocates is to provide timely access to information, and to employ improved techniques for communicating and managing program evaluation results.

Grand challenges for public health: what is the future?

Health practitioners need an opportunity to think about public health futures, the trends and challenges, and the possible ways forward. Can health professionals anticipate and react to potential future scenarios, or can they, in fact, act to shape futures? What are the implications of global warming and ecological sustainability on public health and the health of the population? What do we currently know about likely futures, and how can we take this information into account in making decisions that range from the local to the global level, to pursue preferred futures (Fairchild et al. 2010)?

Kelly (2011) says that we should transcend disciplines that include climatology, sociology, economics, politics and psychology and biomedicine. This will be difficult, however, because of the dominance of the individual in our thinking, and because a focus on trans-disciplinary work takes many of us out of our comfort zone and our training. In conclusion, what we need to be able to do is use a variety of disciplinary perspectives in an integrated fashion without the dominance of a single method or approach (Kelly 2011).

If major public health goals are for global sustainability, and equity and wellbeing are to be achieved, Hanlon et al. (2012) suggest that public health will need to incorporate all of the following approaches: integrative; ecological; ethical; creative; imaginative; embodied in change; and reflexive.

The progress that was made in public health during the twentieth century has been remarkable in many respects, particularly in wealthy countries. However, progress in the health of subpopulations within these countries, such as Indigenous peoples in Australia, and within developing countries, where basic sanitation and food supply are still inadequate, remains a major challenge for public health.

What challenges will public health face in the twenty-first century? Some of those challenges were already emerging late in the twentieth century, such as the development of new infectious diseases and the fundamental question of ecological sustainability. Schneider (2011) believes that the most important challenge facing public health in the twenty-first century will be to have the conversation about the allocation of public resources to improve population health (Schneider 2011). Many authors (Butler & McMichael 2010, Hanlon et al. 2012, Kelly 2011), however, clearly see our future as one of a focus on sustainability, about ensuring positive (and equitable) human experience, of which health is fundamental (see Activity 17.2 and Reflection 17.2).

Public health faces many challenges. As we have seen in this chapter, issues such as ecological sustainability, inequitable resource distribution, and political conditions impact on health, and there seems to be limited political will to restructure resources and infrastructure to ensure the equitable distribution of health in our society. In addition, we face issues of social isolation, an ageing population, and problems of overweight and obesity, particularly among young Australians.

However, the future of public health is an exciting one. Health professionals of the future working to improve the public's health will need to be trans-disciplinary in approach, multiskilled, flexible and adaptable to meet the challenges they will face. Challenges in public health are there to be met, and we are all well placed to make a difference to the health of the population.

A final word

This introductory text to the principles and practices of public health has been designed to help you understand the central issues that have shaped public health in the past, and the emerging issues that will shape public health into the future. We hope that as a result of reading this book you have a fundamental understanding of the nature and scope of public health, the factors that provide the evidence that underpins public health activity, the range and scope of public health interventions, and the emerging issues that will challenge public health into the twenty-first century and beyond. In the face of developments that are outside the current scope of public health, but that impact on the wellbeing of the population, we wish you luck as you travel your professional journeys.

REVIEW QUESTIONS

1   Draw up a chart that displays developments that have advanced the health of the Australian population in the twentieth century, and then the beginnings of this century.

2   What are the major challenges? For example, is over-consumption a problem across the world?

3   How do these challenges differ for wealthy countries compared with poor countries?

4   What part has globalisation played in the emerging patterns of mortality and morbidity?

5   How important is ecological sustainability and, if it is important, for what reasons is it important?

6   What is translational research, and how might it provide evidence of success for public health activity?

7   What skills and expertise do the health workforce of the twenty-first century need that might not have been as important in the previous century?

References

Australian Bureau of Statistics, 2013a. Life Tables for Aboriginal and Torres Strait Islander Australians, 2010–2012. ABS Cat. No. 3302.0.55.003. ABS, Canberra. Online. Available: <http://www.abs.gov.au/ausstats/abs@.nsf/latestProducts/3302.0.55.003Media%20 Release12010-2012> (4 Jun 2014).

Australian Bureau of Statistics, 2013b. Population by Age and Sex, Regions of Australia, 2012. ABS Cat. No. 3235.0. ABS, Canberra. Online. Available: <http://www.abs.gov.au/ausstats/ abs@.nsf/Products/3235.0~2012~Main+Features~Main+Features?OpenDocument#PARAL INK2> (12 Jun 2014).

Australian Institute of Health and Welfare, 2000. Australia's Health 2000. AIHW Cat. No. AUS 19. AIHW, Canberra.

Australian Institute of Health and Welfare, 2010. Australia's Health 2010. AIHW Cat. No. AUS 122. AIHW, Canberra.

Australian Institute of Health and Welfare, 2012. Australia's Health 2012. AIHW Cat. No. AUS 156. AIHW, Canberra.

Baum, F., 2008. The New Public Health, third ed. Oxford University Press, Melbourne.

Baum, F., Fisher, M., Trewin, D., et al., 2013. Funding the 'H' in NHMRC. Australian and New Zealand Journal of Public Health 37 (6), 503–505.

Bauman, A., Nutbeam, D., 2014. Evaluation in a Nutshell: A Practical Guide to the Evaluation of Health Promotion Programs. McGraw-Hill, North Ryde.

Beaglehole, R., Bonita, R., 2004. Public Health at the Crossroads: Achievements and Prospects, second ed. Cambridge University Press, Cambridge.

Butler, C.D., McMichael, A.J., 2010. Population health: where demography, environment and equity converge. Commentary. Journal of Public Health 32 (2), 157–158.

Centers for Disease Control, 1999. Ten great public health achievements—United States, 1900–1999. MMWR Weekly 48 (12), 241–243.

Department of Health website, 2014. Sedentary behaviour. Online. Available: <http://www.health.gov.au/internet/main/publishing.nsf/Content/sbehaviour> (11 June 2014).

Fairchild, A.L., Rosner, D., Colgrove, J., et al., 2010. The exodus of public health: what history can tell us about the future. American Journal of Public Health 100 (1), 54–63.

Friel, S., 2010. Climate change, food insecurity and chronic diseases: sustainable and healthy policy opportunities for Australia. NSW Public Health Bulletin 21 (5–6), 129–133.

Friel, S., Marmot, M.G., 2011. Action on the social determinants of health and health inequities goes global. Annual Review of Public Health 32, 225–236.

Genat, B., Robinson, P., Parker, E., 2009. Foundation Competencies for Masters of Public Health Graduates in Australia. Australian Network of Public Health Institutions, Brisbane.

Gostin, L.O., 2010. Redressing the unconscionable health gap: a global plan for justice. Lancet 37 (9725), 1504–1505.

Gruszin, S., Hetzel, D., Glover, J., 2012. Advocacy and Action in Public Health: Lessons from Australia Over the 20th Century. Australian National Preventive Health Agency, Canberra.

Hancock, T., 2007. Creating environments for health—20 years on. IUHPE—Promotion and Education (Suppl. 2), 7–8.

Hanlon, P., Carlisle, S., Hannah, M., et al., 2012. A perspective on the future public health: an integrative and ecological framework. Perspectives in Public Health 132 (6), 313–319.

Institute of Medicine, 2012. For the Public's Health: Investing in a Healthier Future. National Academies Press, Washington DC.

Katzmarzyk, P.T., 2010. Physical activity, sedentary behavior, and health: paradigm paralysis or paradigm shift? Diabetes 59 (11), 2717–2725.

Kawachi, I., Takao, S., Subramanian, S.V., 2013. Global Perspectives on Social Capital and Health. Springer, New York.

Kelly, M.P., 2011. The future of public health: the lessons of modernism. Commentary. Journal of Public Health 33 (3), 334.

Magnusson, R.S., 2009. Rethinking global health challenges: towards a 'global compact' for reducing the burden of chronic disease. Public Health 123, 265–274.

McMichael, A.J., 2006. Population health as the 'bottom line' of sustainability: a contemporary challenge for public health researchers. European Journal of Public Health 16 (6), 579–582.

McMichael, A.J., Butler, C.D., 2007. Emerging health issues: the widening challenge for population health promotion. Health Promotion International 21 (Suppl. 1), 15–24.

National Public Health Partnership, 1998. Public Health in Australia: The Public Health Landscape—Person, Society, Environment. NPHP, Melbourne.

Rotem, A., Walters, J., Dewdney, J., 1995. The public health workforce education and training study. Australian Journal of Public Health 19 (5), 437–438.

Schneider, M.J., 2011. Introduction to Public Health, third ed. Jones and Bartlett Learning, Sudbury, MA.

Shilton, T., Howat, P., James, R., et al., 2006. Revision of Health Promotion Competencies for Australia: Final Report. Western Australian Centre for Health Promotion Research and The National Heart Foundation of Australia (WA Division), Perth.

Spaulding, D.T., 2014. Program Evaluation in Practice: Core Concepts and Examples for Discussion and Analysis. Jossey-Bass, San Francisco.

United Nations, 2014. Millennium Development Goals and Beyond. Online. Available: <https://sustainabledevelopment.un.org/post2015/summit> (20 Apr 2015).

Watterson, A. (Ed.), 2003. Public Health in Practice. Palgrave Macmillan, Basingstoke.

World Health Organization, 1986. The Ottawa Charter for Health Promotion First International Conference on Health Promotion, Ottawa, 21 November 1986. Online. Available: <http://www.who.int/healthpromotion/conferences/previous/ottawa/en/> (20 May 2014).

Glossary

Acquired immunity Immunity specific to a single organism or group of organisms that is acquired through either active or passive mechanisms.

Active immunity Immunity that is produced by a person's own immune system.

Additional precautions Additional infection control practices taken for patients known or suspected to be infected or colonised with disease agents that may not be contained by standard precautions alone.

Advocacy for health 'A combination of individual and social actions designed to gain political commitment, policy support, social acceptance and systems support for a particular health goal or programme' (World Health Organization (WHO) 1998).

Anthropogenic 'Originating from the activity of humans' (Greenfacts website).

Biodiversity The variability among living organisms from all sources, including terrestrial, marine and other aquatic ecosystems, and the ecological complexes of which they are part. This includes diversity within species, between species and of ecosystems.

Body Mass Index (BMI) (kg/m^2) Underweight less than 18.5; normal weight over 18.5 and less than 25; overweight (but not obese) 25 and above, but less than 30; obese 30 and above (Australian Institute of Health and Welfare 2013).

Chronic conditions 'Health problems that persist across time and require some degree of health care management', including: non-communicable conditions (e.g. cardiovascular disease, diabetes); persistent communicable conditions (e.g. HIV/AIDS, TB), long-term mental disorders (e.g. schizophrenia, depression), and ongoing physical/structural impairments (e.g. blindness, amputation) (WHO 2002).

Chronic disease 'Chronic disease is a subset of chronic conditions and refers to a specific medical diagnosis. It may be more likely to have a progressively deteriorating path than other chronic conditions' (Lawn and Battersby 2009 p 7).

Commensal relationship In communicable terms, one in which the microorganism and the human coexist for mutual benefit.

Communicable (or contagious) disease A disease that can spread from one individual to another.

Community empowerment 'An empowered community is one in which individuals and organizations apply their skills and resources in collective efforts to address health priorities and meet their respective health needs' (WHO 1998 p 354).

Critical appraisal The process of determining how useful the evidence is.

Cultural competence The 'ongoing process a health care provider continuously strives to achieve through the ability to effectively work within the cultural context of the client. This involves the integration of cultural awareness, cultural knowledge, cultural skill, cultural encounters and cultural desire' (Campinha-Bacote 2002 p 182).

Cultural safety '… more or less—an environment, which is safe for people; where there is no assault, challenge or denial of their identity, of who they are and what they need. It is about shared respect, shared meaning, shared knowledge and experience, of learning together with dignity, and truly listening' (Williams 1998 p 2).

Determinants of health 'The range of personal, social, economic and environmental factors which determine the health status of individuals or populations' (WHO 1998 p 6).

Disability-adjusted life years (DALYs) 'A health gap measure that extends the concept of potential years of life lost (PYLL) due to premature death to include equivalent years of "healthy" life lost in states of less than full health, broadly termed disability. One DALY represents the loss of one year of equivalent full health' (WHO 2008).

Disease An abnormal condition of an organism that impairs bodily functions and is associated with specific symptoms and signs.

Dose–response assessment A step in the risk assessment process in which information on the toxicity of the hazardous agent is considered to determine the relationship between various exposure levels and their effects.

Ecological footprint A measure of sustainability that is based on the concept of 'appropriate carrying capacity' and is defined as 'the land area which is needed exclusively to produce the natural resources that population consumes and to assimilate the waste that it generates indefinitely' (Wackernagel et al. 1993).

Ecology The branch of biology that deals with the interrelationships between organisms and their environment.

Ecosystem A dynamic complex of plant, animal and microorganism communities and the non-living environment interacting as a functional unit. Humans are an integral part of ecosystems, with ecosystems varying enormously in size—for example, from a temporary pond in a tree hollow to an entire ocean basin.

Ecosystem services All ecological systems perform essential functions for humans, and 'ecosystem services' are essential for sustaining human life. In addition to providing goods (e.g. food and medicine), ecosystems provide 'services', such as purification of air and water, accumulation of toxins, decomposition of wastes, mitigation of floods, stabilisation of landscapes and regulation of climate.

Empowerment for health 'In health promotion, empowerment is a process through which people gain greater control over decisions and actions affecting their health' (WHO 1998 p 6).

Endemic disease A disease that occurs at low or consistent levels within a community.

Environmental determinant of health Any external physical, chemical and microbiological exposure or process that impacts on the health of individuals and the community at large, and that is beyond their immediate control (i.e. is involuntary).

Environmental health Those aspects of human health, including quality of life, that are determined by physical, chemical, biological and social factors in the environment (enHealth Council 1999).

Environmental health practice The assessment, correction, control and prevention of environmental factors that can adversely affect health, as well as the enhancement of those aspects of the environment that can improve human health (enHealth Council 1999).

Epidemic An excess of cases in the community from that normally expected, or the appearance of a new infectious disease (Webber 2005).

Evaluation 'The process by which we decide the worth or value of something' (Suchman 1967).

Evidence-based medicine The conscientious, explicit and judicious use of current best evidence in making decisions about the care of individual patients.

Evidence-based practice (EBP) Uses various methods (e.g. summarising research, educating professionals in how to understand and apply research findings) to encourage, and in some instances to force, professionals and other decision-makers to pay more attention to evidence that can inform their decision-making.

Exposure assessment A step in the risk assessment process that involves determining the magnitude, frequency, extent, character and duration of exposures in the past, at present and in the future. It also includes identifying the exposed populations and potential exposure pathways (e.g. exposure through the air, food, water or soil).

False negative Where a screening test fails to indicate the presence of disease.

False positive Where a screening test falsely indicates the presence of disease.

Global climate change A change of climate that is attributed directly or indirectly to human activity, alters the composition of the global atmosphere, and is in addition to natural climate variability observed over comparable time periods (United Nations 1992).

Goal What you ultimately want to achieve by implementing your program plan.

Greenhouse gases '… are those gaseous constituents of the atmosphere, both natural and anthropogenic, that absorb and emit radiation at specific wavelengths within the spectrum of infrared radiation emitted by the Earth's surface, the atmosphere and clouds. This property causes the greenhouse effect. Water vapour (H_2O), carbon dioxide (CO_2), nitrous oxide (N_2O), methane (CH_4) and ozone (O_3) are the primary greenhouse gases in the Earth's atmosphere. Moreover there are a number of entirely human-made greenhouse gases in the atmosphere, such as the halocarbons and other chlorine and bromine containing substances, dealt with under the Montréal Protocol. Beside CO_2, N_2O and CH_4, the Kyoto Protocol deals with the greenhouse gases sulphur hexafluoride (SF_6), hydrofluorocarbons (HFCs) and perfluorocarbons (PFCs)' (Intergovernmental Panel on Climate Change 2007).

Hawthorne effect A term referring to the tendency of some people to work harder and perform better when they are participants in an experiment. Student participants may change their behaviour based on the attention they receive from researchers rather than because of any manipulation of independent variables (Anonymous 2006).

Hazard assessment A key stage in the risk assessment process that consists of two parts: hazard identification and dose–response assessment.

Hazard identification A step in the risk assessment process that involves determining what types of adverse health effect might be caused by the implicated agent, and how quickly the adverse health effects might be experienced.

Health education The provision of learning experiences that encourage voluntary modifications of behaviour that are conducive to health.

Health impact assessment A process that systematically identifies and examines, in a balanced way, both the potential positive and potential negative health impacts of an activity (e.g. policy, program, project or development) (enHealth Council 2001).

Health promotion The process of encouraging and enabling individuals and communities to increase their control over the determinants of health, and thereby improve their health (WHO 1986).

Human capital '… the value of skills, education, health, and training of individuals for the economy and society' (Becker 1993).

Human wellbeing There are a range of components that interact to produce human wellbeing, and these include the basic material for a good life, freedom and choice, health, good social relations, and security. Wellbeing is considered to be at the opposite end of a continuum from poverty, which has been defined as a 'pronounced deprivation in wellbeing' (World Bank 2001 p 15).

Incubation period The period of time between contact with a pathogen and the onset of symptoms of a disease. It is during this period that the disease is difficult to detect and may easily spread to other people before symptoms are evident.

Infectious diseases Diseases caused by pathogenic microorganisms, such as bacteria, viruses, parasites or fungi.

Infective period The length of time a patient is infectious and so can transmit a pathogen to another susceptible host. This infective state often commences before the onset of symptoms and may stop before the symptoms cease. It is during the period before the onset of symptoms, and when the patient is infective, that the risk of transmission to others is the highest (also known as 'period of communicability').

Innate or non-specific immunity Immunity present from birth, which includes physical barriers (e.g. intact skin and mucous membranes), chemical barriers (e.g. gastric acid, digestive enzymes and bacteriostatic fatty acids of the skin), phagocytic cells, and the complement system.

Intergovernmental Panel on Climate Change An international body that was established by the World Meteorological Organization (WMO) and the United Nations Environment Program (UNEP) to assess scientific, technical and socioeconomic information relevant for the understanding of climate change, its potential impacts, and options for adaptation and mitigation.

Interpandemic period Describes the time when the particular disease is not affecting humans although there may be a risk.

Intersectoral collaboration 'A recognised relationship between part or parts of different sectors of society which has been formed to take action on an issue to achieve *health outcomes* or *intermediate health outcomes* in a way which is more effective, efficient or sustainable than might be achieved by the *health sector* acting alone' (WHO 1998).

Isolation Separating sick people while they are infectious.

Latent period The period of time between contact with a pathogen and when the patient becomes infective.

Lay beliefs about health and illness Commonsense understandings and personal experience, imbued with professional rationalisation (Blaxter 2007).

Medical microbiology The study of microbes that cause diseases in humans (Irving et al. 2005).

Meta-analyses Identify relevant primary research studies and aggregate the results, and come up with a quantitative estimate of the overall effect (Naidoo & Wills 2005).

Meta-ethnography The systematic synthesis of qualitative research studies.

Mode of transmission The way in which a communicable disease may be spread from one source to another.

Modern environmental health hazards Any hazards that are related to any rapid development that lacks health and environment safeguards, and also to the unsustainable consumption of natural resources.

Morbidity State of illness, or the occurrence of illness in a population.

Mortality Death, or death rates, in a population.

Neutral relationship In communicable terms, one in which the organisms and the humans live in harmony without any adverse or mutual beneficial effects.

Nipah virus A member of the family *Paramyxoviridae*, Nipah virus is a newly recognised zoonotic virus. The virus was 'discovered' in 1999. It has caused disease in animals and in humans.

Objectives Specific statements about the changes you want to see as a result of a program (adapted from Hawe et al. 1990 p 42). For example, the proportion of students who eat a healthy lunch at school.

Organisation for Economic Co-operation and Development (OECD) A Paris-based intergovernmental organisation of 30 wealthy nations whose purpose is to provide a forum for governments to compare experiences to achieve the highest sustainable economic growth and employment and improvement of living standards in member and non-member states.

Outbreak The sudden occurrence of a disease in a community.

Pandemic The occurrence of an epidemic in multiple communities.

Pandemic alert period The time when a disease may be causing isolated human disease or small clusters of patients without rapid spread or significant outbreak.

Pandemic period The situation when there is a pandemic with human-to-human spread and significant numbers of affected persons.

Passive immunity The protection that is provided by the transfer of antibodies derived from immune people.

Pathogen A disease-producing microorganism.

Pathogenic relationship In communicable terms, one in which a microorganism causes disease in a larger organism.

Plan Overall structure of intended set of activities to get you to what you want to achieve.

Policy The process by which governments translate their political vision into programs and actions to delivery 'outcomes'—desired changes in the 'real world' (Cabinet Office 1999 in Naidoo & Wills 2005). For example, the national policy on diabetes.

Population health The study of health and disease in defined populations.

Precautionary approach/principle When credible scientific evidence or concern is raised regarding activities or agents that may harm human health or the environment, this principle states that precautionary measures should be taken even when there is uncertainty and where the cause and effect relationships have not yet been fully established.

Primary care '… is socially appropriate, universally accessible, scientifically sound first-level care provided by a suitably trained workforce supported by integrated referral systems and in a way that gives priority to those most in need, maximises community and individual self-reliance and participation, and involves collaboration with other sectors. It includes the following:
- health promotion
- illness prevention
- care of the sick
- advocacy
- community development' (Australian Primary Health Care Research Institute).

Primary health care '… curative treatment given by the first contact provider and including promotional, preventive and rehabilitative services provided by multi-disciplinary teams of health-care professionals working collaboratively' (WHO 1978).

Prion An infectious agent.

Program A grouping of resources including people, funds, equipment and supplies performing activities that enable the scope of the program and its activities to be measured, fulfilling a definable set of goals and objectives (adapted from Health and Welfare, Canada 1977). Sometimes called an intervention.

Programme Logic Model A graphical depiction of relationships between all planned program components and the desired results.

Propagated exposure Occurs when affected people pass on a disease to other people.

Propagated source Spread from person to person rather than from a single common source.

Quarantine Separating possibly exposed healthy people from non-exposed healthy people.

Repeated exposure Occurs when a community is repeatedly exposed to the cause of an outbreak, as may occur when people continue to drink from an infected water source.

Risk assessment The process of estimating the potential impact of chemical, physical, microbiological or psychosocial hazards on a specified human population or ecological system under a specific set of conditions and for a certain timeframe (enHealth Council 2004).

Risk characterisation Final step in the risk assessment process that seeks to integrate the information from the hazard assessment and exposure assessment steps, and to describe the risks to individuals and populations in terms of the nature, extent and severity of potential adverse health effects.

Risk communication An interactive process involving the exchange between individuals, groups and institutions of information and expert opinion about the nature, severity and acceptability of risks and the decisions taken to combat them (enHealth Council 2004).

Risk management The process of evaluating alternative actions, selecting options and implementing them in response to risk assessments. The decision-making process will incorporate scientific, technological, social, economic and political information. The process requires value judgement, such as on the tolerability and reasonableness of costs (enHealth Council 2004).

Risk transition Used to describe the reduction in 'traditional environmental health risks' and increase in 'modern environmental health risks' that takes place with advances in economic development.

Settings for health 'The place or social context in which people engage in daily activities in which environmental, organizational and personal factors interact to affect health and wellbeing' (WHO 1998).

Single-point exposure Occurs when the source of an outbreak can be traced to a single event or focus, as may occur with an episode of food poisoning.

Social capital Social resources developed through networks, relationships, reciprocity, exchange and connectedness.

Social cohesion The connections and relations between societal units, such as individual, groups and associations, or the 'glue' that holds communities together (AIHW 2005).

Stakeholders Everyone who has an interest in a program, particularly decision-makers and the community for whom the program is planned.

Standard precautions Involves a series of systems and structures that should always be used in patient management so as to minimise the risks associated with infection.

Strategies The methods employed to assist you to reach your objectives—for example, providing healthy foods in a tuckshop. This is about what your plan is going to provide and/or deliver—for example, education programs, brochures, media campaigns, action by parents to change the tuckshop menu and advocacy to ban 'junk' food advertisements during children's television programs.

Sustainability A balance that integrates: the protection of the ecological processes and natural systems at local, regional, state and national levels; economic development; and the maintenance of the cultural, economic, physical and social wellbeing of people and communities (Queensland Government 1997).

Sustainable development Defined by the Brundtland Commission as development that meets the needs of the present without compromising the ability of future generations to meet their own needs.

Target group The group of people a program is aiming to reach—for example, teenage students in Years 9 and 10.

Traditional environmental health hazards Hazards that are often associated with poverty and a lack of development, and include a lack of access to safe drinking water and inadequate basic sanitation in the household and the community.

Urban sprawl A land use/urban planning term to describe haphazard growth or extension outward, especially that resulting from real estate development on the outskirts of a city.

Vector A carrier, especially one that transmits disease.

Zoonotic diseases Infectious diseases of animals that can cause disease when transmitted to humans.

References

Anonymous, 2006. Letter to the editor. Occupational Medicine 56 (3), 217. doi:10.1093/occmed/kqj046.

Australian Institute of Health and Welfare, 2005. Australia's Welfare 2005. AIHW Cat. No. AUS 65. AIHW, Canberra.

Australian Institute of Health and Welfare, 2013. Overweight and obesity website. Online. Available: <http://www.aihw.gov.au/body-weight/> (22 Jan 2015).

Australian Primary Health Care Research Institute. What is primary health care? APHCRI, Australian National University, Canberra. Online. Available: <http://aphcri.anu.edu.au/about-us/what-primary-health-care> (22 Jan 2015).

Becker, G., 1993. Human Capital: A Theoretical and Empirical Analysis, With Special Reference to Education. The University of Chicago Press, Chicago.

Blaxter, M., 2007. How is health experienced? In: Douglas, J., Earle, S., Handsley, S., et al. (Eds.), A Reader in Promoting Public Health. Sage, London.

Campinha-Bacote, J., 2002. The process of cultural competence in the delivery of healthcare services: a model of care. Journal of Transcultural Nursing 13 (3), 181–184.

enHealth Council, 1999. National Environmental Health Strategy. enHealth Council. Commonwealth Department of Health and Aged Care, Canberra.

enHealth Council, 2001. Health Impact Assessment Guidelines, enHealth Council. Commonwealth Department of Health and Aged Care, Canberra.

enHealth Council, 2004. Environmental Health Risk Assessment: Guidelines for Assessing Human Health Risks from Environmental Hazards. Department of Health and Ageing and enHealth Council, Canberra.

Greenfacts website. Online. Available: <http://www.greenfacts.org/glossary/abc/anthropogenic.htm> (23 April 2011).

Hawe, P., Degeling, D., Hall, J., 1990. Evaluating Health Promotion. MacLennan and Petty, Sydney.

Health and Welfare Canada, 1977. Evaluation Guidelines. Health and Welfare Canada, Ontario.

Intergovernmental Panel on Climate Change, 2007. Climate change 2007: Working Group I: The physical science basis. Online. Available: <http://www.ipcc.ch/publications_and_data/ar4/wg1/en/annexessglossary-e-o.html> (23 Jan 2015).

Irving, W.L., Ala'Aldeen, D., Boswell, T., 2005. Medical Microbiology. Taylor and Francis, New York.

Lawn, S., Battersby, M., 2009. Capabilities for Supporting Prevention and Chronic Condition Self-Management: A Resource for Educators of Primary Health Care Professionals. Flinders University. Australian Government Department of Health and Ageing, Adelaide. <http://dspace.flinders.edu.au/jspui/bitstream/2328/26152/3/Lawn%20Capabilities>.

Naidoo, J., Wills, J., 2005. Public Health and Health Promotion: Developing Practice. Baillière Tindall, Edinburgh.

Queensland Government, 1997. Integrated Planning Act 1997. GoPrint, Brisbane.

Suchman, E.A., 1967. Evaluative Research. Russell Sage Foundation, New York.

United Nations, 1992. United Nations Framework Convention on Climate Change. United Nations, New York.

Wackernagel, M., McIntosh, J., Rees, W.E., et al., 1993. How Big is Our Ecological Footprint? A Handbook for Estimating a Community's Appropriated Carrying Capacity. Task Force on Planning Healthy and Sustainable Communities, Vancouver.

Webber, R., 2005. Communicable Disease Epidemiology and Control: A Global Perspective, second ed. CABI Publishing, Oxfordshire, p. 22.

Williams, R., 1998. Cultural safety—what does it mean for our work practice? Online. Available: <http://www.utas.edu.au/__data/assets/pdf_file/0010/246943/RevisedCulturalSafetyPaper-pha.pdf> (23 Jan 2015).

World Bank, 2001. World Development Report 2000–2001: Attacking Poverty. Oxford University Press, New York.

World Health Organization, 1978. Declaration of Alma-Ata. International Conference on Primary Health Care, Alma-Ata, USSR, 6–12 September 1978. WHO, Geneva. Online. Available: <http://www.who.int/publications/almaata_declaration_en.pdf> (23 Jan 2015).

World Health Organization, 1986. The Ottawa Charter for Health Promotion First International Conference on Health Promotion, Ottawa, 21 November 1986. Online. Available: <http://www.who.int/healthpromotion/conferences/previous/ottawa/en/> (6 Nov 2007).

World Health Organization, 1998. Health Promotion Glossary. WHO, Geneva. Online. Available: <http://whqlibdoc.who.int/hq/1998/WHO_HPR_HEP_98.1.pdf> (19 Sep 2014).

World Health Organization, 2002. Innovative Care for Chronic Conditions: Building Blocks for Action: Global Report. WHO, Geneva.

World Health Organization, 2008. Disability Adjusted Life Years (DALYs). WHO, Geneva. Online. Available: <http://www.who.int/healthinfo/boddaly/en/>.

Index

Page numbers followed by '*f*' indicate figures, '*t*' indicate tables, and '*b*' indicate boxes.

Q

R